Prentice Hall Advanced Reference Series

Physical and Life Sciences

Cytokines

Anthony Meager

Prentice Hall
Englewood Cliffs, New Jersey 07632

Library of Congress Cataloging-in-Publication Data

MEAGER, ANTHONY.
    Cytokines / Anthony Meager.

    p.   cm. — (Prentice Hall advanced references series)
    Includes bibliographical reference and index.
    ISBN 0-13-194267-0
    1. Cytokines.   I. Title.
    DNLM: 1. Cytokines—physiology.   QW 568 M482c]
    QR185.8.C95M43   1991
    616.07 '9—dc20
    DNLM/DLC   91-3747
    for Library of Congress   CIP

Cover design: *Karen Stephens*
Prepress buyer: *Kelly Behr*
Manufacturing buyer: *Dave Dickey*

Prentice Hall Advanced Reference Series

First published by Open University Press
Milton Keynes, England

This edition for sale in North America only.

Copyright © 1991 by Anthony Meager

 North American edition published by Prentice Hall
A Division of Simon & Schuster
Englewood Cliffs, New Jersey 07632

Printed in the United States of America

10 9 8 7 6 5 4 3 2 1

ISBN   0-13-194267-0

ISBN 0-13-194267-0

9 780131 942677

PRENTICE-HALL INTERNATIONAL (UK) LIMITED, *London*
PRENTICE-HALL OF AUSTRALIA PTY. LIMITED, *Sydney*
PRENTICE-HALL CANADA INC., *Toronto*
PRENTICE-HALL HISPANOAMERICANA, S.A., *Mexico*
PRENTICE-HALL OF INDIA PRIVATE LIMITED, *New Delhi*
PRENTICE-HALL OF JAPAN, INC., *Tokyo*
SIMON & SCHUSTER ASIA PTE. LTD., *Singapore*
EDITORA PRENTICE-HALL DO BRASIL, LTDA., *Rio de Janeiro*

Contents

Preface

Developments in molecular biology, particularly in recombinant DNA (rDNA) technology, has led to a rapid rise in the number and characterization of biologically active proteins available for scientific studies and clinical investigation. Many of these proteins are secreted in response to specific stimuli and act themselves, via cell-surface receptors, to modulate cellular metabolism which in turn regulates proliferative and functional responses. They may be considered to have hormone-like activities, but since, unlike classical hormones, they are mostly directly mitogenic and act at short range in local cellular environments, they have been designated as a new category of intercellular mediators, now collectively known as cytokines. The latter are usually subdivided into well-characterized classes including 'growth factors', 'colony stimulating factors', 'interleukins', 'tumour necrosis factors', 'interferons', 'chemotactic factors', etc. Nevertheless, all of these molecules have a 'sameness', both in their polypeptide nature and in the way they activate cellular responses through binding to cell-surface receptors. Further, they are all pleiotropic mediators, i.e., they can act on many different cell types or on cells of the same lineage at different stages of development. It is clear that, following receptor occupancy, intracellular signalling pathways are activated to effect metabolic changes, gene induction, and structural alterations leading to proliferative, differentiating, or functional responses. Different cell types respond differently, or seem to do so, to the same cytokine in many instances and thus cytokines may be said to exhibit pleiotypic activities. Understanding why cells respond in particular ways to cytokine stimulation is a central research problem, and while knowledge of receptors and the nature of the downstream intracellular components of signalling pathways is fast accruing, there remains much to be resolved.

There is a strong association between the products of certain genes known as proto-oncogenes and the elements of cellular proliferation-inducing pathways, which include cytokines, receptors, intracellular signal-transducing enzymes, and factors which regulate gene induction. It has also become evident that 'oncoproteins', the products of dysregulated or mutated proto-oncogenes, commonly known as oncogenes, are responsible for loss of growth control and predispose cells to oncogenesis (tumour cell formation). Many cytokines directly regulate cellular proliferation, and thus are not only important to processes of tissue generation and repair, but are also relevant to oncogenic mechanisms.

When applied separately, cytokines markedly affect cellular processes studied *in vitro*, but it is likely that *in vivo* they are involved in complex interactions, both among themselves and with other regulatory substances, e.g. hormones, which underlie embryogenesis, neonatal development, and maintenance of adult tissues. Many cytokines have antiviral, antimicrobial, or antitumour activities, strongly suggesting they play protective roles in the defence of the organism against infectious pathogens and invasive diseases. In this respect, several cytokines have special significance for the regulation of the immune system. For instance, the proliferation, oncogenic development, maturation, and activation to immunologic function of leukocytes is regulated to a large degree by certain cytokines. These, in the form of haemopoietic growth factors, may control steady-state haemopoiesis, the continuous replacement of red blood cells and leukocytes in the circulation from the bone marrow, and increase the overall rate of haemopoietic cell production from stem cells in times of crisis, e.g. when the organism is invaded by pathogenic microbes. Other cytokines, particularly interleukins, specifically regulate the proliferation, differentiation, and function of lymphocytes, both from the antibody-producing B-cell lineage and the antigen-recognizing T-cell lineage. T-lymphocytes themselves produce a range of cytokines which specifically affect other leukocytes and may also have activities in cells outside the immune system, e.g. in vascular endothelial cells which provide the inner lining of blood vessels. While normally co-ordinating immune responses such cytokines, in excess, probably also contribute towards inflammatory reactions, tissue degradation, and potentially lethal systemic effects. Thus, some cytokines are probably associated with the pathogenesis of certain diseases and in certain circumstances may underlie both the symptoms and the pathology manifested.

Based on the putative protective roles of particular cytokines, there has been a great effort in recent years to evaluate clinically the efficacy of interferons and other cytokines in the treatment of human diseases. It has become clear that current therapeutic regimes using these potent pharmacologically active substances are not without complications, e.g. toxic side-effects, and despite some beneficial effects do not in most cases provide cures, especially in cancer. There are, however, a limited number of infections and malignant diseases for which cytokine therapy has shown promise in retarding disease progression. In addition, there are hopes that particular cytokines will be useful in adjunctive therapy, e.g. in restoring leukocyte numbers following high-dose chemotherapy or X-irradiation.

This book attempts to define and classify cytokines, to propose a concept of cytokine stimulation including intracellular signal transmission, and to show that while cytokines act at the cellular level, usually in specific tissue environments, the outcome of their activities may profoundly affect bodily homeostatic and defence mechanisms and link many functions within the various physiological systems. As much up-to-date information as possible about the structures of individual cytokines and their receptors is included, together with comprehensive reviews of the biological activities of cytokines. The relationship between their activities at the cellular and molecular levels and their potential physiological and pathophysiological roles is fully explored. The clinical application of cytokines is also briefly covered. Basic knowledge of biology, molecular biology, and immunology is assumed, but the contents should be of interest and appeal to advanced undergraduates taking a biology degree course, postgraduate biologists, immunologists, biochemists, and clinicians with a specialist interest in cytokines. The book will also provide a handy reference text for those many research scientists engaged in cytokine studies.

In writing this book, which has taken many months to complete, I was sustained by my wife Monique and aided by my colleagues in the Division of Immunobiology at NIBSC. I should like to thank Dr R Thorpe (Head of Immunobiology) particularly for advice and encouragement in the preparation of the book, and Dr A. Gearing (Division of Immunobiology) and Dr S. Poole (Division of Endocrinology) for helpful discussions and comments. I am especially grateful to Miss L. Hudson for typing the draft of the entire book. My thanks also to Mr A. Davies for his help in preparing illustrations.

A. Meager
NIBSC South Mimms Herts

1

The cytokine concept

1.1   Introduction

The multicellular organism, as its complexity has increased, has evolved highly elaborate and interactive communication systems at the cellular and molecular levels. These latter are necessary for

1   co-ordinated cell growth and division in the formation of tissues and organs,
2   maintenance of tissues and organs throughout development into the adult state and beyond,
3   integrated control of the various physiological systems, e.g. digestive, nervous, immune, etc.,
4   recognition and elimination of harmful environmental stimuli and invasive, disease-causing entities — principally viruses, bacteria, and parasitic unicellular organisms.

Two types of cellular interaction underlie these communication systems: cell-to-cell contact and cell-to-cell signalling mediated by electrical impulses and various (bio-) chemical substances. Intracellular interactions mediated by biologically active substances are particularly well developed in higher animals, e.g. mammals, and are especially important for the functioning of the endocrine and immune systems.

In the multicellular, multi-organ animal, the endocrine system functions to regulate and synchronize certain aspects of cellular metabolism and to establish the harmonious operation of different organs throughout daily life. It does this by means of messenger substances, known as hormones. These are produced by highly specialized cells contained in various endocrine

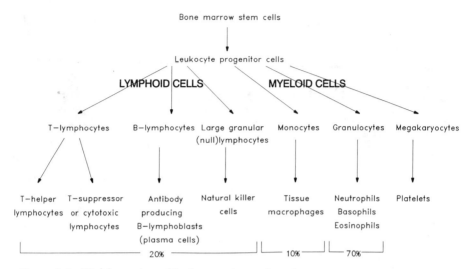

Figure 1.1   The formation of leukocyte classes from bone marrow.

glands, and intermittently released into the bloodstream for transport and eventual action at the target-cell or -tissue level. In comparison, the immune system has evolved from a primitive recognition system whereby self was distinguished from non-self. It functions to protect animals from invasive diseases, caused mainly by numerous, replicating, potentially pathogenic organisms and other entities, e.g. viruses, present in the environment. The immune system may be thought of as a mobile disseminated organ composed mainly of white cells, known as leukocytes, which circulate within the bloodstream and which are also present in the spleen and lymph nodes. Leukocytes are divided into lymphoid cells, the lymphocytes (20 per cent of the total) and myeloid cells, the phagocytic monocyte/macrophages, polymorphonuclear granulocytes, and platelets (Figure 1.1). Leukocytes communicate among themselves and with other cell types both by cell-to-cell contact and by the secretion of biochemical substances that trigger cellular responses in cells to which they specifically bind. These leukocyte-derived, biochemical messengers, which might legitimately be called 'immuno-hormones', form part of a broader group of substances that affect growth, maturation, and behaviour of cells in general. This group of intercellular messengers contains both small and large molecules of various kinds, but the present book is concerned only with a class of soluble, proteinaceous mediators now widely known as *cytokines*.

1.2   What cytokines are

The word 'cytokine', which was first used by Dr S. Cohen in 1974, was originally coined to describe any soluble substance produced by lymphoid and/or non-lymphoid cells that exercises specific effects in its target cells. The term therefore embraces 'lymphokine', a word proposed by Dr D. Dumonde in 1969 to describe soluble mediators produced by lymphoid cells, i.e. lymphocytes, and 'monokine', used to describe soluble mediators produced by cells of the monocyte–macrophage lineage. However, the definition of cytokine to include all secreted soluble mediators is probably too wide in the current context, because it would include substances such as classical hormones and many biologically active small molecules such as histamine, prostaglandins, leukotrienes, and platelet activation factor (PAF). Classical hormones may be peptides and proteins, derivatives of aromatic amino acids, steroids, or prostaglandins, and include sex steroids, adrenocorticoids, thyroid hormones, hypophysial hormones, insulin, glucagon, etc. For simplicity, and because of limitations of space, classical hormones and other small mediators mentioned above will be excluded here, as too will be immunoglobulins, complement, enzymes, and mediators of plant and microbial origin. For the purposes of the present book, therefore, cytokines are defined as a class of inducible, water-soluble, heterogeneous proteinaceous mediators of animal origin of molecular weight (MW) greater than 5000 that exercise specific, receptor-mediated effects in target cells and/or in the mediator-producing cells themselves. In general, these cytokine-mediated effects partly underlie the normal physiological control of

(a) *mitogenesis* (cell division) which is required for cell proliferation and thus tissue development and repair, and
(b) *cell function* which is required for the maintenance of homeostatic and defence mechanisms, and the integrated control of different physiological systems.

Such a class of mediators therefore includes, in contrast to classical hormones, several directly mitogenic factors such as the soluble proteins designated as interleukins or colony-stimulating factors and other well-defined protein growth factors. In addition, it includes cell differentiation or maturation factors and cell growth inhibitory factors such as a family of proteins known as interferons.

Nevertheless, it is virtually impossible to define cytokines precisely, and the proposed definition may give rise to problems in classifying certain mediators. For example, erythropoietin, a mediator produced by the kidney which stimulates red blood cell growth, is most often referred to as a hormone, but both molecularly and biologically it shares many properties with cytokines and thus could probably be considered to be one. However, most cytokines are not normally considered to act at long range in an 'endocrine' manner, as do most classical hormones, although this is possible under certain circumstances. Cytokines, once secreted, diffuse through intercellular spaces and act locally on their target cells in what is known as 'paracrine' action or, if the mediator-producing cells themselves are affected, as 'autocrine' action. Another feature that may be used to distinguish classical hormones and cytokines is that, whilst both classes of mediators elicit their effects by interaction with specific cell receptors, hormone receptors appear generally to be much more restricted in their tissue distribution than are cytokine receptors, which can often be found in virtually all cell types. Thus, many cell types can have receptors for several different cytokines. It must be recognized that the dividing line between hormones and cytokines (see Table 1.1 for their comparison) is very fine, and that the distinction between these classes of mediators is often blurred.

1.3   Naming of cytokines

The existence of cytokines gradually gained credence with the opening up of the field of cellular immunology in the 1960s. The advent of routine leukocyte culture and the development of *in vitro* assays for investigating different aspects of cellular immune reactions produced the first firm evidence of cytokine involvement. However, with only one or two exceptions, the nature of cytokines was unknown at that time. For this reason, such uncharacterized cytokines were quite reasonably referred to as 'factors' of some defined biological activity. In many cases, the naming of these factors was governed by the effects in particular experimental, cell-based systems, usually involving leukocytes. Thus, there was T-cell growth factor (TCGF), B-cell growth factor (BCGF), lymphocyte activating factor (LAF), macrophage activating factor (MAF), macrophage migration inhibition factor (MIF), tumour necrosis factor (TNF), etc. However, the naming of cytokines has not been

Table 1.1   Comparison of the characteristics of classical hormones and cytokines

Classical hormones	*Cytokines*
Small to large polypeptides, proteins, derivatives of aromatic amino acids or steroids	Large polypeptides, proteins or glycoproteins (MW > 5000)
Produced by specialized cells of endocrine glands to act at a distance (endocrine action) on target cells and organs	Produced by specialized and unspecialized cells of many tissues and organs to act locally (paracrine or autocrine action), but can act at a distance if released into the blood supply
Receptors restricted to one or a few target cell type(s)	Receptors usually found on many cell types other than predicted target cells
Rarely directly mitogenic (causing cell division) *in vitro*, with the notable exception of insulin	Many are directly mitogenic *in vitro*
Low overlap of biological activities	Frequent high overlap of biological activities

entirely logical or predictable; often words have been introduced as 'jargon' and subsequently adopted for scientific reporting. For instance, in 1957 Isaacs and Lindemann discovered a factor produced by virally infected cells that transferred virus resistance to fresh tissues, for which they coined the term 'interferon'. More recently, the word 'interleukin' has been introduced as a generic name for cytokines released by leukocytes which also have specific effects in other leukocytes. Therefore, for example, LAF has become interleukin-1 (IL-1) and TCGF is now known as interleukin-2 (IL-2). Several others factors have been re-designated as interleukins after their molecular structures have been ascertained by modern recombinant DNA methods. For example, BCGF activity can be attributed to at least two distinct cytokines, now known as interleukin-4 (IL-4) and interleukin-6 (IL-6). Further, recent findings concerning the activities of interferons (IFN) would also make it valid to refer to them as interleukins. It is clear, though, that interferons are not simply interleukins; they can be produced by a wide variety of cells and are known to act on many different cell types. Moreover, the original names of several other cytokines are now so widely accepted and familar to scientists and clinicians alike that to re-name at this stage would be inappropriate and would almost certainly create more confusion than already exists! For this reason, certain cytokines have retained their 'factor-name', e.g. granulocyte-colony stimulating factor (G-CSF), transforming growth factor (TGF), and fibroblast growth factor (FGF).

Further problems in the nomenclature of cytokines have arisen where knowledge of molecular characteristics of particular cytokines has increased in recent times. This has been emphasized dramatically with IFN, a term first used to designate a substance able to transfer virus resistance, whose meaning has subsequently had to be extended to cover both different types of IFN and molecular sub-species (subtypes) contained within each type. Without going into detail at this point, it can be said that such problems have to some extent been resolved (by international nomenclature committees) by giving each type of IFN a Greek letter as a suffix, starting logically with α, with the further addition of an arabic numeral for individual subtypes, e.g. IFN α-1, IFN α-2, etc. IFN β-1, etc. Another example of molecular heterogeneity in particular cytokines is to be found in interleukin-1 (IL-1) which is composed of two structurally distinct types now known as interleukin-1 α (IL-1α) and interleukin-1 β (II-1β). Table 1.2 sets out to illustrate the range of substances which have been or may be classified as cytokines. The left-hand column gives the most recent designation of each cytokine and the one now most frequently used in scientific reporting, and the right-hand column shows former or alternative names, some of which are still commonly used. The list of cytokines is not comprehensive; it includes only those which have been fully or partially characterized on a molecular basis. Many other factors mediating specific biological effects have been described, but are as yet molecularly uncharacterized; no doubt some of these will eventually be classified as cytokines.

Table 1.2   Cytokine designations

Modern name and abbreviation	Former or alternative name
Epidermal growth factor (EGF)	Urogastrone
Insulin-like growth factor-I (IGF-I)	Somatomedin C
Insulin-like growth factor-II (IGF-II)	Multiplication stimulating activity
Transforming growth factor alpha (TGF$_\alpha$)	—
Transforming growth factor beta (TGF$_\beta$)	—
Platelet-derived growth factor (PDGF)	—
Acidic fibroblast growth factor (aFGF)	Prostatropin, endothelial cell growth factor (ECGF), eye-derived growth stimulating factor-1 (EDGSF-1)
Basic fibroblast growth factor (bFGF)	
Nerve growth factor (NGF)	—
Erythropoietin (EPO)	—
Granulocyte-colony stimulating factor (G-CSF)	Pluripoietin, D-or diff factor (DF), macrophage granulocyte inducer-type 2 (MGI-2)
Macrophage-colony stimulating factor (M-CSF)	Colony stimulating factor-1 (CSF-1), macrophage granulocyte inducer-type 1M (MGI-1M)
Granulocyte-macrophage-colony stimulating factor (GM-CSF)	Colony stimulating activator–granulocyte macrophage (CSA-GM), Macrophage granulocyte inducer-type 1G (MgI-1G)
Interleukin-1 alpha (IL-1α)	Lymphocyte activating factor (LAF), haemopoietin-1 (HP-1), endogenous pyrogen (EP)
Interleukin-1 beta (IL-1β)	
Interleukin-2 (IL-2)	T-cell growth factor (TCGF)
Interleukin-3 (IL-3)	Multi-colony stimulating factor (multi-CSF), persisting cell-stimulating factor (PSF), mast cell growth factor
Interleukin-4 (IL-4)	B-cell growth factor-1 (BCGF-I), B-cell stimulating factor 1 (BSF-1)
Interleukin-5 (IL-5)	Eosinophil differentiation factor (EDF), B-cell growth factor-II (BCGF-II)
Interleukin-6 (IL-6)	B-cell stimulating factor-2 (BSF-2), hybridoma-plastocytoma growth factor (HPGF), interferon beta-2 (IFNβ2), 26K protein, hepatocyte stimulating factor (HSF)
Interleukin-7 (IL-7)	Lymphopoietin-1 (LP-1)
Interleukin-8 (IL-8)	Monocyte-derived neutrophil activating protein (MONAP), macrophage

Table 1.2 (Con't)

Modern name and abbreviation	Former or alternative name
	inflammatory protein (MIP), neutrophil activating factor (NAF)
Tumour necrosis factor alpha (TNFα)	Cachectin
Tumour necrosis factor beta (TNFβ)	Lymphotoxin (LT)
Leukaemia inhibitory factor (LIF)	Macrophage differentiation factor (MDF), human interleukin with differentiating activity (HILDA)
Interferon alpha subclass I (IFNαI) Interferon alpha subclass II (IFNαII)	Leukocyte interferon, acid-stable interferon, type I interferon (IFNαII also called IFN omega (ω))
Interferon beta (IFN β)	Interferon beta-1 (IFNβ$_1$), fibroblast interferon, acid-stable interferon, type I interferon
Interferon gamma (IFNγ)	Immune interferon, acid-labile interferon, type II interferon, macrophage activating factor (MAF)

1.4 Cytokine biology

Before going on to describe individual cytokines, it is worth considering some general aspects of cytokine biology in order to provide a conceptual framework for understanding how cytokines act, and why and when an organism requires particular cytokine-mediated activities.

Molecular nature of biologically active cytokines

As previously mentioned, cytokines may be regarded as inducible, soluble, heterogeneous proteinaceous mediators (MW > 5000) produced by animal cells, which exercise specific, receptor-mediated effects in target cells and/or in the mediator-producing cells themselves. Despite the heterogeneity in molecular structure, there is an overall 'sameness' about cytokines. They are all proteins or glycoproteins, mostly in the molecular weight range 5000–50 000. In some cases, individual monomeric cytokine proteins are active, whereas in other cases, covalent or non-covalent association between monomeric proteins to form dimers, trimers, or possibly even higher oligomers is required to produce the active form of the cytokine. The intactness or integrity of cytokine structure has been shown to be necessary for efficient receptor-binding and hence biological activity. Generally speaking, with few exceptions, it has not been possible to produce fragments of cytokine molecules that are biologically active, although some fragments may compete for binding to receptors with intact whole cytokine molecules.

Cytokine induction and production

The nuclear genes coding for cytokines mostly appear to be very tightly regulated, and most of the time little or no transcription into messenger RNA (mRNA) or subsequent translation of mRNA on polyribosomes into cytokine molecules is taking place. A specific stimulus is usually required for induction or de-repression of cytokine genes. The exterior surface of all cells is continually exposed to an ever-changing, potentially hostile, environment which contains a myriad of substances and entities having the capacity to act as exogenous stimuli. In many instances, a number of these substances and entities act by binding to the cell surface, in a way much resembling the binding of cytokines to their cell receptors (see p. 10), to stimulate cytokine synthesis. For example, part of the cell wall of pathogenic Gram-negative bacteria known as lipopolysaccharide (LPS) binds to the cell surface of macrophages and induces the synthesis of a number of cytokines (Figure 1.2).

In the immune system, leukocytes have acquired the ability to recognize foreign, non-self molecules, also known as antigens, and to present these to 'responder' cells (Figure 1.2) to cause eventual elimination of these antigens. In this process, cytokine synthesis is invariably induced. These cytokines act on other cells, including leukocytes, to stimulate cell proliferation and the activation of defence mechanisms. Cytokines themselves can also act as stimuli for the induction of cytokine synthesis (Figure 1.2), and this can promote amplification of the initial response (see p. 16) which is important,

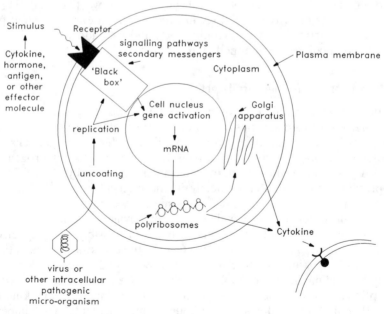

Figure 1.2   Induction of cytokine synthesis.

for example, in the development of inflammatory responses at sites of tissue injury.

In contrast, viruses, some bacteria and some other classes of micro-organisms replicate inside cells, i.e. they are intracellular pathogens. Replication of these pathogens, or more precisely of certain molecules produced during the replicative process, causes the induction of cytokine synthesis (Figure 1.2). Double-stranded RNA, for instance, which is often produced as an intermediate of virus genome transcription is associated with the activation of IFN α and IFN β genes. Additionally, some viral and bacterial proteins may be expressed at the cell surface and will be recognized as foreign antigens by certain leukocytes. The subsequent intercellular interactions lead to cytokine induction (Figure 1.2), as mentioned in the previous paragraph.

The process or processes by which induction of cytokine synthesis occurs are as yet poorly understood. There is often said to be a 'black box' between the cell surface and the cell nucleus; this denotes a lack of understanding concerning the mechanism of signal transmission between the point of receipt of the stimulus and the de-repression (activation) of particular cytokine genes. However, it appears that intracellular signalling pathways involving the phosphorylation and dephosphorylation of particular regulatory enzymes are critical to the induction process (see p. 13 and Chapter 2 for more details). Furthermore it is clear that cytokine genes contain regulatory elements of DNA which are found upstream from the coding DNA sequence and which control initiation of transcription. Details of the structure of particular cytokine genes will be found in succeeding chapters. In addition, there is evidence of factors, as yet undefined, that regulate translation of cytokine mRNAs on polyribosomes. The co-ordination of gene activation, synthesis, processing, and secretion in cytokine production is also governed by a number of variable genetic factors.

The primary translation products of cytokine mRNAs are precursor proteins composed of a leader or signal amino acid sequence at the N-terminus covalently linked through a peptide bond to the native (mature) protein amino acid sequence. As for nearly all secreted proteins, the signal sequence is required to deliver the cytokine protein through the endoplasmic reticulum and is cleaved off before secretion of cytokine from the cell (Figure 1.2). From the endoplasmic reticulum the cytokine protein passes through the Golgi apparatus where it may be glycosylated before being secreted (Figure 1.2). However, a few cytokines, e.g. IL-1 and TNF, probably exist in precursor form as membrane-bound proteins prior to proteolytic cleavage and exit of the mature form from the cell.

Why do cells use relatively large polypeptides and proteins as intercellular messenger molecules, when their production is so expensive in terms of cell energy and substrate resources? This may be answered, although not completely satisfactorily, in the following way. First, as already mentioned, protein synthesis can be very tightly controlled: many cytokine genes are transcribed for a very limited interval following activation and are then shut down again completely. Second, proteins have complex structures that can confer a high degree of specificity in interactions with cell receptors and therefore, perhaps relatedly, they are biologically active at very low concentrations. Third, and lastly, proteins when secreted in excess can be readily denatured, inactivated, and eliminated from the body. These reasons are not sufficient to account for the seemingly wasteful biochemical redundancy where two or more different cytokines have considerable overlap of biological activities. This will be discussed later in this chapter (see pp. 14–15) and referred to again later in the book.

Cytokine binding to cell surface receptors

Cytokines may be viewed as informational or messenger protein molecules which, like hormones, exercise their effects at extremely low molar concentrations via cell receptors. An individual cytokine interacts in a highly specific manner with its cell receptor. It is generally assumed, although often not proven, that there is a single, structurally homogeneous cell-surface receptor population, varying in number from a few hundred up to several thousands per cell. Presumably, each cytokine molecule contains a structural element whose conformation allows close-fit binding to a complementary structure, e.g. a pocket or groove, present in the receptor molecule (Figure 1.3).

The event of a cytokine binding to its receptor is a necessary first step for the effective transmission of the 'informational content' of particular cytokines to the interior of the cell. Presently, however, it is not clear how the level of cytokine receptor occupancy is linked to the production of cellular responses. For example, is there a cytokine concentration at which a threshold level of receptor occupancy is reached for triggering a cellular response — in other words, an all-or-none phenomenon? Or is the magnitude of the cellular response linked to increasing cytokine concentration and hence to increasing levels of receptor occupancy? For instance, it is known that the antiviral activity of IFN is apparently manifested at lower doses than its anticellular (anticell-proliferation) activity. If, however, virus multiplication is regarded as a form of pathological growth of a foreign, cell-like, component within a cell and at its expense, replication of viral proteins, which is usually rapid, can therefore be envisaged to be more sensitive to IFN action than the slower and more complex cellular growth. Thus triggering of a cell response may occur at a single threshold level of receptor occupancy, dependent upon a certain cytokine concentration being reached, but the extent of the response will depend upon operational levels of multifactorial intercellular processes.

Structure of cytokine receptors

Receptor molecules themselves are known to be mostly integral plasma membrane glycoproteins, and the structures of several of these have already been elucidated. In general terms, they may be pictured as complex molecules with up to three distinct domains (Figure 1.3). First, there is a recognition domain which protrudes outwards from the plasma membrane and which confers specificity with regard to the binding of particular cytokines. This

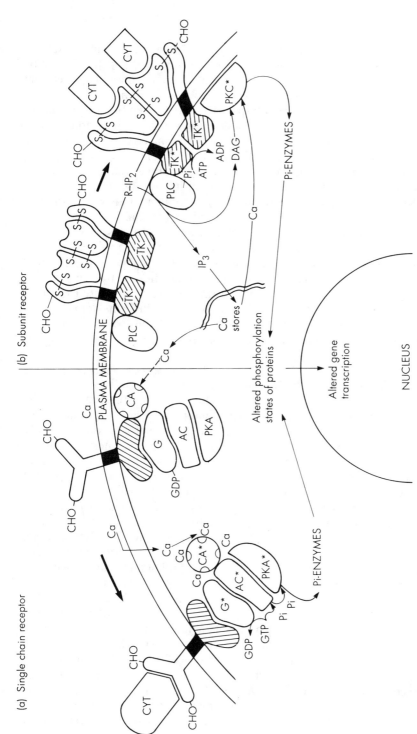

Figure 1.3 Cytokine receptors and proposed signal transmission pathways. Abbreviations: R-IP$_2$, diacylglycerophospho (1) inositol 4, 5-bisphosphate; IP$_3$, inositol 1, 4, 5-triphosphate; DAG, diacylglycerol; ATP, adenosine triphosphate; ADP, adenosine diphosphate; GTP, guanosine triphosphate; GDP, guanosine disphosphate; P$_i$, inorganic phosphate; CYT, cytokine; G, G-protein; CA, calmodulin; AC, adenylate cyclase; PKA, protein kinase A; PKC, protein kinase C; PLC, phospholipase C; Ca, calcium ions; CHO, carbohydrate; TK, tyrosine kinase. * indicates activation.

region of the molecule is usually heavily glycosylated, i.e. it contains several covalently linked sugars or oligosaccharide side chains, and these may be involved in the actual receptor binding site or in maintaining its correct conformation. Second, there is a region of receptor molecule which is relatively hydrophobic in nature and spans the plasma membrane lipid bilayer from its outer to its inner surface. This domain, which has been found to be structurally similar for different hormone and cytokine receptors, anchors the receptors to the plasma membrane. Finally, a third domain of the receptor is located on the inner surface of the plasma membrane and functions as a signalling device to other molecules located in its vicinity. This part of the molecule has been found in many instances to contain an enzyme, usually a tyrosine kinase, which is able to phosphorylate tyrosine residues both of itself (autophosphorylation) and of other protein molecules to which it is closely associated. While these three structural domains are common to most receptors that have been characterized, it should be pointed out that individual receptors have distinctive structures and are frequently composed of subunits (Figure 1.3). In some cases the three domains are fused together in one large receptor molecule, and in other cases different domains may be found in separate, but closely associated, subunits. More details of the structures of individual cytokine receptors will be given in subsequent chapters.

Signal transmission across the plasma membrane
The mechanism by which the recognition domain of the receptor transmits the signal occasioned by specific cytokine binding through the plasma membrane to activate the functional domain of the receptor is rather poorly understood. Recently, however, some clues have been emerging. First, it has been shown that mere receptor occupancy may be insufficient for signal transmission. For example, small antagonist molecules that bind to receptors frequently do not elicit the expected cellular response. Thus, it is probable that the overall size and orientation of the cytokine molecule with respect to the receptor binding site are important for efficient signalling. Second, cleavage of the extracellular recognition domain with a proteolytic enzyme such as trypsin sometimes elicits the same cellular response, e.g. mitogenesis (cell division), as does bona fide cytokine–receptor binding. This implies that the recognition domain also contains a control element which prevents signal transmission in the absence of cytokine binding. It is presumed therefore that when a cytokine occupies its receptor binding site it somehow modifies the recognition domain such that the control element is removed and signalling to the intracellular functional domain ensues (Figure 1.3). What happens when the control element is lost, and what is the nature of the signal, are matters for speculation. Probably, structural changes occasioned by cytokine occupancy of the receptor binding site have 'knock-on' effects which lead to alterations in plasma membrane mobility and permeability and to the juxtaposition of membrane components, including molecules that are closely associated with

receptors. As yet it remains unclear to what extent these alterations are necessary for signal transduction.

Intracellular signal transmission
The means by which cytokine–receptor interactions connect further with intracellular signalling pathways whereby information is transmitted elsewhere within the cell, e.g. to the cell nucleus, are also incompletely understood. However, there is a growing volume of experimental work strongly implicating the requirement for calcium ions (Ca^{2+}), high-energy nucleotide intermediates, e.g. GTP, cyclic AMP, phospholipid derivatives, and protein kinases and phosphatases (enzymes that respectively add and remove phosphate groups on many intracellular protein substrates), in the transmitting process. It is known that altered phosphorylation states of proteins, in particular those with enzymic activity, govern whether they are activated or de-activated and thus can significantly affect the functioning of various metabolic pathways. Rather less is known about how nuclear gene transcription is altered in cytokine-treated cells, and why subsequently the stimulation or inhibition of the synthesis of particular proteins happens. Obviously such changes do occur, and can contribute substantially to modification of cellular activities.

At the present time, at least two signal-transmitting or activation pathways have been described that appear to relate directly to hormone- or cytokine-mediated cellular responses. One of these involves the calcium-binding protein calmodulin, GDP-binding proteins (G-proteins), and the enzymes adenylate kinase and protein kinase A (Figure 1.3). The latter phosphorylates several well-defined regulatory enzymes involved in metabolic pathways, e.g. glycogen synthase, pyruvate kinase. In the other activation pathway, the receptor molecules themselves contain a tyrosine kinase which, when activated, subsequently activates phospholipases, possibly also through G-protein intermediates (Figure 1.3). The latter are responsible for the breakdown of plasma membrane inositol phopholipids to inositol triphosphate and diacylglycerol which are active intermediates for intracellular Ca^{2+} release and protein kinase C activation, respectively. Protein kinase C has a number of potential protein substrates, although these have not yet been defined, and thus probably activates many intracellular enzymes. More details will be given in Chapter 2 when cell proliferation is considered.

Internalization of cytokine–receptor complexes
Following cytokine binding the cytokine–receptor complexes are taken up into the cell by a process of plasma membrane invagination, and probably degraded by lysosomal enzymes. It is generally unknown whether the internalized cytokines and their degradation products have any additional effects on cellular metabolism which could then further modify cellular responses. This potential route of activation is, however, difficult to study, and for this

reason is often excluded from playing a major role at least in the causation of cytokine-mediated effects, although probably it should not be ignored.

Cytokine activities

It is probably true to say that cytokines function only as intercellular (and possibly intracellular) messenger molecules, albeit relatively complex ones. They do not appear to have any other functions, e.g. as enzymes or carrier molecules. However, it is very common to read about this or that cytokine activity, action, or function. While this is undoubtedly due to a confusion of terms, the practice of assigning activities to certain cytokines is now so widespread that it would be inappropriate to discontinue it. For example, IFNs are frequently described as having antiviral activity. In reality, antiviral activity is a cellular response to IFN, measured as the degree of inhibition of viral replication in IFN-treated cells. Therefore, cytokines should be considered to have particular activities only by association with the cellular responses they evoke. In a few instances, the association of a particular biological activity with an individual cytokine is straightforward, i.e. on a one-to-one basis. However, more often than not a particular biological activity is associated with two or more different cytokines. For instance, there are several examples of two or more cytokines, which are molecularly only rather distantly related, binding to the same surface receptor and therefore evoking the same cellular response(s). Obviously here, while there may be very large differences in amino acid sequences, common structural features between the two different cytokines must be conserved, at least sufficiently to allow specific binding to the receptor they share. In other cases, two or more cytokines which are apparently entirely molecularly unrelated and bind to distinct cell-surface receptors may also produce an apparently identical cellular response. It should be pointed out, though, that it can be difficult to ascertain whether an observed cellular response is the result of a primary cytokine–receptor interaction, or of auto-activation by the induced secretion of 'secondary' cytokines, or of multiple cytokine–receptor interactions exercising synergistic or antagonistic effects.

Most interestingly, it has also been found that an individual cytokine can, in many instances, be associated with the production of several apparently unrelated cellular responses, although some of these may be peculiar to distinct cell types and thus may not occur in every cell treated with a particular cytokine. Since, following cytokine stimulation, pleiotypic cellular responses are often observed, several cytokines have thus been described as pluripotent, polyfunctional, or pleiotropic mediators. The explanation for these pleiotypic responses appears to stem mainly from the diversity of intracellular signalling pathways that may be activated by a single population of cytokine receptors. It has also been speculated that there may be more heterogeneity in receptor populations than is readily apparent, and that different permutations of receptor structure and connections largely underlie the varied responses observed (Figure 1.4).

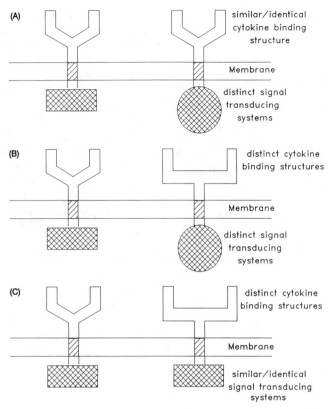

Figure 1.4 Diversity of receptors and interfacing signal transducing systems.

The fact that there are so many different cytokines with so much overlap of biological activity or function raises some important issues. From a biological standpoint, it is fair to say that the apparent biochemical redundancy of cytokines is not completely understood. However, the multitude of growth factors, for example, is partly explained by the varying cell type specificities of different growth factors. It is also known that in many instances multiple growth factors are required for maximum stimulation of cell growth and proliferation, for example, by acting at successive stages of the cell cycle (see Chapter 2).

With classical hormones, a balance of actions is obtained by the constant interaction of hormones with opposing actions: oestrogens–androgens, insulin–glucagon, parathyroid hormone–calcitonin, prostaglandin E–prostaglandin F_2, and prostacyclin–thromboxane, are readily identifiable pairs with opposing actions. For cytokines, the identification of pairs with opposing actions is not usually as clear cut. It may be considered, however, that cytokines fall into two mutually antagonistic groups; those with growth-promoting or mitogenic activity and those with growth-inhibitory or antimitogenic activity. On this basis, some pairs of cytokines with opposing actions are recognizable. For example, PDGF and IFN β could be one pair since the former can induce the latter: PDGF stimulates cell growth and proliferation, whereas IFN β inhibits this and therefore institutes negative feedback control of PDGF-stimulated growth (Figure 1.5).

Other growth factors and colony stimulating factors (CSF) also appear to form mutually antagonistic pairs with either IFN α or IFN β. Such negative feedback loops are important in the regulation of cell proliferation which, for obvious reasons, must normally be tightly controlled. In addition, exposure of a cell to one cytokine may raise the threshold for activity of a second cytokine. This can occur, for example, if the first cytokine leads to the down-regulation of receptors for the second one. In other circumstances, e.g. during an episode of acute infection with a virus, amplification of particular cellular responses is required and it has been shown that certain cytokines

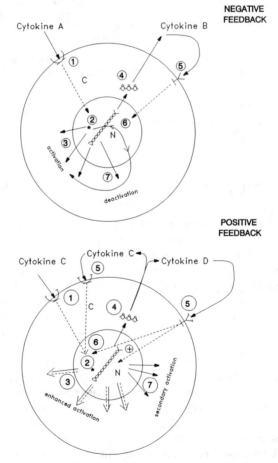

Figure 1.5 Negative and positive feedback of cell activation/proliferation by cytokines.

(e.g. TNF and IFN) can act synergistically to produce such amplified states (Figure 1.5). Furthermore, some cytokines are able to induce the production of others which also have stimulatory (agonistic) effects and thus exert positive feedback in responder cells (Figure 1.5). Interactions among cytokines will be discussed more fully in succeeding chapters.

The complexity of cytokine actions and interactions has only recently been brought to light, but it should be borne in mind that under physiological conditions a number of other exogenous (non-cytokine) factors, together with variable environmental conditions and genetic characteristics, may all have a bearing on cytokine-mediated cellular responses, making the real-life situation more complex than ever. Thus, it should be recognized that in reality cytokines seldom, if ever, act alone. It is important to remember this fact when experimental laboratory research on cytokine action is considered, because in most experiments particular cytokines are used alone, often at non-physiological concentrations, or used in rather selective combinations. Much of the data reviewed in the subsequent chapters has been obtained from such experimental systems, mainly from *in vitro* work, and thus should be read and interpreted with caution. The following quotation from René Dubos succinctly sums up the need for this caution: 'In the most common and probably the most important phenomena of life, the constituent parts are so interdependent that they lose their character, their meaning, and indeed their very existence when dissected from the functional whole' (Dubos, 1965).

The role of cytokines in the whole organism

It is probable that many cytokines are derivatives of products of primitive cellular recognition systems. Such recognition systems evolved to regulate cell-to-cell contact, including distinction of self from non-self, and to counteract noxious environmental influences that disturb homeostasis. Thus, it may be reasonably believed that cytokines have important roles in the growth, development, and maintenance of advanced multicellular, multi-organ species (e.g. mammals) where the orderly and unharmed assembly and functioning of cells is vital to normal morphogenesis, not only during embryogenesis and neonatal development but also through to adolescence and adulthood.

All exogenous stimuli cause localized perturbations in cells, resulting in imbalances in cellular metabolism. If not corrected, these may lead to pathological consequences, not only to the receiving cells, but also to neighbouring cells and possibly to the whole organism. In most circumstances, cells receiving exogenous stimuli respond rapidly to counteract any subsequent imbalances by internal adjustment of metabolic processes and by the secretion of mediators to communicate the nature of the imbalance to other cells and stimulate such cells to respond accordingly.

During morphogenesis, the orderly proliferation of cells and their differentiation to form specialized organs and tissues is essential. This process of development, it may be reasonably conjectured, must be largely dependent upon and controlled, both temporally and spatially, by the episodic and often cyclical release of many different hormones and cytokines and their subsequent concerted actions. Such episodic production and action of these intercellular mediators will be expected to continue throughout development until adulthood is reached; thereafter it will be used for maintenance and repair of organs and tissues and the integrated control of the various physiological systems. Superimposed upon the processes of self development, maintenance, and control is the requirement of the organism, at all times during life, to respond antagonistically to any noxious stimuli (e.g. chemical insult) and to any non-self forms, particularly foreign, replicating cell (or cell-like) entities such as bacteria and viruses. Cytokines have a crucial role in the defence of the organism, especially in the regulation of the immune system. For example, some cytokine-mediated actions probably help protect the fetus *in utero* from rejection by the mother, whose cells recognize embryonic cells as foreign. At birth, the external surfaces of the newborn go from a sterile to a non-sterile environment and the skin, orifices, and gut are rapidly colonized by bacteria and other micro-organisms. This engenders immune responses, regulated by cytokine release and actions, to control the proliferation of potentially pathogenic micro-organisms. Occasionally, micro-organisms temporarily evade the host immune defence mechanisms and cause disease. In these circumstances, the immune system reacts to the proliferation of such infective agents by production of relatively high levels of cytokines to amplify the overall immune response and to prevent the infection from spreading and having pathological consequences. In the process, excess levels of cytokines may be produced at the site of infection or inflammation, or may be released systemically and act on distant organs and tissues; in both cases they may have toxic effects. In fact, cytokines appear to contribute both to disease symptoms, such as fever, and to pathology, for example causing tissue damage. In this sense, cytokines can be thought of as 'two-edged swords'. At certain levels their actions are protective, but at overproduced high levels they are toxic and instigate deleterious or pathological changes in organs and tissues, even resulting in death in some cases. However, more often than not, acute illnesses due to infection are overcome and normal health gradually returns. Cytokines continue to play a part during recovery and probably act to 'damp down' the immune responses once the infectious agent has been eradicated.

It can also be envisaged that cytokines can influence the outcome of chronic and invasive diseases, but here the situation is probably more complex than in the case of acute infections. Cytokine overproduction can, as has just been mentioned, prolong inflammatory immune reactions and cause tissue injury. Thus, cytokines have often been found in association with chronic diseases, especially autoimmune diseases such as diabetes mellitus and rheumatoid arthritis, where activated, sensitized leukocytes attack certain apparently uninfected tissues. The cause of this leukocyte sensitization is usually unknown, but there is often circumstantial evidence that prior infection by a micro-organism, which may have occurred several years previous to the onset of auto-immune disease, has provided the trigger. In certain cancers, the unregulated proliferation of tumour cells may be due to the overproduction of a particular cytokine acting as a stimulatory growth factor for the tumour cells. In fact, it has been found that some cancer cells themselves are capable of producing a cytokine that can act as an autocrine (autostimulatory) growth factor. They may often also show a reduced requirement for growth factors and/or have abnormalities in their growth factor receptors, and this may also contribute to unregulated cell proliferation (see Chapter 2).

On the other hand, the absence or reduced levels of certain cytokines, in terms of their production and actions, can also lead to chronic infections and/or auto-immune disease, and/or cancer. This is now commonly observed in acquired immunodeficiency syndrome (AIDS), where infection with human immunodeficiency viruses leads to the destruction of major cyto-kine-producing leukocytes, the T-helper lymphocytes (see Chapter 4), in-volved in protective cellular immunity. As a result, AIDS patients may suffer from frequent chronic opportunistic infections, dementia caused by auto-immune destruction of brain (nerve) cells, a relatively rare skin cancer known as Kaposi's sarcoma, and possibly malignant lymphomas. Such observations, and others from the field of cancer biology, have given rise to the belief that many cytokines can have a therapeutic potential in the treatment of diseases including cancer and auto-immune disease. In some cases, they would act as simple replacement therapies. In others, since they are biologically very active, they could act as 'biological response modifiers' (BRMs) — cytokines are now often referred to as such — to increase immune and other physio-logical reactions and thus produce beneficial effects.

In conclusion, the balanced, episodic production and actions of cytokines are essential in maintaining an organism in a state in which it will survive and flourish in what is presumably a foreign and potentially hostile environment. Such a state in humans and animals is referred to as 'good health'.

Further reading

Bocci, V. (1988) Roles of interferon produced in physiological conditions. A speculative review. *Immunology* **64**, 1.

Cohen, P. (1985) The role of protein phosphorylation in the hormonal control of enzyme activity. *European Journal of Biochemistry* **151**, 439.

Cohen, S., Pick, E., and Oppenheim, J.J. (eds) (1979) *Biology of the Lymphokines*. Academic Press, New York.

De Maeyer, E. and De Maeyer-Guignard, J. (1988) *Interferons and Other Regulatory Cytokines*. Wiley, New York.

Dubos, R. (1965) *Man Adapting*. Yale University Press, New Haven.

Goustin, A.S., Leof, E.B., Shipley, G.D., and Moses, H.L. (1988) Growth factors and cancer. *Cancer Research* **46**, 1015.

Hamblin, A.S. (1988) *Lymphokines*. In Focus Series, IRL Press, Oxford.

Inglot, A.D. (1983) The hormonal concept of interferon. *Archives of Virology* **76**, 1.

Maizel, A.L. and Lachman, L.B. (1984) Biology of disease: control of human lymphocyte proliferation by soluble factors. *Laboratory Investigation* **50**, 369.

Metcalf, D. (1984) *The Hemopoietic Colony Stimulating Factors*. Elsevier, Amsterdam.

Michell, R. and Houslay, M. (1986) Pleiotypic responses: regulation by programmable messengers or by multiple receptors? *Trends in Biochemistry* **11**, 239.

Mortsyn, G. and Burgess, A.W. (1988) Hemopoietic growth factors: a review. *Cancer Research* **48**, 5624.

Oppenheim, J.J., Matsushima, K., Yoshimiera, T., and Leonard, E.J. (1987) The activities of cytokines are pleiotropic and interdependent. *Immunology Letters* **16**, 179.

Powanda, M.C., Oppenheim, J.J., Klager, M.J., and Dinarello, C.A. (1988) *Monokines and Other Non-lymphocytic Cytokines*. Alan R. Liss, New York.

Sachs, L. (1987) The molecular control of blood cell development. *Science* **238**, 1374.

Ullrich, A. and Yarden, Y. (1988) Molecular analysis of signal transduction by growth factors. *Biochemistry* **27**, 3113.

Webb, D.R. and Goeddel, D.W. (eds) (1982) *Lymphokines, Volume 13: Molecular Cloning and Analysis of Lymphokines*. Academic Press, New York.

Cell proliferation, growth factors, and oncogenes

2.1 The cell cycle

Many cell types of the adult animal do not undergo cell division. For example, mature nerve cells do not generally divide, although such cells continue actively to synthesize RNA and protein throughout life. However, during development, with the formation of tissues and organs, and for tissue repair involving cell replacement, cells are required to grow and multiply. In addition, several cell types, e.g. red blood cells (erythrocytes) and leukocytes, are produced continuously from precursor or stem cells. Such cells grow, proliferate, and mature into cells with specialized functions, e.g. macrophages and lymphocytes. Besides nutritional conditions, many aspects of the cell growth and division process are positively regulated by production of appropriate growth factors and expression of their cell receptors.

Evidence to show that cells which are committed to divide go through a programme or cycle of specific metabolic events has been gained from the study of cells in culture, which divide rapidly. The latter, under suitable conditions, may be synchronized with respect to the growth and division cycle, of which there are four distinct stages. The first stage is characterized by a lack of any DNA synthesis, but synthesis of RNA and protein synthesis actively takes place. It is of 8–10 hours duration depending on nutritional status, and is known as the Gap$_1$- or G$_1$-phase (Figure 2.1). The second stage, the so-called S-phase, encompasses a period of active DNA synthesis, again of 8–10 hours duration. Both RNA and protein synthesis are maintained during the S-phase. In the third stage, DNA synthesis ceases whilst RNA and protein synthesis continue for a further 3–4 hours. This stage is known as the G$_2$-phase. Finally, in the fourth stage, mitosis occurs, i.e. condensed chromo-

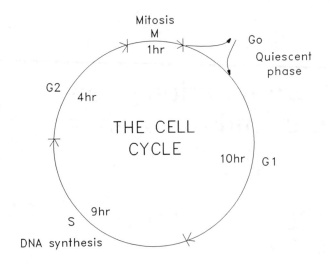

Figure 2.1   The cell cycle. The intervals for each phase are for a typical animal cell, but they will vary greatly among different cell types.

some pairs separate and subsequently the cell divides. The mitotic phase is known as the M-phase and lasts only about 1 hour. In contrast to other phases, little or no DNA, RNA, or protein synthesis occurs in the M-phase. Following cell division, this cycle, occupying about 24 hours, can be repeated. Alternatively, a cell may apparently leave the cycle in G_1 and become growth-arrested. This quiescent phase is often referred to as G_0 (Figure 2.1). It might seem obvious that, in the absence of growth factors and necessary nutritional substances, a cell would simply not grow or divide. However, recent evidence points to the growth-arrested state being positively controlled by the expression of certain inhibitory proteins.

2.2   Cell proliferation requirements

For cells in culture that continue to grow and multiply, it has become clear that is it necessary not only to provide all essential nutritional factors for maintaining cell metabolism and physiology, but also to provide the necessary factors that stimulate cells to grow and divide. Such 'growth factors' are present in animal blood sera, and preparations of animal sera, often of bovine origin, are commonly used to supplement defined cell-growth media. Serum contains a very complex mixture of proteins, carbohydrates, lipids, and other metabolites, and it has proved extremely difficult to isolate individual growth factors in any amount from this mixture. The relative concentrations of particular growth factors are usually very low, and fractionation and purification of serum components tends to yield individual factors that alone are insufficient to stimulate cells to proceed right through the cell cycle to cell division. Many cells in culture therefore appear to require several growth factors acting sequentially or in concert to stimulate growth and division. For instance, a growth-arrested cell in G_0 will presumably require a stimulus to (re-)commit it to enter the cell cycle in G_1. Following receipt of an appropriate stimulus occasioned by interaction of an exogenous growth factor with its receptor, it may be envisaged that inhibitory proteins will be removed or inactivated with the possible subsequent induction of another set of proteins, known as 'competence' (preparedness to enter the cell cycle) factors, which commit the cell to growth. It is then probable that the 'committed' cell will require a series of further external stimuli mediated by other growth and intracellular 'progression' factors for it to proceed through G_1-phase into S-phase (DNA synthesis), G_2-phase, and M-phase, after which cell division occurs. It can be pointed out here that cancer or tumour cells, or more commonly cell lines adapted to grow in culture from tumour cells, generally have:

1 a lower requirement for growth factors, or
2 an abnormal synthesis of competence/progression factors, or
3 both, than do normal diploid cells grown *in vitro*.

Tumour cell lines will, for example, proliferate at a lower serum concentration than normal cells. In other words, the proliferation of tumour cells is less well regulated than that of normal cells. As is well known, the abnormal unregulated proliferation of tumour cells *in vivo* may ultimately lead to cancer. The growth of tumour cells will be more fully discussed in relation to oncogenes later in this chapter (see Section 2.4).

From Chapter 1, it is apparent that many cytokines have or are associated with growth factor activity. Some of these growth-promoting cytokines, e.g. epidermal growth factor (EGF), act on many diverse cell types while others, e.g. nerve growth factor (NGF), appear more specific for certain cell types. Furthermore, some cytokines, e.g. TGFβ, are able to induce competence or progression factors, but alone may not promote growth through to cell division. The rest of this chapter is devoted to the exploration and discussion of various aspects of the activities of certain growth-promoting cytokines concerning their molecular structure and induction, the structure–function relationship of interactions with their cell surface receptors, the pathways of signal transduction and the induction of competence and progression factors, together with the relationship of cytokines, their receptors and competence/progression factors to oncogenes. This chapter will confine itself to the following cytokines:

- epidermal growth factor (EGF), transforming growth factors alpha and beta (TGFα, TGFβ) and related polypeptides
- insulin and insulin-like growth factors-I and II (IGF-I, IGF-II)
- platelet-derived growth factor (PDGF)

- acidic and basic fibroblast growth factors (aFGF, bFGF)
- nerve cell growth factor (NGF)

that is, cytokines which are not specifically involved in either haematopoiesis or immune responses, although they may affect either or both of these processes.

2.3 Cell activation

A speculative and probably oversimplified model of cell activation has already been sketched in outline in Chapter 1 (p. 13). Before going further, however, it is necessary to return to the process of cell activation and to re-emphasize its probable functional components. It is known that different cytokines bind to distinct cell-surface receptors. These receptors, while specific for individual or molecularly related cytokines, have structural elements in common and probably function in rather similar ways. Thus, while there is a diversity of cytokines and receptors, there are probably relatively few ways in which signals may be transduced across the cell plasma membrane. Further transmission of signals to internal compartments of cells is dependent upon the presence and activation of

1 functional elements of receptors themselves, e.g. tyrosine kinase
2 functional proteins associated with receptors, e.g. G-proteins
3 enzymes responsible for the production of secondary messengers
4 protein kinases and phosphatases responsible for the activation and de-activation of intracellular enzymes
5 metal ion (e.g. Ca^{2+}) transport systems.

All of these functional components are interlinked and interdependent. Together they provide a variable response network which is dependent on

(a) the strength of stimulus and ensuing signal(s)
(b) cell type and degree of maturation or specialization
(c) the stage of the cell cycle
(d) environmental, nutritional, and genetic factors.

They may be seen to mediate the early events, taking place in seconds or minutes from receipt of stimulus, of the cellular response.

Signal transmission to the cell nucleus results in the de-repression or activation of particular genes. In the present context of cell growth and division, the activation of genes coding for competence proteins is especially important. This is because the protein products of competence genes are able to regulate further nuclear and cytoplasmic events and to enable the cell to respond appropriately to other growth-stimulating factors. In most cases, the identity of competence proteins is not yet known, but it is expected that this group of proteins will contain several nucleus-located proteins that bind directly or indirectly to DNA. These appear to enhance the transcription of a number of other genes, probably including those specifying some competence proteins, while suppressing the transcription of others. The competence/progression proteins also appear likely to include components of the cell-surface receptor system, either elements of receptors themselves or functional proteins associated with receptors or even secreted cytokines which may act in an autocrine way. They probably also include regulators of DNA synthesis and further (late) gene transcription. Thus, it may be envisaged that there are two or more classes of competence/progression proteins which act sequentially, and that for each stimulus there will be a corresponding wave of specific gene modulation and competence/progression protein synthesis (Figure 2.2). Accordingly, there may well be several waves of gene modulation and competence/progression protein synthesis during the cell cycle, each wave being occasioned by successive, different stimuli at the cell surface mediated by cytokine (growth factor)–receptor interactions. For instance, by analogy, it might be imagined that cytokines, their receptors and competence/progression proteins could each be signified by a single letter of the alphabet, e.g. G for growth factor, R for receptor, etc. If in sequential combination these spelt a word, e.g. G-R-O-W-T-H, then this would translate into the appropriate response of cell growth and division (Figure 2.2). If, however, a word could not be spelt, or was mis-spelt, then either there would be no response, e.g. cells halted at certain stages of the cell cycle, or the response would be inappropriate, e.g. unregulated proliferation as in tumour cells. Actual breakdown of cell growth regulation might therefore be conceived of as resulting from defective competence/progression proteins or their faulty synthesis.

The synthesis and action of competence/progression proteins takes place in hours rather than minutes from the time of stimulation, although gene transcription may start within minutes. It covers the intermediate events of

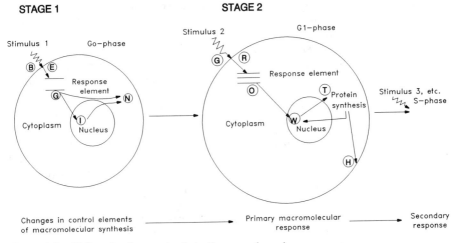

Figure 2.2 Cell activation: entry into the growth cycle.

the cellular response to growth factors, and probably occurs mainly in the G_1-phase of the cell cycle. Late stage events happen in S-phase and G_2-phase, where DNA synthesis and synthesis of structural proteins and other components of the cell respectively take place.

It seems probable that early, intermediate, and late stage events of the cellular response are mostly positively regulated. It should not, however, be forgotten that there must necessarily be negative feedback mechanisms to ensure that transcription of genes, synthesis of proteins, etc. are shut down at appropriate times and that de-activation of regulatory enzymes occurs as required. There is, for example, growing evidence for the existence of a set of inhibitory proteins with opposing action(s) to those of competence proteins. Furthermore, some cytokines, e.g. interferons, appear to have analogous, growth-inhibitory actions.

2.4 Oncogenes

It is clear that for commitment to growth and for progression through the cell cycle there must be underlying operational communicative intracellular pathways, e.g. pathways of signal transmission and gene modulation. Although the details of these are as yet only understood in a rather fragmented, rudimentary way, there is growing experimental support for the basic features of the current model as proposed in the preceding section. However, much of this evidence came originally not from the study of cells in culture, but from virological studies, in particular those pertaining to a group of enveloped viruses known as *retroviruses* (retroviridae). Viruses in general, in comparison to cells, are rather simple organic entities and encode relatively few proteins in their genomes. Retroviruses have an RNA genome, and their replication involves an unusual step whereby this RNA genome is first transcribed into DNA by a virion-associated enzyme called reverse transcriptase (Figure 2.3). This double-stranded DNA copy of the genome is then inserted or integrated into the host cell nuclear DNA where it serves as a template for viral mRNA synthesis and new genomes (Figure 2.3). Subsequently, new viral structural proteins are synthesized and finally progeny virus particles are assembled and bud out through the plasma membrane (Figure 2.3). However, the viral DNA inserted into nuclear DNA frequently remains intact and is replicated when a cell divides.

Perhaps more importantly, certain retroviruses, e.g. avian retroviruses such as Rous sarcoma virus (RSV), are known to transform normal cells in culture. Transformation here means that the cell becomes 'immortalized' and may lose normal growth control. This is associated with a loss of growth factor requirements and a marked increase in tumorigenic potential, i.e. when injected into animals these cells may form tumours. In other words, retroviruses must carry in their small genomes the information necessary to transform a normal cell into a tumour cell. The gene or genes encoding this 'oncogenic' (cancer-forming) information are now known as viral oncogenes, or v-*onc* for

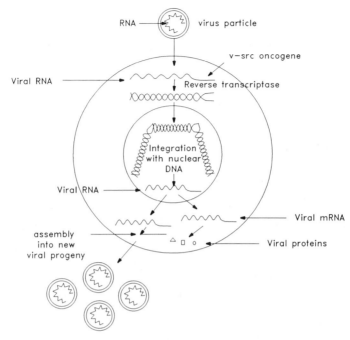

RNA — virus particle

v—src oncogene

Viral RNA — Reverse transcriptase

Integration with nuclear DNA

Viral RNA —

Viral mRNA

assembly into new viral progeny

Viral proteins

Figure 2.3 Retrovirus replication.

short. The first of these v-*onc* genes to be studied in detail was the so-called v-*src* oncogene (all oncogenes are designated in three-letter, lower-case, codes) of RSV in the early 1970s. It was established that besides coding for viral structural proteins, the RSV genome also coded for a non-structural protein of MW 60000. By accident, it was then discovered that this protein, now called pp60v-*src*, was a protein kinase and more specifically a tyrosine kinase. Furthermore, the location of pp60v-*src* was shown to be the inner surface of the plasma membrane, a position where it could phosphorylate other regulatory enzymes. It is now known, as has been discussed previously (see Chapter 1), that protein phosphorylation probably plays a major role in cell activation, and that several receptors for cytokine and other mediators contain tyrosine kinases. Thus, a clear link between cytokine-induced and v-*onc*-induced cell growth and proliferation was established. The reason why the expression of v-*onc* leads to cell transformation and unregulated cell proliferation is probably that pp60v-*src* tyrosine kinase is made in relatively large amounts and, in contrast to cytokine receptors, does not appear to have a control element and so is 'switched on' all the time.

Following the discovery of the v-*src* oncogene and the characterization of its protein product, a number of other v-*onc* have been found in other retroviruses. Some 20 or more distinct v-*onc* have been described in different retroviruses (Table 2.1). Most commonly, tyrosine kinase proteins are the products of v-*onc*, e.g. v-*fps*, v-*yes*, and v-*ros*, but several other v-*onc* specify

Table 2.1   Connections between oncogenes, growth factors, and growth control response elements

	(Proto)-oncogenes (cellular or retroviral)
Growth factors:	
Platelet-derived growth factor B-chain	*cis*
Fibroblast growth factor-like proteins	*int-2, hst, fgf-5*
Growth factor receptor tyrosine kinases:	
Epidermal growth factor receptor (EGF-R)	*erbB*[a,d]
Related to EGF-R	*neu (erbB2)*
Insulin receptor	—
Insulin-like growth factor-I receptor	—
Platelet-derived growth factor receptor	—
Macrophage-colony stimulating factor (M-CSF-R)	*fms*
Related to M-CSF-R	*kit*[a]
Atrial natriuretic factor receptor[b]	—
Receptor-less tyrosine kinases:	
'src-like family' includes:	*src, fgr, fyn, hck, lck, lyn, yes*
miscellaneous[c] includes:	*trk, ros, abl, fps/fes, pim-1, rel, ret, sea, bcl-2*
Plasma membrane-associated transducing proteins	
RAS membrane GTPase p21	*H-ras, K-ras, N-ras*
G-proteins	—
Cytoplasmic response elements	
Serine kinases	*mos, mil/raf*
Nuclear transcription factors	
Miscellaneous	*jun, fos, myc, myb*
Viral only	*Ela* (adenovirus)
	T-Ag (simian virus 40, polyoma virus)
	tat (human immuno-deficiency virus)

a, retroviral v-*erb* B and v-*kit* encode truncated receptors missing most of extracellular domains; *b*, ANF-R is guanylate cyclase containing intracellular tyrosine kinase; *c*, functionally related, but not belonging to 'src-like' family; *d*, *erbA* is T3 thyroid hormone receptor located in nuclear chromatin.

proteins that have different functions and/or occur in different intracellular compartments. Many appear to be components of the cytokine-receptor signal transmission pathway, or are highly analogous to them. For instance, the v-*ras* oncogenes, of which there are three different types, specify proteins of MW 21 000 which bind GDP/GTP and are located on or in association with the intracellular face of the plasma membrane. Functionally, therefore, they appear to be highly analogous to the more complex G-proteins. The latter are heterotrimers with subunits α, β, and γ of which the more variable α-subunit (MW 39 000–52 000) has GDP-binding and GTPase activities. The G-proteins appear to be important intermediaries in the adenylate cyclase pathway, and may also have a role in the transmission of signals from tyrosine kinase receptors. By analogy, v-RAS proteins (upper-case letters signify the protein coded by *onc*) might therefore perform the same task, but this has not been rigorously proved. Other v-*onc* specify proteins that are located in the nucleus and which bind directly or indirectly to DNA, e.g. v-FOS, v-MYC. These are probably involved in control of transcription of particular sets of nuclear genes. In fact, there are yet other v-*onc* present in DNA genome viruses such as polyoma virus and adenovirus which are functionally analogous to 'v-*myc*-like' oncogenes from retroviruses (Table 2.1). It should be pointed out that, in contrast to the 'v-*src*-like' oncogene products, generally neither v-RAS nor 'v-MYC-like' proteins can alone transform cells, but their combination will often achieve full transformation.

At first it was thought that v-*onc* were peculiar to retroviruses and certain DNA viruses. However, it was a puzzle why many retroviruses contained these genes. There appeared to be no requirement for v-*onc* since those retroviruses without v-*onc* were able to replicate as well. It also came as quite a surprise when it was found, in about 1976, that there was a cellular gene homologous to v-*src*. In the following years, cellular homologues of all the retroviral v-*onc* have been discovered and found to exist in the cells of virtually all animals and insects. Since these cellular genes have been conserved throughout evolution, it is assumed that they code for important functional proteins, especially those regulating cell growth and proliferation. For this reason, they were first known as proto-oncogenes. Presumably, retroviruses have acquired proto-oncogenes, or parts thereof, from cells in which they replicated by a process of recombination with adjacent nuclear genes following integration of retroviral DNA into host cell DNA (Figure 2.3). Subsequent to such recombination, v-*onc* emerged from proto-oncogene modifications, e.g. point mutations, deletions, or insertions, and because the modified proto-oncogene was placed in tandem with a strong transcriptional promotor of viral gene transcription leading to high levels of expression of oncogene mRNA and thence oncoprotein. Originally it was not thought that the cellular proto-oncogenes could be responsible for cell transformation, but investigation of tumour cells in the last decade or so, and in particular the transfer of DNA from transformed, tumour cells to untransformed, 'normal' cells in culture, has readily established that proto-oncogenes can be oncogenic. Thus, they are now more commonly called, rather confusingly, cellular oncogenes or c-*onc* for short. Again the reason they become oncogenic is because of mutations, deletions, or insertions causing synthesis of defective oncogene proteins and/or because they are translocated from their normal chromosomal location to a position in the genome where they are subject to 'abnormal' transcriptional control, e.g. in tandem with a strong promotor of transcription of genes coding for proteins normally made in large amounts. In the latter case, overproduction of the oncoprotein results and it is assumed that transformation ensues partly because of the relatively high abnormal dosage of enzymatic or regulatory function. For instance, in many malignant lymphomas the tumour cells, which are neoplastically transformed antibody-producing B-lymphocytes, have a translocation of c-*myc* to the chromosomal location of antibody (immunoglobulin) genes which are normally highly transcribed and thus c-MYC protein is constitutively produced at high levels being no longer subject to normal regulation by exogenous stimuli. In normal B-lymphocytes, c-MYC protein appears only to be transiently produced early in the cell cycle following stimulation by growth-promoting cytokines or mitogens. In contrast to c-*myc*, c-*ras* oncogenes in tumour cells are more likely to be the result of point mutation in the proto-oncogene leading to a single amino acid substitution in the c-RAS protein. Approximately 15 per cent of all human tumours contain mutated c-*ras* oncogenes, and the transforming c-RAS proteins most commonly have a substitution at amino acid residue 12 or 61 with resulting reduced GTPase activity. Transforming c-*ras* genes and oncoproteins occur only in tumour cells and are not found in normal cells.

Summarizing thus far, many retroviruses and certain DNA viruses can neoplastically transform, or at least immortalize, cells on account of the expression of v-*onc* they carry in their genomes. Cellular proto-oncogenes become c-*onc* once they are subject to abnormal expression or if they are modified. Generally speaking, the expression of oncogenes is necessary, but not always sufficient, to induce neoplastic transformation. It has been found that, at several different stages of development, the cells of different tissues can express high levels of proto-oncogene protein at certain times, particularly at stages of rapid cell proliferation. Thus, proto-oncogene expression could be seen as opening important 'permissive' growth or differentiation pathways during normal development. Oncogene (v-*onc*, c-*onc*) expression might also therefore be conceived of as rendering cells 'permissive' for growth or differentiation, but in the process rendering them also susceptible to the action of factors that cause neoplastic transformation, which is known to be multi-step process.

Strong links between expression of proto-oncogenes/ oncogenes and cytokine-receptor signal transmission pathways have been established (Table 2.1). Proto-oncogenes and their oncogenic counterparts appear mostly to code for normal or abnormal components, or their functional analogues, of cytokine-receptor signal transmission pathways (Figure 2.4). Oncoproteins containing analogous functional moieties of:

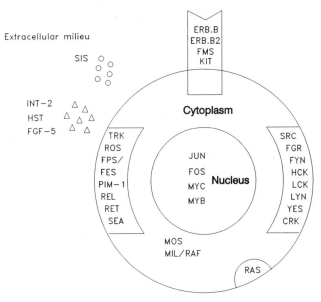

Figure 2.4   Location of oncoproteins along the growth-factor-mediated mitogenic pathway.

(a)   cytokine receptors, e.g. pp60 v-*src* tyrosine kinase
(b)   signal transducing G-proteins, e.g. p21 RAS GTPase, and
(c)   DNA-binding transcription factors, e.g. FOS, MYC proteins,

have already been mentioned.

Further, more recent, findings have cemented this relationship. For example, the protein products of c-*sis*, c-*erb B*, and c-*fms* have been shown to exhibit extensive amino acid sequence homology with PDGF, the EGF receptor, and the macrophage-colony stimulating factor (M-CSF) receptor, respectively (Figure 2.4). In addition, three recently discovered oncogenes, c-*int-2*, c-*hst/ks3*, and c-*fgf-5*, have all been shown to code for proteins that show considerable homology to FGFs, cytokines which induce division in a wide variety of cells. There has also been the discovery of further oncogenes that specify nuclear proteins, e.g. c-*jun*. Rather interestingly c-*jun* specifies a protein, JUN, which is identical to a transcription factor previously known as AP-1. JUN (AP-1) has been shown to associate with FOS, and the JUN–FOS complex binds to a specific transcription enhancer in DNA. In quiescent (G_0) cells, both c-*jun* and c-*fos* are rapidly induced without prior protein synthesis by cytokines such as EGF, and thus JUN and FOS are probably 'early' competence proteins. In addition to enhancing transcription, the JUN–FOS complex probably also acts as a transcription repressor, possibly down-regulating transcription of c-*jun* and c-*fos*, i.e. causing feedback inhibition.

In conclusion, experimental evidence is accumulating to support a conceptual model of cell growth, proliferation, and differentiation, features of which have been discussed above, in which proto-oncogene products are essential components of cytokine-receptor signal transmission pathways, including trophic factors *per se*, their receptors and elements of a connecting intracellular regulatory network. Together they control cellular responses to cytokines and other exogenous factors, which may have both stimulatory (growth-promoting) and inhibitory (differentiating) activities, depending on the target cell. They probably regulate episodic rapid cell proliferation as occurs at different developmental stages of embryogenesis as well as in, for example, haematopoiesis and tissue repair. Normally, these periods of rapid cell proliferation are self-limiting, presumably the results of negative feedback mechanisms which probably include inhibition of cytokine production, down-regulation of receptors, and repression of proto-oncogenes. Abnormalities in the sequences and regulation of expression of proto-oncogenes frequently disturb these tightly regulated growth control mechanisms and predispose cells to neoplastic transformation. There are a variety of ways in which such disturbances can be effected; some of these have been previously alluded to, e.g. overproduction of oncoproteins, but a fully detailed description of these several oncogenic mechanisms is beyond the scope of this book (see Further reading, pp. 60–61). Returning to the simple analogy of designating elements of the cytokines receptor-signal transmission pathways by a single letter (p. 25), disturbances might be illustrated simply as mis-spelt or deformed words, e.g. GRRROWTH, GЯOWTH (Figure 2.5). However, it should also be realized that loss of growth control will result not only from positive, aberrant oncogene expression and products, but also from the loss of negative

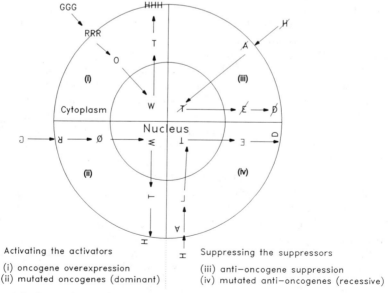

Activating the activators   Suppressing the suppressors

(i) oncogene overexpression   (iii) anti–oncogene suppression
(ii) mutated oncogenes (dominant)   (iv) mutated anti–oncogenes (recessive)

Figure 2.5   Loss of growth regulation.

control mechanisms. Some of the elements inhibiting cell growth have been called 'anti-oncogenes', and if these are suppressed, or mutated then unregulated cell proliferation may ensue (Figure 2.5). In this respect, certain cytokines, e.g. TGFβ, which can act on cells in an autocrine growth inhibitory way, could be viewed as anti-oncogene products. When their expression is suppressed, or when they are inactivated by mutation, they could also be said to be 'oncogenic by defect'. Thus, in conclusion, loss of growth control may be the result of either activating the activators, or suppressing the suppressors (Figure 2.5).

2.5   Growth factors

Introductory comments

Much of what follows is based on extensive reading of the voluminous literature on the so-called growth factors. There are thousands of scientific reports for each growth factor, and it is not possible to give detailed reviews of all aspects of individual growth factors. This chapter and those to follow therefore attempt to summarize the nature and biology of the growth factors which I have defined as cytokines (see Table 1.1).

Growth factors, and indeed cytokines in general, have a history going back many years. The discovery of several of them predates the advent of the DNA technological revolution which began in the mid- to late-1970s. Before that time growth factors were usually isolated from various natural sources, i.e. cells, tissues, body fluids, and were not in general available as highly purified proteins. In fact, in some cases it could be said that such preparations were mixtures of soluble proteins 'contaminated' by growth factors! At the time researchers genuinely believed that the effects they observed using 'crude' growth factor preparations were due to the specific growth factor(s) they contained, but the validity of some (although not all) such observations may now be questioned in retrospect. The work of the pioneers in this field was, however, of great value: the biology, or at least certain biological parameters, characteristic of many diverse growth factors was established in early research investigations and has paved the ground for the later gene cloning and expression of individual growth factors by rDNA technological methods.

Advances made in molecular genetics and nucleic acid chemistry in the late 1970s and early 1980s now enable the genes coding for natural, biologically active proteins to be identified, analysed in fine detail, transferred between organisms, and expressed under controlled conditions so as to obtain synthesis of the polypeptide which they encode. Thus, the genes coding for many cytokines, including growth factors, have been identified, analysed, and expressed to give high yields of biologically active product in suitable heterologous prokaryotic or eukaryotic cells. The means of enabling this process to work efficiently often necessitates the following common strategy:

a naturally occurring or synthetic nucleotide sequence is inserted into an appropriate DNA vector this is subsequently introduced into a suitable host organism to ensure that the desired product, i.e. that coded by the inserted polynucleotide, is expressed in high yield.

The various steps required for RNA and DNA isolation, their copying, linking, and insertion operations, transduction/transfection of recombinant vectors into heterologous host organisms, and expression of the protein product will not be described here.

The main outcome of the rDNA technological revolution is that polypeptides and proteins such as cytokines which were previously difficult to prepare from natural sources can now be manufactured in relatively large amounts, and can be purified to virtual homogeneity in many cases. The ready availability of recombinant cytokines has led to a surge in interest in these mediators, and to an exponential rise in the number of scientific and clinical investigations, and subsequent publications. Unlike the situation that existed before cytokines were cloned, where cytokine preparations were often of low purity and probably contained mixtures of biological mediators, researchers can now be confident that what they are applying to their various experimental systems is a single, biologically active cytokine, and that the biological effects they observe are attributable to the action(s) of the cytokine in question. This has enabled the biology of individual cytokines to be described much more fully, and further rapid progress in this area is likely. One of the aims of this chapter, and of this book as a whole, is to be as up to date as possible, but it is only too likely that new facts will emerge concerning particular cytokines which unfortunately cannot be incorporated before publication. I hope readers and authors will excuse this inevitable shortcoming, and also the rather limited scope of the following reviews.

Epidermal growth factor, transforming growth factor alpha and vaccinia growth factor

The discovery of EGF dates from around 1960 and was the outcome of acute observation, and perhaps a little serendipity. Stanley Cohen and colleagues were studying NGF activity in snake venom extracts. They reasoned that the submaxillary glands of mice might provide a more readily available, and safer, source of NGF. This proved to be the case, and Cohen was able to purify NGF from an extract of the mouse submaxillary gland. However, he also noticed that some fractions from the NGF purification, which were devoid of NGF activity, caused the precocious opening of the eyelids of newborn mice. On this basis, Cohen was then able to purify the factor responsible for this effect, which he named epidermal growth factor because it was also found that it would induce cell proliferation in the basal cells of skin.

The structure of mouse-derived EGF was published in 1972 by Cohen's group; subsequently in 1975 a polypeptide, urogastrone, purified from urine and shown to inhibit gastric secretion, proved to have the same amino acid sequence. The native form of EGF consists of 53 amino acids (MW~6000).

There is extensive amino acid sequence homology (approximately 70 per cent) between human and mouse EGFs, and in particular the positions of three internal disulphide bonds are highly conserved (Figure 2.6). It is now known that a much larger precursor polypeptide (MW~130 000) containing the native EGF sequence is synthesized initially, and this is apparently proteolytically cleaved to yield EGF following plasma-membrane insertion. Cloning and analysis of the gene coding for the EGF precursor has shown it to be a surprisingly large gene with many exons and potential to code for a sequence of up to 1217 amino acids. Obviously, mature EGF accounts for a small proportion, residues 977–1029, of this deduced sequence. The EGF gene has been found to occur in a large variety of tissues, but the EGF precursor polypeptides may not always be processed to yield mature EGF molecules, e.g. in kidney tubules, although EGF itself is to be found in virtually all body fluids. EGF is, however, not known to be synthesized by tumours.

TGFα was discovered in about 1978 by George Todaro's group as a product of cultured retrovirus-transformed fibroblastic cells. Its name derives from its capacity to induce the anchorage-independent proliferation of normal cells in soft agar. (Normally, fibroblastic cells in culture stick or anchor themselves to the glass or plastic surface of the vessel they are grown in and will only proliferate in an anchorage-dependent way. If these cells are transferred to soft agar where they will effectively remain unattached (unanchored) in suspension, they will not divide. However, the addition of TGFα to the soft-agar medium causes certain cells to multiply and form colonies in the agar, i.e. to exhibit anchorage-independent growth.) Mature TGFα appears to be a polypeptide of 50 amino acids (MW~5600), although it is probable that there are additional multiple heterogeneous forms of higher molecular weight. It shows distinct structural homology (30 per cent relatedness at the amino acid level) to EGF. In particular, TGFα contains three internal disulphide bonds which are identically placed to those of EGF (Figure 2.6). Similarly to EGF, TGFα is synthesized as an internal polypeptide of a larger precursor (MW 160 000), which is probably initially a transmembrane protein before cleavage to release native TGFα. The TGFα gene is also correspondingly large, but is non-identical and completely separate from the EGF gene; the human TGFα gene is located on chromosome 2 whereas the EGF-gene is on chromosome 7. TGFα synthesis has been mainly associated with a variety of tumours, e.g. carcinomas, and tumour-derived or transformed cells, and TGFα has been implicated in maintaining the transformed phenotype of cell lines. However, there is growing evidence that TGFα is produced by non-malignant cells and tissues, especially during embryogenesis, e.g. in the developing kidney or in the placenta. It has been conjectured that TGFα may represent the fetal analogue of EGF which is widely found in adult tissues, but not as commonly in embryonic ones. TGFα has the potential to stimulate the growth and proliferation of many cell types, but its exact physiological role remains enigmatic.

Rather curiously, a third member of the EGF/TGF family has turned up;

	1				5					10					15					20					25
mEGF			N	S	Y	P	G	C	P	S	S	Y	D	G	Y	C	L	N	G	G	V	C	M	H	I	E	S
hEGF			N	S	D	S	E	C	P	L	S	H	D	G	Y	C	L	H	D	G	V	C	M	Y	I	E	A
rTGF	V	V	S	H	F	N	K	C	P	D	S	H	T	Q	Y	C	F	H	-	G	T	C	R	F	L	V	Q
hTGF	V	V	S	H	F	N	D	C	P	D	S	H	T	Q	F	C	F	H	-	G	T	C	R	F	L	V	Q
VGF			P	A	I	R	L	C	G	P	E	G	D	G	Y	C	L	H	-	G	D	C	I	H	A	R	D

				30					35		40						45					50
mEGF	L	D	S	Y	T	C	N	C	V	I	G	Y	S	G	D	R	C	Q	T	R	D	L	R	W	W	E	L	R
hEGF	L	D	K	Y	A	C	N	C	V	V	G	Y	I	G	E	R	C	Q	Y	R	D	L	K	W	W	E	L	R
rTGF	E	E	K	P	A	C	V	C	H	S	G	Y	V	G	V	R	C	E	H	A	D	L	L	A
hTGF	E	D	K	P	A	C	V	C	H	S	G	Y	V	G	I	R	C	E	H	A	D	L	L	A
VGF	I	D	G	M	Y	C	R	C	S	H	G	Y	T	G	A	R	C	Q	H	V	V	L	V	D	Y	Q	R	S

(a)

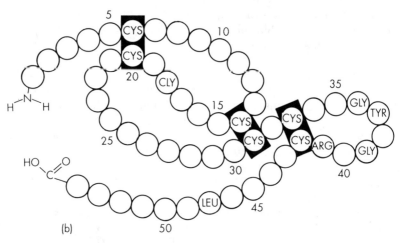

(b)

Figure 2.6 A. Amino acid sequences of growth factors related to EGF. The sequences of the individual polypeptides are taken from references cited at the end of the chapter and are shown in comparison with mouse EGF. B. Representation of strictly conserved amino acid residues in the EGF family of growth factors and the positioning of disulphide bonds. (Reprinted with permission from Carpenter and Zendegui, 1986; copyright Academic Press.)

this is the result not of practical research investigations but of a fishing expedition into a computer base of DNA sequences. By this means, three groups of researchers simultaneously 'hooked' a DNA sequence coding for a polypeptide showing 36 per cent overall homology with human EGF and containing the central core peptide with its highly conserved cysteine residues and internal disulphide bonds (Figure 2.6). This DNA sequence occurs in a large DNA virus, vaccinia virus of the poxvirus group (of which smallpox virus is also a member), and it appears that the growth-factor-like polypeptide is produced during viral replication in host cells. The polypeptide binds to the same cell surface receptor as that recognized by EGF and TGFα, and appears to have similar growth-promoting activity to these mediators. It has therefore been named vaccinia growth factor (VGF). However, just why a virus requires such a growth factor, and whether VGF plays a role in vaccinia pathogenesis, remain obscure. The presence of VGF in vaccinia infections probably accounts for the benign hyperplasia (rapid cell proliferation) associated with virus-containing skin lesions.

It has already been pointed out that EGF and TGFα, despite being only 30 per cent structurally homologous, together with VGF, bind to the same cell-surface receptor. Experiments initiated in the early 1970s when purified EGF became available demonstrated the presence of a single population of saturable, high-affinity receptors in EGF-responsive cells. These receptors have now been found to exist in virtually all cell types, but biochemical characterization of EGF receptors (EGF-R) remained almost impossible owing to the fact that cells contained relatively low numbers of EGF-R and yielded miniscule amounts of receptor molecules. The breakthrough came in around 1978 with the finding that a tumour-derived cell line designated A-431, originating from a human epidermoid carcinoma, markedly overproduced EGF-R. The EGF-R was purified from A-431 cells and shown to be an integral plasma-membrane glycoprotein (MW 170 000). It was subsequently shown to contain a large N-terminal, glycosylated, extracellular binding domain specific for recognition of EGF, a short hydrophobic transmembrane region, and a third C-terminal domain associated with the intracellular face of the plasma membrane and which contains a tyrosine kinase. Since then, EGF-R has become one of the most studied and best characterized growth factor receptors, serving as a paradigm in structure and function for other cytokine and hormone receptors. It has become apparent that different receptors for a diversity of mediators share the three-domain configuration of EGF-R, but vary considerably in how each domain is composed. This class of receptors is now often referred to as 'the family of receptor tyrosine kinases (RTK)'. In contrast, the 'src-like' oncogenes give rise to 'receptor-less tyrosine kinases', so called because these proteins have no extracellular domain (Table 2.1).

The amino acid sequence of EGF-R has been deduced and shown to display marked homology with the v-ERB B oncoprotein (see Table 2.1). The latter is a truncated form of EGF-R lacking a considerable portion, nearly all, of the extracellular domain and a smaller fragment from the intracellular domain (Figure 2.7). The v-ERB B oncoprotein is therefore an incomplete receptor, and is not subject to stimulation by EGF/TGFα.

An insight into how the EGF-R functions and is regulated comes mainly from recent elegant studies involving site-directed mutagenesis of the c-erb B proto-oncogenes, or more correctly the cDNA coding for EGF-R, and the expression of mutant EGF-R in cells not previously containing any EGF-R.

Without going into any detail, the main conclusions of these studies are as follows:

1   the level of cell response to EGF/TGFα is governed by the numbers of EGF-R expressed at the cell surface;
2   oligomeric EGF-R, which binding of ligand promotes, have a higher affinity for EGF and probably have a more active tyrosine kinase through allosteric (conformational) interactions occasioned by close association of intracellular receptor domains;
3   the activity of the intrinsic tyrosine kinase is indispensible for eliciting the mitogenic effect of EGF, but is not necessary for its binding;
4   autophosphorylation by the intrinsic tyrosine kinase of tyrosine residues in the intracellular C-terminal domain of EGF-R is probably not essential for either ligand binding or signal transduction;
5   phosphorylation of a threonine residue, position 654 (Thr^{654}), by the Ca^{2+}-dependent protein kinase C (a kinase that phosphorylates serine and threonine residues, but not tyrosine) is responsible for de-activation or down-regulation of EGF-R (possibly by preventing the formation of high-affinity oligomeric EGF-R) and thus probably provides a negative control mechanism for EGF-induced mitogenesis (Figure 2.7);
6   over-expression of v-*ERB* B oncoprotein, rather than deletions in its N-terminal and C-terminal domains, is probably likely to account for its transforming capacity. In addition, over-expression of c-*erb* B, which codes for complete EGF-R, or of a related but distinct proto-oncogene c-*erb* B2 (also known as *neu* or *her2*), which codes for a plasma-membrane receptor (p185) (MW 185 000) of the tyrosine kinase class whose cognate ligand remains unknown, probably also leads to transformation. Further, by comparison, a single point mutation in the c-*erb* B2 proto-oncogene converts it into a potent oncogene by inducing a single amino acid change in the receptor molecule, p185.

All the foregoing well illustrates the complexity of the functional EGF-R and related homologous oncoproteins, and just how complicated the study of such receptors and their regulation has become.

Besides being stimulated by ligand (EGF/TGFα) binding, EGF-R can also be modulated by other growth factors. For example, PDGF (see Section 2.5) probably stimulates phosphorylation of thr^{654} in EGF-R by protein kinase C and blocks the mitogenic effect of EGF/TGFα. Another example of this sort of 'transmodulation' that occurs among growth factors and their receptors comes from the recent observation that binding of EGF to EGF-R induces not only autophosphorylation of its own tyrosine kinase domain but also of the *neu* p185 product. This kind of 'cross-talk' among receptors is thus probably one way a cell has of governing their functional capacity to transmit signals.

Once the EGF-R has been activated by binding of either EGF or TGFα, a

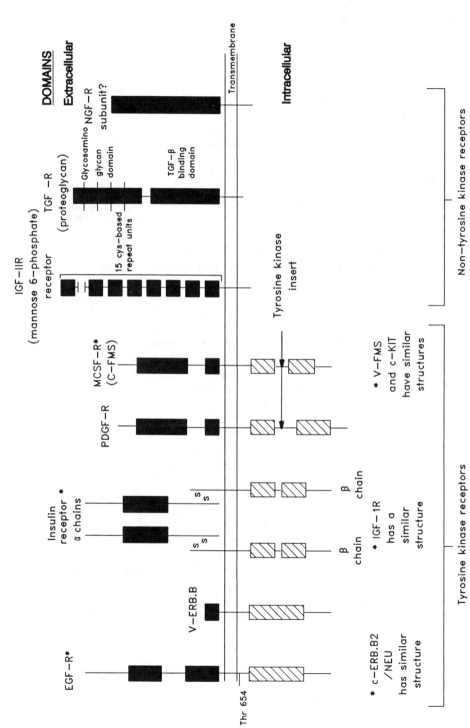

Figure 2.7 Growth factor receptors: basic structures.

number of changes in cellular metabolism and architecture take place. Principal among these are

1   an increase in Na/H$^+$ exchange leading to intracellular alkalinization (i.e. raising of intracellular pH);
2   physical effects in the plasma membranes including activation of ruffling and pinocytosis;
3   changes in the cytoskeleton;
4   increased Ca^{2+}ion mobilization and activation of Ca^{2+}-dependent proteins and protein kinases;
5   elevated expression of c-*fos* and c-*myc* proto-oncogenes.

It is assumed that it is the functioning of EGF-R tyrosine kinase which triggers off these changes, but the details of the underlying biochemical reactions are unknown; nor is it known which of these several induced changes are crucially involved in the mitogenic effect of EGF, although it must be presumed that gene depression is a prerequisite for cell division. It is clear, however, that the critical cellular response elements must pre-exist in cells having no EFG-R, since transfection of such cells with genes coding for EGF-R renders them susceptible to the mitogenic effect of EGF.

EGF and TGFα have mitogenic and differentiating activity in a wide variety of cell types *in vivo*. For example, EGF accelerates proliferation and differentiation of skin, corneal epithelium, and tracheal tissue. Rather interestingly, EGF has also been shown to promote bone resorption and inhibit bone formation and collagen synthesis. It may therefore play a role in tissue and bone re-modelling during development. TGFα has also been found to stimulate bone resorption and bone formation *in vitro*, but is quantitatively superior to EGF. Since many tumours produce TGFα, its elevated presence in some cancer patients may possibly underlie the observed osteolysis (bone degradation) that often accompanies progression of their disease. It is also possible that TGFα synthesis by tumour cells stimulates their proliferation in an autocrine or paracrine fashion and thus promotes oncogenesis and tumour growth. On the other hand, the fact that macrophages and keratinocytes in the skin produce TGFα and respond to it suggests a role for TGFα in wound healing and thus one possible therapeutic application.

In summary, EGF and TGFα appear to play similar, but probably non-identical, roles for the stimulation of cell proliferation and differentiation in a wide variety of tissues during embryogenesis and neonatal development. Additionally, they probably contribute to cell-replacing processes in tissue regrowth following injury, and possibly have other roles in the adult animal.

Insulin and insulin-like growth factors

Insulin is the primary hormone involved in the control of blood glucose levels.

It acts in cells via plasma membrane receptors to stimulate glucose, protein, and lipid metabolism, and in addition can act as a mitogen. The insulin receptor, unlike the single polypeptide chain EGF-R, is composed of four subunits, two α-chains (MW 135 000) which are glycosylated and form the extracellular insulin-binding domain, and two β-chains (MW 95 000) which are bound to α-chains on the extracellular face of the plasma membrane by disulphide bridges, span the plasma membrane lipid bilayer, and contain intracellular tyrosine kinase domains (Figure 2.7). Despite the seemingly increased structural complexity of the insulin receptor, it nevertheless conforms to the three-domain configuration characteristic of most hormone and cytokine receptors. Further, similarities in amino acid sequence between the insulin receptor α-chain and the extracellular domain of EGF-R and between the insulin receptor tyrosine kinase located in the β-chains and members of receptorless tyrosine kinases, particularly ROS, have been revealed by sequencing the cDNA coding for the insulin receptor precursor polyprotein (1370 amino acids). Binding of insulin to its receptor appears to remove the inhibitory effect of the α-chains on the β-chains and leads to tyrosine kinase activation, autophosphorylation, and phosphorylation and activation of key intracellular kinases and enzymes controlling metabolic pathways. In other words, the insulin receptor appears to function in a very similar way to EGF-R and this, in part, possibly explains why insulin can have mitogenic activity.

Insulin is a classical hormone produced by the islet cells of the pancreas, and acts at long range in a typical endocrine way. However, growth factors which structurally resemble insulin have been subsequently discovered. These are produced by many mammalian tissues, and can act locally in a paracrine (or autocrine) fashion; they could thus be classified as cytokines. Two insulin-like growth factors (IGF) have been characterized; they are IGF-I, also commonly called somatomedin C (originally described as a 'sulphation factor'), and IGF-II, widely known as 'multiplication–stimulating activity'. Both IGF-I and IGF-II have been found in human and animal plasma, and are believed to mediate the mitogenic effects of growth hormone upon which their production is dependent. Among growth factors, IGF-I and IGF-II are somewhat unusual in that they occur in plasma bound to specific carrier proteins and are probably inactive in the bound state.

IGF-I is a single-chain polypeptide of 70 amino acids containing three intrachain disulphide bonds (Figure 2.8). It is 43 per cent homologous in amino acid sequence to pro-insulin; like the latter, it is synthesized as a large precursor protein, i.e. pre-pro IGF-I of 130 amino acid residues. Similarly, IGF-II, a 67-amino acid polypeptide with three intrachain disulphide bonds (Figure 2.8) which is 62 per cent homologous to IGF-I, is synthesized as a precursor protein of 180 residues. The cDNAs for both IGF-I and IGF-II have been isolated and their respective genes located on human chromosomes 12 and 11. The IGF-II gene is closely linked to the insulin gene.

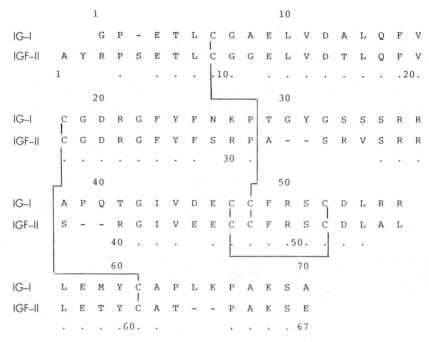

Figure 2.8 Primary structures of human IGF-I and IGF-II. Solid lines indicate cysteine pairings to form disulphide bridges. Dots indicate amino acid positions of identity between IGF-I and IGF-II.

Despite their structural similarities, IGF-I and IGF-II have distinct cell-surface receptors. The IGF-I receptor (IGF-IR) has been shown to resemble the structure and configuration of the insulin receptor (Figure 2.7). IGF-IR is composed of two α-chains and two β-chains showing a high degree of homology to the insulin-receptor β-chains, i.e. in the tyrosine kinase domain. Insulin may bind to IGF-IR besides its own receptor, but appears to be required at a higher concentration than IGF-I, the cognate ligand, for mitogenic action. Conversely, IGF-I and IGF-II cross-react with low potency on the insulin receptor. In contrast, the IGF-II receptor (IGF-IIR) appears to be a single polypeptide chain (MW 250 000) having preferential specificity for IGF-II, although IGF-I may also bind to it. Insulin, on the other hand, appears not to be able to bind to IGF-IIR. Interestingly, it has been recently reported that IGF-IIR is identical to the receptor for mannose-6-phosphate. The latter receptor appears to be involved in the targeting of lysosomal enzymes to lysosomes, and may also be involved in the transport and targeting of other proteins containing mannose-6-phosphate. Thus, the IGF-IIR appears peculiar in that it can function both intracellularly and as an integral plasma membrane receptor for a growth factor. The binding sites on IGF-IIR for mannose-6-phosphate and IGF-II are separate, and indeed the structure of this receptor, while maintaining the three-domain configuration, is also somewhat unusual. It consists of a very large extracellular domain made up almost exclusively of 15 cysteine-based repeat amino acid sequences, plus a short hydrophobic transmembrane region and a relatively small hydrophilic cytoplasmic domain (Figure 2.7). The cytoplasmic domain contains no enzyme such as the tyrosine kinase found in several other growth factor receptors. It is not clear how transmembrane signalling occurs in such a receptor. Many of the effects of IGF-II could be mediated by its binding to IGF-IR or insulin receptors, and it remains to be established what effects are mediated by the second class of receptors; i.e. IGF-IIR that bind IGFs.

The mechanism of signal transmission by insulin receptors, IGF-IR, or IGF-IIR remains to be elucidated. It is apparent that in the case of insulin receptors and IGF-IR that the heterotetramer, involving both pairs of α- and β-chains, is required for high-affinity binding of insulin and IGF-I, respectively. Dissociated heterodimers have much lower binding affinity for their respective ligands. This finding therefore suggests that association of receptor 'halves' may be an important mechanism for modulating receptor function. Binding of the cognate ligands to these heterotetrameric receptors appears to release an inhibitory effect of the α-chains on the β-chains. As in the case of EGF-R, the tyrosine kinase domain of insulin receptors and IGF-R is essential for signal transmission. Following ligand binding, autophosphorylation of the tyrosine kinase occurs, but exactly how the receptor kinase transmits its signal remains uncertain. Activation of the kinase by autophosphorylation and its subsequent initiating action in the phosphorylation cascade of a number of key regulatory enzyme substrates appears to be the most attractive and likely pathway, but there is little rigorous proof to support this model. There is some experimental evidence for the involvement of G-proteins or RAS proteins; for example, pertussis toxin (from the bacterium which causes whooping cough) blocks guanyl nucleotide binding to a G-protein and inhibits some of insulin's effects. Receptor-mediated activation of calcium channels in the plasma membrane and influx of Ca^{2+} ions may also be involved in the mitogenic effects of IGFs. Other intracellular events following cell activation, e.g. activation of nuclear genes and DNA synthesis, appears to be similar to those found following EGF-R stimulation (see p. 40). It is not known whether the genes coding for insulin- or IGF-receptors can become oncogenes by way of overexpression in the manner of the EGF-R gene.

The physiological roles of insulin and IGFs are apparently quite different. Insulin is well known to regulate anabolic (synthetic) pathways in which glucose is taken up into muscle and fat cells (adipocytes), glycogen synthesis occurs in the liver, and fat is built up in adipocytes. In contrast, IGF-I appears to mediate the growth-promoting activity of growth hormone (GH), and IGF-I has been shown to promote skeletal cartilage growth *in vitro*. IGF-I probably also mediates GH action on the mammary gland and increases lactation. The role of IGF-II appears less clear, although its expression in rat embryos suggests that, in comparison with IGF-I which probably functions to promote growth of neonatal and adolescent tissues, IGF-II is the fetal counterpart of IGF-I. Virtually all tissues that have been analysed synthesize IGF-I, and its receptors are equally widespread; they have been identified in fibroblasts, muscle cells, Leydig cells, lymphocytes and monocytes, neuronal cells, mammary gland, and placenta. IGF-IIR is also produced by many cell lines in culture, of which some also express IGF-IR. Tumour cells, particularly those isolated from breast carcinomas, appear both to produce and to respond to IGF-I, and possibly IGF-II. Thus, the potential autocrine and paracrine action of IGFs may increase oncogenesis of breast carcinoma cells. The observation that sex hormones, e.g. estrogen, appear to promote the synthesis of IGFs and their receptors suggests another mechanism by which the oncogenic process may be augmented. Another finding that oestrogen induces IGF-I expression in the uterus confirms that regulation of IGF synthesis extends beyond that related to growth hormone.

Several IGF-binding proteins, which are not homologous to IGF receptors and do not bind to insulin, have now been identified. The role of these in the regulation or IGF activities is now the subject for intensive research. In general, the binding proteins are much larger than the IGFs and thus may inhibit binding of IGFs to their receptors. Other roles for these binding proteins have been proposed, e.g. protection of IGFs from proteolytic cleavage, prolonging the half-life of IGFs in the circulation. It is confidently predicted that this area will continue to provide fascinating insights into the growth regulatory activities of IGFs.

Fibroblast growth factors

It has been known since the early 1940s that extracts of brain tissue contain potent mitogenic substances. A number of these growth factors have subsequently been isolated and purified, yielding a class of heterogeneous proteins with diverse biological actions. In fact, it was not until comparatively recent times that any kind of family relationship among these brain-derived growth factors was established. Gene-cloning of the relevant FGF genes and their expression in heterologous micro-organisms has revealed that several biologically active substances, variously referred to previously as endothelial cell growth factor, eye-derived growth factors, heparin-binding growth factors, chondrosarcoma-derived growth factor, prostatropin, etc., may be accounted for by two structurally related proteins. These two proteins, now most commonly referred to as acidic fibroblast growth factor (aFGF) and basic fibroblast growth factor (bFGF), are the products of two distinct genes, located on human chromosome 5, coding for polypeptides of similar length which are approximately 55 per cent related in amino acid sequences. The mature form of aFGF contains 140 amino acids (MW~16 000), and that of bFGF, 146 amino acids. There are, however, several reports indicating microheterogeneity at both the N-terminal and C-terminal ends of these molecules when isolated and purified from different tissues. Both fibroblast growth factors also show a distinct sequence homology to IL-1, suggesting that FGF and IL-1 share a common ancestral gene. The lack of an N-terminal signal sequence preceding the mature FGF proteins is also similar to IL-1 proteins, although the latter do contain very long N-terminal 'leader' sequences (see Chapter 4), whereas FGFs do not.

Most natural FGFs have been isolated from brain tissue, in particular the pituitary gland. It is probable, however, that FGFs can be synthesized by a number of cell types, contained for example in brain, adrenal gland, retina, corpus luteum, and kidney. They may also be produced by tumour cells derived from chondrosarcomas. It is as yet unclear how FGFs are secreted; since they lack a signal sequence, it has been conjectured that they leak out of cells, or are released following cell lysis, or leave the cells by some other unknown means. Nevertheless, it is certain that once outside the producing cells, FGFs are very potent mitogens for a wide variety of cell types. Rather interestingly, both FGFs bind heparin, a mucopolysaccharide released by mast cells which has anticoagulant properties. Endothelial cells, for example those lining the inner surfaces of blood vessels, appear also to contain heparin and heparin-like polysaccharides and these may enhance binding of FGFs to their cell surface receptors in such cells. Heparin has been shown to increase the activity of aFGF, but apparently has little or no effect on bFGF.

FGFs are known to stimulate DNA synthesis in many cell types. The cell-surface receptors for FGFs, however, remain only partially characterized. There appear to be distinct classes of high-affinity and low-affinity binding sites, but interference with the binding of radiolabelled FGF to specific receptors by cell-associated, non-receptor, heparin binding sites for FGF has precluded definitive enumeration of FGF-receptors (FGF-R). There is, however, some evidence for the presence of a 130–170 kDa membrane-protein, which could be the cognate receptor for FGF (for new information see Chapter 7), in cells in culture or brain tissue. It is hypothesized that aFGF and bFGF share a common receptor, but this has not yet been verified.

Physiological roles for FGF remain uncertain, although from work *in vitro* it is clear that FGFs induce the proliferation and/or differentiation of neuroectodermal cells and therefore could be involved in the regulation of nerve cell growth in the central nervous system. Besides neural tissues, FGFs promote the growth of mesodermal cells such as vascular endothelial cells (as has been previously mentioned) and fibroblasts, and has also been shown to be angiogenic, i.e. to cause blood capillaries to grow *in vivo*. This suggests that FGFs have a role in the vascularization of tissues and may have a therapeutic application for wound-healing. Possibly, FGFs may also aid the healing of other tissues, such as bone, and be useful in lens and limb regeneration.

A relationship of FGFs to oncogenes has only very recently been revealed. This has come through the discovery in separate research investigations of a family of proto-oncogenes coding for proteins with distinct sequence homology to FGFs. The first '*fgf*-like' proto-oncogene, *int-2*, was isolated following mouse mammary tumour virus (MMTV) infection and transformation of mouse cells. MMTV itself does not contain an oncogene, but by insertion of its DNA into nuclear DNA at particular integration sites it is able to activate *int-2* proto-oncogene transcription and hence expression. Based on other methods of identifying oncogenes, two additional related proto-oncogenes *hst* (also called *KS3*) and *fgf-5* have subsequently been discovered (Table 2.1). All three of these proto-oncogenes code for proteins which share marked amino acid sequence homology with FGFs, ranging from 35–55 per cent identity (Figure 2.9), and have similar mitogenic actions. Interestingly, in contrast with FGFs, the precursors of the FGF-like proteins contain typical N-terminal signal sequences necessary for secretion.

The expression of *int-2* proto-oncogene is normally tightly regulated, and no *int-2* mRNA transcripts have been found in adult tissues. However, *int-2* mRNA is found in mouse embryos and in embryonal carcinomas, suggesting that the INT-2 protein has a physiological role during embryogenesis. The relationship of INT-2 and the other *hst* and *fgf-5* proto-oncogene products and the potential roles of the latter are the subject of intense study. It is apparent, however, that *int-2*, *hst*, or *fgf-5* may be activated and act as oncogenes in several different tumour types, including hepatomas, colon carcinoma, stomach tumour, and Kaposi's sarcoma. The latter is associated with AIDS, and is usually classified as an angiogenic tumour. Genetic changes in such tumour cells can presumably lead to an overproduction of 'FGF-like' growth factors which could both enhance tumour cell proliferation by persistent autocrine stimulation and promote neovascularization by their angiogenic effects on blood capillaries. Paracrine stimulation of cells in adjacent tissues may result in their hyperplasia, which is often found accompanying the development of carcinomas.

The probability that some members of the FGF family can act as oncogenic

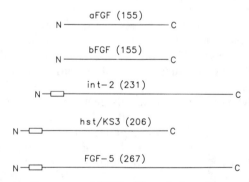

Figure 2.9 Schematic alignments of FGFs. The relative alignments of the five gene products are shown with their names, lengths in amino acid residues, with amino (N) and carboxy(C) terminal ends labelled. The locations of homology among the five proteins are contained in the common overlapping regions. Hydrophobic leader sequences are denoted as open boxes. (Reprinted with permission from Thomas, 1988; copyright Elsevier Science Publications, UK).

growth factors is in keeping with the overall scheme of cell growth control where, as has already been seen (pp. 30–3), malfunction and overexpression of key elements in the signal-receptor pathways may lead to unregulated rapid cell proliferation. This oncogenic mechanism in which growth factors are over-produced is not unique to FGF-like proteins and is certainly shared by PDGF — see below — and possibly other growth factors.

Platelet-derived growth factor

The significance of the existence of several heterogeneous FGF molecules and their extended FGF-like homologues with regard to biological potency and specificity is presently not understood. It does, however, seem likely that such molecular heterogeneity could provide a mechanism for varying both potency and specificity. A clearer understanding of the way in which the heterogeneity of the molecular form of growth factors affects their biological activities has recently come from the elucidation of the structure of PDGF and its related molecular isoforms. PDGF is synthesized by platelets and several other cell types, and in humans consists of a disulphide-bonded dimer of two different, but markedly homologous (60 per cent related), polypeptide chains, designated A- and B-chains. The gene coding for human A-chains is located on chromosome 7 and that for B-chains on chromosome 22, and they appear to be independently regulated. The PDGF-A and -B mRNAs encode large precursor A- and B-chains containing secretory signal sequences, and the precursors are proteolytically cleaved following dimerization (Figure 2.10). The resulting heterodimer has a molecular weight in the range 30–32 000 and is composed of a 14–18 kDa A-chain and a 16 kDa B-chain. The heterogeneity of size of the A-chain probably reflects differential degradation of A-chain termini and varying glycosylation levels. Interestingly, the B-chain is now known to be coded by the c-*sis* proto-oncogene (Table 2.1) and is almost identical to the product of v-*sis* oncogene found in simian sarcoma virus (SSV). However, in SSV-infected cells the production of B-chains predominates with the formation of homodimers. The PDGF-like B-chain homodimer (also referred to as PDGF-BB) retains potent mitogenic activity, and probably acts as an autocrine growth factor in the oncogenic transformation of SSV-infected cells. Curiously, the main form of PDGF produced by porcine platelets is also PDGF-BB (Figure 2.10) and not the heterodimer as in human PDGF. PDGF-like proteins have also been shown to be produced by vascular endothelial cells, smooth muscle cells, and cells of the cytotrophoblastic shell. The latter are among the most invasive and proliferative cells known, and invade uterine tissue to attach the developing embryo. It is clear that cytotrophoblastic cells must also contain specific receptors for PDGF, and it has been established that several other cell types, particularly certain tumour cells, both produce and respond to PDGF or PDGF-like molecules. A common finding, however, is that normal cells, such as endothelial cells or activated macrophages, and tumour cells, e.g. from gliomas, produce PDGF-like proteins, but do not themselves respond to it.

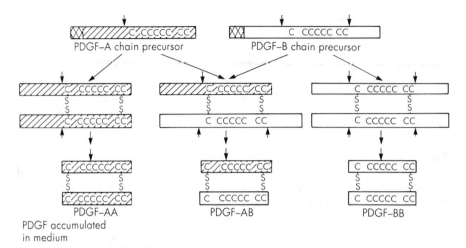

Figure 2.10   Schematic illustration of the biosynthesis, assembly and processing of the dimeric forms of PDGF. The A chain (hatched bars) and the B chain (open bars) of PDGF are synthesized as precursor molecules with signal peptides (crossed parts). After assembly into disulphide-bonded dimers proteolytic processing occurs (arrows). It is not known exactly which cysteine residues (C) participate in interchain disulphide bonds. (Reprinted with permission from Östman *et al.*, 1988, *J. Biol. Chem.* **263**, 16202; copyright The American Society for Biochemistry and Molecular Biology.)

Instead, it is believed that such PDGF-like proteins act in a paracrine manner on neighbouring cells. For instance, PDGF-like proteins secreted by activated macrophages could be involved in the stimulation of connective tissue cells, a response often observed in chronic inflammatory processes. Further, the normal counterparts of tumour cells, e.g. of gliomas, respond to PDGF-like proteins and may thus account for accompanying hyperplasia in tissues adjacent to growing tumours. Interestingly, the predominant PDGF-like protein produced by tumour cells appears to be the A-chain homodimer, PDGF-AA (Figure 2.10), and this, in contrast to PDGF-AB and PDGF-BB, has been reported to have low mitogenic activtiy and no chemotactic activity. The significance of this in relation to tumour cell growth is not known.

Originally it was thought that PDGF-AA, PDGF-AB, and PDGF-BB all shared the same cell surface receptor. Although this may still be true, the existence of other classes of receptors recognizing individual PDGF isoforms has become a distinct possibility. For instance, it would appear that human dermal fibroblasts express receptors for the PDGF-BB isoform in greater numbers than a receptor class binding all three isoforms. However, the receptor glycoprotein that has been cloned is probably the one recognizing all three PDGFs. The gene encoding the human PDGF receptor (PDGF-R) is located on chromosome 5, and is contained in a cluster of genes specifying various growth factors and receptors. PDGF-R is a 185 kDa glycoprotein with a large glycosylated external domain involved in binding of PDGF, a transmembrane segment, and a tyrosine kinase-containing intracellular domain (Table 2.1; Figure 2.7). It thus resembles the structure of EGF-R, but there are notable differences in both the extracellular and intracellular domains between EGF-R and PDGF-R which put the latter in a distinct receptor class. For example, the distribution of extracellular domain cysteine residues in the two receptors is different and there is an insertion sequence in the tyrosine kinase domain of PDGF-R which is absent in EGF-R. These distinctions apart, however, the stimulation of tyrosine kinase autophosphorylation following PDGF binding to PDGF-R is now a familiar observation in the activation of growth factor receptors in general. There also appears to be some similarity in the early effects triggered by PDGF-R activation to those previously discussed for EGF-R and IGF-IR. These include membrane ruffling, intracellular alkanization and increased Ca^{2+} ion mobilization, increased inositol phosphate turnover and activation of protein kinase C, and the induction of specific nuclear genes. Since PDGF acts at an early stage of the growth cycle, probably on cells leaving G_0, it is not surprising that nuclear *fos* and *myc* proto-oncogenes, whose products are involved in transcriptional control of other genes, have been shown to be strongly induced. Thus, PDGF may be viewed as a competence factor enabling commitment to enter the cell growth cycle. In fact, the mitogenic signal provided by PDGF is sometimes so strong as to drive cells through the cell cycle to division without the apparent requirement of additional growth factors in some cases. In order to sustain the proliferative response, PDGF must therefore induce other proliferation-related elements besides the early *fos* and *myc* proto-oncogenes. An important PDGF-inducible gene in this respect is the glucose transporter gene. The glucose transporter protein regulates the uptake of glucose across the plasma membrane. Increased glucose metabolism is essential for proliferation, and PDGF has been shown to increase both glucose entry into cells and the amount of glucose transporter protein present in plasma membranes in cultured cell lines. Therefore, the glucose transporter protein might also be seen as a competence factor, its function presumably and necessarily extending throughout the growth cycle. It is also known that other growth factors, e.g. IGF-I acting as a progression factor, induce the glucose transporter system, and thus such induction will have particular relevance to growth factor-driven oncogenesis. Tumour cells are known to have higher levels of glucose metabolism than normal cells, and the overexpression of glucose transporter could presumably contribute to unregulated tumour cell proliferation.

PDGF isoforms have many potential normal physiological roles. Their potent mitogenic action on connective tissue cells suggest a role in tissue repair and wound healing. The presence of PDGF-like proteins in early *Xenopus* embryos also suggests that endogenous PDGF acts in the early stages of embryogenesis and is involved in the development of particular tissues. Interestingly, PDGF, which usually stimulates DNA synthesis in mesodermal cells, has been found to stimulate the postnatal rat lens, an epidermal tissue of ectodermal origin. PDGF also stimulates the proliferation of glial cells which are the precursors of oligodendrocytes, the myelin-producing cells of the central nervous system, and type-2 astrocytes which contact nerve axons at the gaps between adjacent myelinated regions. This would suggest a role for PDGF in the development of the central nervous system. The diversity of cells responding to PDGF indicates that its target cell populations and its long-term biological effects need reassessment. It is expected that future developments in this research area will provide clarification of the biological roles of individual PDGF isoforms and whether they act through distinct receptor classes (see Chapter 7).

Transforming growth factor beta and related proteins

TGFβ is very different molecularly to the previously discussed TGFα (see p. 35) and probably functions in a rather different way. Like PDGF, it is dimeric in structure and exists as a family of three or more isoforms. The subunit chains of TGFβ have been designated β1 and β2, and these combine through interchain disulphide bridges to form homodimers (MW 25 000), TGF-β1 (2 × β1) and TGF-β2 (2 × β2) or the rare heterodimer, TGF-β1.2 (1 × β1, 1 × β2). It has turned out that the TGFβ originally discovered as a regulator of cell proliferation is TGF-β1. Both β1 and β2 chains are encoded by genes containing seven exons, coding for much large secretory precursor polypeptides of about 390 amino acids (Figure 2.11). Both mature chains are 112 amino acids in length and are derived from the C-terminal domain of precursor polypeptides following proteolytic cleavage. The β1 and β2 chains

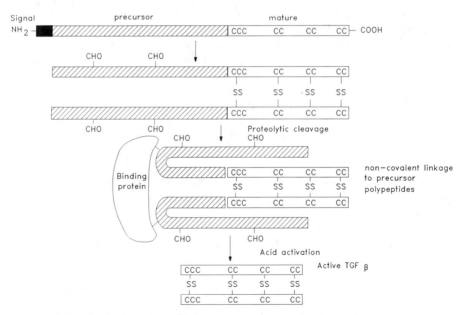

Figure 2.11   Processing of TGFβ from precursor to active homodimer.

are about 70 per cent homologous in amino acid sequence, and the positions of nine cysteine residues, which determine disulphide bond formation, are highly conserved. A high degree of species conservation of β1 and β2 chains is also manifest: there is only one amino acid difference in β1 between mouse and human TGF-β1. This striking conservation argues strongly for a critical biological role of TGF-β1.

The very recent discovery of a third TGF-β precursor chain, β3, which is approximately 80 per cent homologous to β1 and β2 chains, increases the probability of the existence of further TGFβ isoforms. The mature form of β3 contains 112 amino acids, identical in length to the β1 and β2 chains, but the length and sequence of the precursor polypeptide is different to that of the β1 and β2 precursors. The three genes encoding β1, β2, and β3 chains are located on different human chromosomes and thus it is likely that their common ancestral gene is of particularly ancient origin. Structural similarities at the polypeptide level have been maintained by the probably highly conserved function(s) of TGFβ.

TGFβs are produced by a wide variety of cell types. However, as with PDGF, a major cell source of TGFβ1 is blood platelets. It may also be produced in bone matrices, kidney, placenta, and certain tumour cell lines. Similarly, TGFβ2 has been found in high concentrations in bone extracts, in porcine platelets, and in the supernatant culture fluid of some tumour cell lines. On the basis of the presence of TGFβ mRNA transcripts in cell extracts, TGFβ1 and TGFβ2 are found in both epithelial and mesenchymal cell lines, as well as certain normal tissue cells, e.g. kidney, whereas TGFβ3 appears to be largely confined to mesenchymal cell lines. TGFβs released from certain cells may be inactive, possibly through association with a binding protein (cf. IGF-I): acid treatment has been demonstrated to cause the irreversible activation of such 'latent' TGFβs (Figure 2.11).

The biology of TGFβ actions is very complex indeed. Originally TGFβ, like the completely distinct TGFα, was described as a factor promoting anchorage-independent proliferation in cells that were normally anchorage dependent. Unlike TGFα, however, TGFβ probably requires co-factors to stimulate cell growth and division. For instance, the anchorage-independent growth of normal rat kidney (NRK) cells requires growth medium containing both TGFβ and EGF (or TGFα). NRK cells appear to be unusual in requiring this combination as, in most cells stimulated to grow by TGFβ, the c-*sis* proto-oncogene is expressed. Thus the mitogenic action of TGFβ is indirect and is probably due to PDGF-BB acting in an autocrine manner. This observation adds weight to the model proposed for cell activation in which different growth factors act successively or in concert (see Section 2.3).

Although TGFβ can enhance cell proliferation in some mesenchymal tissues, its main biological activity seems to be the inhibition of proliferation of a wide variety of cell types. Further, in apparent contradiction to the synergistic mitogenic activities of TGFβ and other growth factors just described, it has frequently been shown to antagonize growth factor stimulation. For example, in anchorage-dependent monolayer cultures, TGFβ blocks the actions of PDGF, EGF, and FGFs. In addition, TGFβ antagonizes the effects of proliferation-enhancing cytokines in fat and muscle cells and in the generation of blood cells (haematopoiesis). It also down-regulates the activities of cells involved in the inflammatory response. Thus, the activity of TGFβ is very dependent on cell-type, and appears also to be related to differentiated states. In fact, the antiproliferative action of TGFβ can often be coupled to its stabilizing effect on particular states of cell differentiatioin. For instance, TGFβ blocks the mitogenic effects of insulin and hydrocortisone in kidney epithelial cells, but without inhibiting protein synthesis, thus stabilizing the differentiated state induced by these hormones. In other circumstances, TGFβ may actively promote or inhibit differentiation, again depending on cell type and conditions.

Many tumour-derived cell lines produce TGFβ, and it has been suggested that it could act as an inhibitory or negative autocrine factor. Evidence to support this hypothesis has come from the finding that the proliferation of a monkey kidney cell line is suppressed by TGFβ which is also actively produced by this cell line. Such an autocrine inhibitory loop could have important implications in the development of tumours. As has been previously discussed, some growth factors, e.g. TGFα, IGFs, and PDGF, probably contribute to the oncogenic process by maintaining unregulated tumour cell proliferation. Besides providing strong mitogenic signals to tumour cells, they also appear to up-regulate growth control elements, e.g. glucose transporter, necessary to sustain proliferation. They also induce collagenase and metalloproteases, such as transin (stromelysin), which degrade the extracellular matrix to permit cell division. Levels of transin are much higher in tumour cells than in their normal counterparts, and transin is dramatically overexpressed in carcinomas showing a high propensity for metastasis. TGFβ1 has been recently shown to inhibit EGF-induction of transin mRNA and to decrease transin levels. This finding therefore suggests a molecular mechanism for the autocrine and paracrine antiproliferative action of TGFβ. In breast carcinomas, both the tumour cells and their normal counterparts produce TGFβ and have receptors for it, but there is a progressive loss of TGFβ-responsiveness. This may in part explain subsequent tumour progression, and is in keeping with a model in which loss of a growth inhibitory response has the same consequences as the induction of overactive proliferative responses.

Various receptors for TGFβ have been demonstrated in cultured cell lines. The principal receptor appears to be of relatively high molecular weight, and is composed of subunits of approximately 300 kDa. Other lower-molecular-weight receptors of 60–100 kDa have also been reported, which apparently have a higher affinity for TGFβ1 than for TGFβ2. However, the high-molecular-weight receptor appears to bind all three isoforms of TGFβ equally. Recently, this receptor has been shown to have the characteristics of a proteoglycan, in this case consisting of glycosaminoglycan and oligosaccharide side chains covalently linked to a core polypeptide of 100–120 kDa (Figure 2.7). It is intriguing that a potential regulator of extracellular matrix formation should use as its receptor one component of that matrix, namely proteoglycan. Structurally, this TGFβ receptor is obviously dissimilar to those of other growth factors and the functioning of this receptor is probably also different. It has no tyrosine kinase domain, and thus the mechanism of signal transduction across the membrane remains enigmatic. However, in proliferation-responsive cells TGFβ induces nuclear c-*fos* and c-*myc*, although this is probably initiated by prior induction of c-*sis* and the subsequent autocrine action of the resultant PDGF-BB released. Thus, like other growth factor receptors, TGFβ-R is capable of transmitting signals to the cell nucleus to stimulate gene activation. TGFβ might therefore be envisaged as an early acting competence factor initiating a cascade of gene activation and growth factor stimulation. A hypothetical scheme of events is shown in Figure 2.12. By contrast, in cells in which TGFβ has an antiproliferative effect, c-*myc* has been shown to be repressed. TGFβ may also cause repression of other elements involved in growth control, e.g. down-regulation of EGF-R.

The majority of the findings so far discussed pertaining to the biological actions of TGFβ have come from *in vitro* cell systems. Therefore, the physiological roles of TGFβ are uncertain. However, the association of TGFβ production with platelets and its abundance in bone matrices strongly suggests that TGFβ isoforms could be involved in wound healing/tissue repair and in bone formation/remodelling, respectively. In fact, a potential therapeutic role of TGFβ has been indicated by the finding that bovine TGFβ can significantly accelerate a wound-healing response in a rat *in vivo* model system. Besides promoting connective tissue synthesis in wounds, TGFβ also has chemotactic properties and causes an infiltration of inflammatory cells,

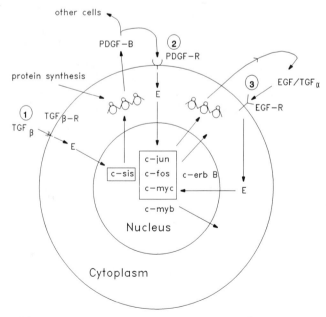

Figure 2.12 Hypothetical growth factor proliferation cascade.

e.g. monocytes, which are known to be involved in physiological wound healing. On the other hand, the observed increasing TGFβ levels in regenerating liver coupled with its known antiproliferative effect on hepatocytes suggest a role of TGFβ in limiting tissue repair processes by a paracrine or autocrine inhibitory loop. This once again emphasizes the bi-functional nature of TGFβ, the outcome of its action being dependent upon cell type and probably local concentrations of TGFβ *per se*.

Two substances originally described as cartilage-inducing factors (CIF) and designated CIF-A and CIF-B have been shown to be identical to $TGF\beta_1$ and $TGF\beta_2$, respectively. These have been demonstrated to enhance synthesis of extracellular matrix components *in vitro* including collagen, fibronectin, and proteoglycans, and to inhibit degradative enzymes such as collagenase and transin. Thus, TGFβs (CIF-A and -B) are possibly involved in cell differentiation, including cartilage production during the first step of bone formation. However, TGFβs have not been demonstrated to induce cartilage and bone *in vivo*. This property may apparently reside in the recently discovered 'TGFβ-like' bone morphogenetic proteins (BMP) (Table 2.2). The derived amino acid sequences of two growth factors designated BMP-2A and BMP-3 show marked homology (~37 per cent) to TGFβ1 and β2 chains and also to the β chain of inhibin (see below). Similar to TGFβ, they are synthesized as large precursor polypeptides and the C-terminal segments are cleaved to produce active dimeric species. A third BMP, designated BMP-1,

Table 2.2 The TGFβ family of growth and differentiation factors

Subclass	Designation	Subunits	Bioactive dimer composition
Transforming growth factor beta	TGFβ1 (CIF-A)	β1	$(\beta 1)_2$
	TGFβ2 (CIF-B)	β2	$(\beta 2)_2$
	TGFβ3	β3	$(\beta 3)_2$
	TGFβ1.2	β1, β2	(β1, β2)
Bone morphogenetic proteins	BMP-2A	2A	Not known whether homodimers or heterodimers
	BMP-2B	2B	
	BMP-3	3	
Inhibins and activins	Inhibin A	α, βA	(α, βA)
	Inhibin B	α, βB	(α, βB)
	Activin A	βA	$(\beta A)_2$
	Activin AB	βA, βB	(βA, βB)
Müllerian inhibitory substance	MIS	MIS	$(MIS)_2$
Vegetalizing factor	Vg-1	Vg-1	$(Vg-1)_2$
Decapenta-plegic transcript complex	DPP-C	DPP-C	$(DPP-C)_2$

is molecularly unrelated to BMP-2A, BMP-3, or TGFβ but may possibly be a binding protein for members of the TGFβ family. BMP-1 contains a protease-containing domain which could be involved in the activation of TGFβ-like proteins (see also nerve growth factor, p. 56, for similar mechanism of activation). Recombinant BMP-2A and BMP-3 both induce cartilage formation in an *in vivo* assay system, and may find clinical applications in bone regeneration and healing. In addition to their potential effects on bone synthesis *per se*, members of the TGFβ family present in the bone marrow probably play a role in regulating the proliferation and differentiation of early progenitor cells of the different populations of circulating blood cells. Its effects on haematopoiesis appear largely inhibitory, although its antiproliferative activity appears to be more pronounced in early immature haematopoietic progenitors than in more mature precursors. It does still, however, effectively inhibit IL-2-driven T-lymphocyte proliferation and antagonize the stimulatory effects of various other cytokines on lymphocytes involved in immune responses, e.g. by inhibiting antibody production by B-lymphocytes. The activation of cytotoxic lymphocytes, e.g. natural killer (NK) cells, and macrophages is also counteracted by the action of TGFβ. Its overall inhibitory effects on haematopoiesis and its immunosuppressive action suggest that TGFβ plays a role in the down-regulation of inflammatory responses. Possibly, initial low levels of TGFβ at sites of inflammation act as a chemoattractant for lymphocytes, macrophages, and platelets with the ensuing build-up of TGFβ concentrations released from these cells subsequently suppressing their activities and feeding-back on the bone marrow to inhibit the production of inflammatory cell types. In tumours, besides loss of responsiveness to TGFβ (see p. 52), local or generalized immunosuppression caused by the continuous secretion of TGFβ from tumour cells may contribute to their 'escape' from normal immune surveillance mechanisms.

The finding that high levels of TGFβ1 mRNA transcripts are found throughout normal mouse embryogenesis strongly suggests that it has an important role in this process. TGFβ1 appears to be more associated with mesenchymal tissues, as one would expect from the discussion above, than other embryonic tissues. However, TGFβ1 is apparently absent from neural crest mesenchymal tissues such as the developing palate at particular times of embryonic development, and its expression in general is both spatially and temporally controlled. In frog (*Xenopus*) eggs a TGFβ-related protein, vegetalizing protein-1 (Vg-1; Table 2.2) also seems to play a role in the very early stages of amphibian embryogenesis. It has been conjectured that the 'TGFβ-like' Vg-1 synergizes with FGF in the formation of germ layers, i.e. the mesodermal and ectodermal layers. Just how TGFβ or Vg-1 regulate cell-differentiating processes involved in embryonic morphogenesis remains to be elucidated.

In addition to the closely related TGFβ isoforms, other more distantly related 'TGFβ-like' proteins, besides BMP-2A and -3, with separate, distinctive functions, have been discovered. The first of these, inhibin (Table 2.2), which occurs naturally as two heterodimeric isoforms, inhibin A and inhibin

B, is a specific, potent inhibitor of the pituitary secretion of follicle stimulating hormone (FSH). Inhibins are present in ovarian and testicular fluids and probably regulate differentiation of cells in the ovarian–pituitary endocrine axis, including controlling FSH release. The action of inhibins is opposed by those of activins which are dimers of the inhibin β-chains (see Table 2.2). Inhibins have different receptors to TGFβ, but it has been speculated that activins might compete for the inhibin receptors to antagonize the action of inhibin. Alternatively, the antagonistic effects of inhibins and activins may be mediated by separate receptor classes. That activins can act as erythroid differentiation factor whereas inhibins cannot, suggests that activins have different receptors and other functions besides those antagonistic to inhibin action.

Another TGFβ-related protein is Müllerian inhibitory substance (MIS, Table 2.2) which is produced by the testis and is associated with the regression of Müllerian ducts during development of the reproductive tract in the male embryo (Table 2.2). Structurally, MIS is a homodimer of two relatively large glycosylated polypeptides (70–72 kDa) of which the C-terminal domains show homology to TGFβ chains.

Lastly, TGFβ-related proteins have been demonstrated in the embryonic forms of amphibians and insects. Vg-1 present in the earliest stages of frog embryogenesis has already been described (see p. 55). In addition, the predicted product of the decapentaplegic gene complex (DPP-C) mRNA in the fruit fly (*Drosophila*) shows amino acid sequence homology to TGFβ (see Table 2.2). DPP-C appears to play a critical regulatory role during the larval stages of morphogenesis.

A detailed review of the biology of inhibins, activins, and other TGFβ-related proteins is beyond the scope of this chapter; the reader should refer to the relevant articles cited in the additional recommended reading listed at the end of the chapter (pp. 63–4).

Nerve growth factor, neuroleukin, and other growth factors

NGF derived from snake venom, and subsequently from mouse submaxillary glands, was first isolated by Stanley Cohen's group in the 1960s (see also the isolation of EGF, p. 34). Active NGF was later shown to be a component of a 7S complex (MW 130–140 000) containing three subunits designated α, β, and γ. The α-subunit (MW 26 000), has no known function. The β-subunit (MW 26 500), a protein encoded by a gene on the short arm of human chromosome 1, is the one that stimulates nerve growth: it is a dimer of two 118-amino-acid polypeptides, these being synthesized as larger 307-residue precursors. Native NGFβ chains are contained in residues 188–305 of the precursor. The dimeric structure of active NGF thus resembles those of PDGF and TGFβ, although there is little sequence homology between NGFβ and these other growth factors. The γ-subunit (MW 27 500), appears to be a member of the general class of serine proteases and may be involved in the proteolytic cleavage of NGFβ chains to produce active NGF (cf. BMP-1 action on latent TGFβ or BMP-2A/3, see pp. 51, 55). The 7S oligomer is composed of two α-, one β-, and one γ-subunit together with one tightly bound zinc ion per molecule. Naturally occurring forms of NGF may, however, be more heterogenous.

The submaxillary gland of male mice is one of the best sources of NGF; it is present in higher concentrations in males than in females because expression of all three subunits is inducible by testosterone, a male sex hormone. It has also been isolated from snake venom, bovine seminal plasma, and the prostate gland of guinea pig. NGF seems to be absent from serum, although it may be produced locally in the placenta. In addition, NGF may be synthesized in parts of the brain and central nervous system.

NGF appears primarily to be a neurotropic protein necessary for the growth and survival of some nerve cells in the brain and in both the central and peripheral nervous systems, including sensory afferent and sympathetic neurons. However, its production in the submaxillary gland and the widespread presence of NGF receptors (NGF-R) in many cells and tissues suggests that NGF may have broader biological functions, in keeping with other growth factors. Cross-linking studies with radiolabelled NGF have identified a 70–80 kDa receptor protein in the rat phaeochromocytoma cell line PC12, and receptor species of similar size have been found in other cells. Both high- and low-affinity NGF-R have been described, but the significance of these in relation to NGF activities is presently unknown. By molecular cloning, an NGF-R cosmid DNA has been isolated which codes for a glycoprotein (MW~75 000). The NGF-R gene is located on human chromosome 17, and contains six exons. So far it has not been possible to prove conclusively that this 75 kDa glycoprotein is responsible for all the NGF-mediated responses, although the induction of c-fos, an NGF-associated cellular response, has been demonstrated. It has been speculated that the receptor is a complex of two or more (glyco) proteins and that the cloned NGF-R is a subunit which without other receptor components may be unable to function as a high-affinity receptor (Figure 2.7).

Besides plasma membrane receptors for NGF, there is growing evidence that internalized NGF, presumably the result of endocytosis of NGF–receptor complexes, binds directly to nuclear chromatin. Similar observations have been made for EGF, PDGF, and FGF. Binding of these growth factors to chromatin suggests that they may mediate additional cellular responses to those they they evoke by occupying plasma membrane receptors. In the case of NGF, specific chromatin receptors have been documented which appear to mediate inhibition of gene transcription and cell growth. It has been speculated that NGF may play a role in the mechanism of growth control in cells of tumours such as melanoma and colorectal carcinoma, which express NGF-specific plasma membrane and chromatin receptors. Thus, NGF might act as a paracrine growth inhibitory factor in much the same way as has been suggested for TGFβ. In support of this hypothesis, NGF has antiproliferative and differentiating effects in rat phaeochromocytoma PC12 cells.

Several observations suggest that the biological effects of NGF extend beyond those relevant for nerve cell maintenance and growth. Thus, NGF has been shown to cause degranulation of rat peritoneal mast cells, to induce changes in shape of platelets and to accelerate wound healing. When injected into neonatal rats, NGF stimulates an increase in mast cell numbers in various tissues. NGF may therefore be an accessory regulatory growth and differentiation factor for mast cells. Mast cells (basophils) and the factors they release are important in allergic inflammation, and thus mast cell/nerve cell interactions may be important in neurogenic inflammation.

In addition to NGF, a further neurotrophic factor, designated neuroleukin (NRL) by Gurney and co-workers, appears to be involved in the development of spinal and sensory motor neurons. NRL has been shown to be produced by a wide variety of tissues and is found in abundance in muscle, brain, and kidney. It can also be produced by T-lymphocytes and act on antibody-producing B-lymphocytes, a fact which contributed to its name, i.e. neuro-'leukin'. An NRL–cDNA isolated from mice salivary glands has led to the deduction of its primary amino acid sequence and the expression of active NRL in mammalian cells. NRL is a single polypeptide chain (MW 56 000), showing no homology to the sequences of known growth factors, but interestingly showing partial homology to a segment of the external envelope glycoprotein, gp120, of human immunodeficiency virus-I (HIV-I). Much more surprisingly, however, has been the recent discovery that NRL shares approximately 90 per cent homology with pig muscle phosphohexose isomerase (PHI), an enzyme which catalyses the conversion of glucose-6-phosphate to fructose-6-phosphate as an intermediate step in the glycolytic pathway. This finding has raised doubts as to whether the properties assigned to NRL actually reside in this molecule or are present in another factor released by NRL-producing cells. Nevertheless, it has been suggested that NRL may represent a processed form of PHI. This processing may change the latter from an enzyme into a trophic factor. For instance, tumour cells have higher levels of PHI than normal cells, and tumour cell-derived PHI is present as 56–57 kDa variants not found in normal cells. This is consistent with the suggested processing of PHI to NRL or NRL-like proteins and may explain the association of NRL with the transformed malignant phenotype. However, NRL has not been shown to be directly mitogenic, although it has been reported to induce proliferation as a late response reaction. While the conversion of an enzyme into a growth factor remains an intriguing possibility with exciting implications, further knowledge of the controversial biology of NRL must be forthcoming before this possibility can be said with any confidence to be a reality.

Numerous other growth factors, besides those covered in this chapter (summarized in Table 2.3), have been reported. Many have been molecularly identified and a discussion of these, e.g. CSFs and ILs, will form the basis of subsequent chapters. Some growth factors have not yet been fully characterized, either from a molecular or biological standpoint. These may include novel growth factors, e.g. amphiregulin (AR), which may either be molecularly related to known growth factors, e.g. TGFα or TGFβ, or whose

Table 2.3   Characteristics of growth factors

Factor	Precursor aa	Mature protein aa	Cell source	Target cell	Receptor
EGF	1217	53	Submaxillary gland and various other tissues (not tumours)	Various epithelial and mesen-chymal cells	C-ERB.B oncoprotein; 170 kDa tyrosine kinase
TGFα	160	50	Transformed/tumour cells, placenta, embryos	Same as EGF, e.g. hepatocytes	Same as EGF
IGF-I	130	70	Adult liver, and many, if not all, body tissues. Tumour cells	Epithelial and mesen-chymal cells. Tumour cells	450 kDa complex (2α + 2β chains) β-chain tyrosine kinase
IGF-II	180	67	Fetal liver, placenta, tumour cells	Same as IGF-I	250 kDa single chain
aFGF	unknown	140	Pituitary gland, brain, adrenal gland, kidney, chondro-sarcoma	Endothelial cells, fibroblasts neuroecto-dermal cells	130–170 kDa glycoprotein
bFGF	unknown	146	Same as aFGF	Same as a FGF	Same as aFGF
PDGF	241 (B-chain) A-chain unknown	16 kDa (B) 14–18 kDa (A) homo- or hetero-dimers of A and B chains	Platelets, endothelial cells, placenta, tumour cells	Mesenchy-mal cells, smooth muscle, placental trophoblast, glial cells	185 kDa tyrosine kinase
TGFβ	390 approx.	112; 25 kDa dimers of	Platelets, bone, placenta, kidney,	Fibroblasts keratino-cytes, haemo-	High MW glycosamino-glycan-containing

Table 2.3 (Con't)

Factor	Precursor aa	Mature protein aa	Cell source	Target cell	Receptor
		β-1, -2, -3 chains	cells in culture, e.g. tumour cells	poietic progenitors, lymphocytes, epithelial cells, etc	membrane protein
NGF	307 (β subunit)	118 26 kDa homodimer	Submaxillary gland, prostate gland, brain and nervous system	Sympathetic and sensory neurones, widespread among other tissues and cells	75 kDa glycoprotein

structure is unique. In some cases, the elucidation of new biological properties of well-characterized biologically active polypeptides, e.g. atrial natriuretic factor, may lead to a reassessment of their functions and may ultimately classify them as having growth factor- or cytokine-like biology.

Further reading

General

Baserga, R. (1985) *The Biology of Cell Reproduction*. Harvard University Press, Cambridge, Mass.

Goustin, A.S., Leof, E.B., Shipley, G.D., and Moss, H.L. (1986) Growth factors and cancer. *Cancer Research* **46**, 1015.

Heldin, C.-H. and Westermark, B. (1989) Growth factors as transforming proteins. *European Journal of Biochemistry* **184**, 487.

O'Keefe, E.J. and Pledger, W.J. (1983) Review: a model of cell cycle control: sequential events regulated by growth factors. *Molecular and Cellular Endocrinology* **31**, 167.

Pledger, W.J., Stiles, C.D., Antoniades, H.N., and Scher, C.D. (1978) An ordered sequence of events is required before BALB/C-373 cells become committed to DNA synthesis. *Proceedings of the National Academy of Sciences, USA* **75**, 2839.

Sporn, M.B. and Roberts, A.B. (1988) Peptide growth factors are multifunctional. *Nature* **332**, 217.

Waterfield, M.E. (ed.) (1989) *Growth Factors. British Medical Bulletin* **45** (2). Churchill Livingstone, New York.

Whitman, M. and Cantley, L. (1988) Phosphoinositide metabolism and the control of cell proliferation. *Biochimica et Biophysica Acta* **948**, 327.

Yarden, Y. and Ullrich, A. (1988) Molecular analysis of signal transduction by growth factors. *Biochemistry* **27**, 3113.

Oncogenes

Alitalo, K. (1985) Amplification of cellular oncogenes in cancer cells. *Trends in Biochemical Sciences*, **10**, 194.

Bishop, J.M. (1982) Oncogenes. *Scientific American* **246**, 69.

Bishop, J.M. (1985) Viral oncogenes. *Cell* **42**, 23.

Green, M.R. (1989) When the products of oncogenes and anti-oncogenes meet. *Cell* **56**, 1.

Kaczmarek, L. (1986) Protooncogene expression during the cell cycle. *Laboratory Investigation* **54**, 365.

Katan, M. and Parker, P.J. (1988) Oncogenes and cell control. *Nature* **332**, 203.

Knudson, A.G. (1985) Hereditary cancer, oncogenes and antioncogenes. *Cancer Research* **45**, 1437.

Lebovitz, R.M. (1986) Oncogenes as mediators of cell growth and differentiation. *Laboratory Investigation* **55**, 249.

Lebovitz, R.M. and Lieberman, M.W. (1986) Modulation of cellular genes by oncogenes, in *Progress in Nucleic Acid Research and Molecular Biology*. **35** (W.E. Cohn and K. Moldave, eds) Academic Press, New York, pp.73–94.

Macara, I.G. (1989) Oncogenes and cellular signal transduction. *Physiological Reviews* **69**, 797.

McCormick, R. (1989) ras GTPase activating protein: signal transmitter and signal terminator. *Cell* **56**, 5.

Marsnall, C.J. (1986) Oncogenes. *Journal of Cell Science Supplement* **4**, 417.

Müller, R. (1985) Proto-oncogenes and differentiation. *Trends in Biochemical Sciences*, March, 129.

Richardson, M. (1988) Molecular associations and conceptional connections. *Nature* **334**, 100–102.

Schneider, C., King, R.M. and Philipson, L. (1988) Genes specifically expressed at growth arrest of mammalian cells. *Cell* **54**, 787.

Westermark, B. and Heldin, C.H. (1984) Growth factors: mechanism of action and relation to oncogenes. *Cell* **37**, 9.

Weinberg, R.A. (1984) Cellular oncogenes. *Trends in Biochemical Sciences*, **9**, 131.

Weiss, R.A. and Marshall, C.J. (1984) DNA in medicine: oncogenes. *The Lancet*, **ii**, 1138.

Epidermal growth factor, transforming growth factor alpha and vaccinia growth factor

Bargmann, C.I. and Weinberg, R.A. (1988) Increased tyrosine kinase activity associated with the protein encoded by the activated neu oncogene. *Proceedings of the National Academy of Sciences USA* **85**, 5394.

Carpenter, G. and Zendegui, J.G. (1986) Epidermal growth factor, its receptor, and related proteins. *Experimental Cell Research* **164**, 1.

Derynck, R. (1988) Transforming growth factor alpha. *Cell* **54**, 593.

Kokai, Y., Dobashi, K., Weiner, D.B., Myers, J.N., Nowell, P.C., and Greene, M.I. (1988) Phosphorylation process induced by epidermal growth factor alters the oncogenic and cellular neu (NGL) gene products. *Proceedings of the National Academy of Sciences USA* **85**, 5389.

Schlessinger, J. (1988) The epidermal growth factor receptor as a multifunctional allosteric protein. *Biochemistry* **27**, 3119.

Spriggs, D.R. (1986) Vaccinia virus growth factor: a surprising catch. *Journal of Infectious Diseases* **153**, 382.

62   Cytokines

Insulin and insulin-like growth factors

Anderson, A.S. (1989) Reception and transmission. *Nature* **337**, 12.
Czech, M.P. (1989) Signal transmission by the insulin-like growth factors. *Cell* **59**, 235.
Daughaday, W.H. and Rotwein, P. (1989) Insulin-like growth factors I and II. Peptide, messenger ribonucleic acid and gene structures, serum and tissue concentrations. *Endocrine Reviews* **10**, 68.
Froesch, E.R., Schmidt, C., Schwander, J. and Zapf, J. (1985) Actions of insulin-like growth factors. *Annual Review of Physiology* **47**, 443.
Gilmour, R.S., Prosser, C.G., Fleet, I.R., *et al.* (1988) From animal to molecule: aspects of the biology of insulin-like growth factors. *British Journal of Cancer* **58**, Supplement IX, 23.
Kahn, R.C. and White, M.F. (1988) The insulin receptor and the molecular mechanism of insulin action. *Journal of Clinical Investigation* **82**, 1151.
Morgan, D.O., Edman, J.C., Standring, D.N., *et al.* (1987) Insulin like growth factor II receptor as a multifunctional binding protein. *Nature* **329**, 301.
Ooi, G.T. and Herington, A.C. (1988) The biological and structural characterization of specific serum binding proteins for the insulin-like growth factors. *Journal of Endocrinology* **118**, 7.
Steele-Perkins, G., Turner, J., Edman, J.C., *et al.* (1988) Expression and characterization of a functional human insulin-like growth factor I receptor. *Journal of Biological Chemistry* **263**, 11486.
Yee, D., Cullen, K.J., Paik, S., *et al.* (1988) Insulin-like growth factor II mRNA expression in human breast cancer. *Cancer Research* **48**, 6691.

Fibroblast growth factors

Barr, P.J., Cousens, L.S., Lee-Ng, C.T. *et al.* (1988) Expression and processing of biologically active fibroblast growth factors in the yeast *Saccharomyces cerevisiae*. *Journal of Biological Chemistry* **263**, 16471.
Bovi, P.D., Curatola, A.M. Kern, F.G., *et al.* (1987) An oncogene isolated by transfection of Kaposi's sarcoma DNA encodes a growth factor that is a member of the FGF family. *Cell* **50**, 729.
Courty, J., Dauchel, M.C., Mereau, A., *et al.* (1988) Presence of basic fibroblast growth factor receptors in bovine brain membranes. *Journal of Biological Chemistry* **263**, 11217.
Folkman, J. and Klagsbrun, M. (1987) Angiogenic factors. *Science* **235**, 442.
Thomas, K.A. (1988) Transforming potential of fibroblast growth factor genes. *Trends in Biochemical Sciences* **13**, September, 327.
Thomas, K.A. and Gimenez-Gallego, G. (1986) Fibroblast growth factors: broad spectrum mitogens with potent angiogenic activity. *Trends in Biochemical Sciences* **11**, February, 81.
Wilkinson, D.G., Peters, G., Dickson, C., and McMahon, A.P. (1980) Expression of the FGF-related proto-oncogene int-2 during gastrulation and neurulation in the mouse. *The EMBO Journal* **7**, 691.

Platelet-derived growth factor

Deuel, T.F. (1987) Polypeptide expression during the cell cycle. *Laboratory Investigation* **54**, 365.
Hart, C.E., Forstrom, J.W., Kelly, J.D., *et al.* (1988) Two classes of PDGF receptor recognise different isoforms of PDGF. *Science* **240**, 1529.

Heldin, C.H., Westeson, A., and Westermark, B. (1985) Platelet derived growth factor. *Molecular and Cellular Endocrinology* **39**, 169.

Heldin, C.H., Hammacher, A., Nister, M., and Westermark, B. (1988) Structural and functional aspects of platelet-derived growth-factor. *British Journal of Cancer* **57**, 591.

Johnsson, A., Heldin, C.H., Westermark, B., *et al.* (1984) The c-*sis* gene encodes a precursor of the B-chain of platelet derived growth factor. *The EMBO Journal* **3**, 921.

Owen, A.J., Pantazis, P., and Antoniades, H.N. (1984) Simian sarcoma virus-transformed cells secrete a mitogen identical to platelet-derived growth factor. *Science* **225**, 54.

Robbins, K.C., Antoniades, H.N., Devare, S.G., *et al.* (1985) Structural and immunological similarities between simian sarcoma virus gene product(s) and human platelet-derived growth factor. *Nature* **305**, 605.

Rollins, B.J., Morrison, E.D., Usher, P., and Flier, J.S. (1988) Platelet derived growth factor regulates glucose transporter expression. *Journal of Biological Chemistry* **263**, 16523.

Ross, R., Raines, E.W., and Bowen-Pope, D.F. (1986) The biology of platelet-derived growth factor. *Cell* **46**, 155.

Yarden, Y., Escobedo, J.A., Kuang, W.J., *et al.* (1986) Structure of the receptor for platelet-derived growth factor helps define a family of closely related growth factor receptors. *Nature* **323**, 226.

Transforming growth factor beta and related proteins

Cheifetz, S., Andres, J.L., and Massagué, J. (1988) The transforming growth factor-β receptor type III is a membrane proteoglycan. *Journal of Biological Chemistry* **263**, 16984.

Derynk, R., Lindquist, P.B., Lee, A., *et al.* (1988) A new type of transforming growth factor-β, TGFβ3. *The EMBO Journal* **7**, 3737.

Kerr, L.D., Olashaw, N.E. and Matrisian, L.M. (1988) Transforming growth factor β1 and cAMP inhibit transcription of epidermal growth factor- and oncogene-induced transin mRNA. *Journal of Biological Chemistry* **263**, 16999.

Ling, N., Ueno, N., Ying, S.Y., *el al.* (1988) Inhibins and activins in *Vitamins and Hormones* **44** (D. B. McCormick, ed.) Academic Press, New York, pp. 1–46.

Massagué, J. (1985) The transforming growth factors. *Trends in Biochemical Sciences*, June, 23.

Massagué, J. (1987) The TGFβ family of growth and differentiation factors. *Cell* **49**, 437.

Mustoe, T.A., Pierce, G.F., Thomason, A., *et al.* (1987) Accelerated healing of incisional wounds in rats induced by transforming growth factor-β. *Science* **237**, 1333.

Roberts, A.B., Flanders, K.C., Kondaiah, P. *et al.* (1988) Transforming growth factor beta: biochemistry and roles in embryogenesis, tissue repair and remodeling and carcinogenesis in *Recent Progress in Hormone Research* **44**. Academic Press, New York, pp. 157.

Roberts, A.B., Thompson, N.L., Heine, U., *et al.* (1988) Transforming growth factor-β: possible roles in carcinogenesis. *British Journal of Cancer* **57**, 594.

Sporn, M.B. and Roberts, A.B. (1985) Autocrine growth factors and cancer. *Nature* **313**, 745.

Sporn, M.B., Roberts, A.B., Wakefield, L.M., and Assoian, R.K. (1986) Transforming growth factor-β: biological function and chemical structure. *Science* **233**, 532.

Woodland, H. and Jones, L. (1988) Growth factors in amphibian cell differentiation. *Nature* **332**, 113.

Wozney, J.M., Rosen, V., Celeste, A.J., *et al.* (1988) Novel regulators of bone formation: molecular clones and activities. *Science* **242**, 528.

Nerve growth factor, neuroleukin, and other growth factors

Baumann, M. and Brand, K. (1988) Purification and characterization of phosphohexose isomerase from human gastrointestinal carcinoma and its potential relationship to neuroleukin. *Cancer Research* **48**, 7018.

Bradshaw, R.A. (1978) Nerve growth factor. *Annual Review of Biochemistry* **47**, 191.

Chao, M.V., Bothwell, M.A., Ross, A.H., *et al.* (1986) Gene transfer and molecular cloning of the human NGF receptor. *Science* **232**, 518.

Chaput, M., Clees, V., Portetelle, D., *et al.* (1988) The neurotrophic factor neuroleukin is 90 per cent homologous with phosphohexose isomerase. *Nature* **332**, 454.

Faik, P., Walker, J.I.H., Redmill, A.A., and Morgan, M.J. (1988) Mouse glucose-6-phosphate isomerase and neuroleukin have identical sequences. *Nature* **332**, 455.

Gurney, M.E. (1987) Neuroleukin: basic biology and functional interaction with human immunodeficiency virus. *Immunological Reviews* **100**, 203.

Hempstead, B.L., Schleifer, S., and Chao, M.W. (1989) Expression of functional nerve growth factor receptors after gene transfer. *Science* **243**, 373.

Lindsay, R.M. and Harmer, A.J. (1989) Nerve growth factor regulates expression of neuropeptide genes in adult sensory neurons. *Nature* **337**, 362.

Matsuda, J., Coughlin, M.D., Bienenstock, J., and Denburg, J.A. (1988) Nerve growth factor promotes human hemopoietic colony growth and differentation. *Proceedings of the National Academy of Sciences USA* **85**, 6508.

Purves, D., Snider, W.D., and Voyvodic, J.T. (1988) Trophic regulation of nerve cell, morphology and innervation in the autonomic nervous system. *Nature* **336**, 123.

Rakowicz-Szulczynska, E.M., Herlyn, M., and Koprowski, J. (1988) Nerve growth factor receptors in chromatin of melanoma cells, proliferating melanocytes, and colorectal carcinoma cells *in vitro*. *Cancer Research* **48**, 7200.

Scott, J., Selby, M., Urdea, M., *et al.* (1983) Isolation and nucleotide sequence of a cDNA encoding the precursor of mouse nerve growth factor. *Nature* **302**, 538.

Young, M., Blanchard, M.H., Sessions, F., and Boyle, D.P. (1988) Subunit structure of high molecular weight mouse nerve growth factor. *Biochemistry* **27**, 6675.

3

Haemopoietic growth factors

3.1 Introduction

The cells that populate the blood are all derived from multipotential (or pluripotential) stem cells present in bone marrow. Multipotential stem cells continually proliferate and renew themselves, but also give rise to common progenitor cells. Once committed, progenitor cells differentiate into immature precursor cells of the various blood cell lineages which, following further differentiation stages, eventually give rise to mature functional blood cells, such as erythrocytes, monocytes, and lymphocytes. Terminally differentiated blood cells generally lose their ability to proliferate — indeed mammalian erythrocytes and platelets contain no nuclei — and thus have finite lifetimes. Granulocytes exist only for a matter of hours, whereas human erythrocytes remain in circulation for over 100 days and some lymphocytes have life-spans measured in years. Therefore, to maintain steady-state numbers of particular blood cell types, there must be a continual production of these from the bone marrow. This process, known as haemopoiesis (haematopoiesis), is as yet poorly understood. The study of multipotential stem cell proliferation and the development of committed progenitor and precursor blood cells has proved extremely difficult. Experimental investigations in this area require the establishment of *in vitro* model systems involving components of bone marrow, including haemopoietic and accessory cells, and although some success has been achieved, much remains to be learned. It is however, clear, that many steps in the haemopoietic process are controlled by certain cytokines, also known as haemopoietic growth factors.

A number of cytokines now fall into the category of haemopoietic growth factors, and this number will probably increase as more knowledge is gained of the mechanisms underlying haemopoiesis. Some of the haemopoietic growth factors appear to be very pleiotropic, i.e. act on many cell types, rather in the manner of the growth factors discussed in Chapter 2, whilst others appear to be restricted to particular blood cell lineages. Thus, IL-1, IL-3, IL-6, and GM-CSF could be considered to form one group of haemopoietic growth factors which is 'promiscuous' regarding cell type, whereas G-CSF, M-CSF, IL-5, and erythropoietin (EPO) form another group of factors with limited target-cell specificity.

This chapter will deal comprehensively with IL-3, GM-CSF, G-CSF, M-CSF, IL-5, and EPO. Only a selective approach towards the biology of IL-1 and IL-6 is given here as these cytokines will be considered in more detail in subsequent chapters.

3.2   The bone marrow and haemopoiesis

Except in early stages of embryogenesis, the first stages of the haemopoietic process are confined to the red bone marrow. In neonatal mammals all marrow is red, but in adults red marrow is found only in breast bone, ribs, clavicles, vertebrae, pelvis, and skull. Red bone marrow has a complex structure. Bone-forming cells (osteoblasts) line the inner surface of the bone cavity and are supplied with nutrients via arterial capillaries. Filling the spaces between the incoming arteries and leaving veins are irregularly branching, interconnected reticular cells and fibres which form a honeycomb type of structure. The pores left in this reticular framework are filled with haemopoietic tissue (Figure 3.1). This latter contains, in addition to the haemopoietic stem and progenitor cells, some fat cells, lymphocytes, macrophages, and mast cells. Initial stages of haemopoietic cell development are extravascular, i.e. they occur outside blood vessels. However, in most cases, secondary differentiation into more mature blood cells occurs intravascularly and this necessitates the progenitor/precursor cells leaving the bone marrow by migrating through blood vessel walls. In many instances, further differentiation of newly produced blood cells occurs following their colonization of specialized organs, e.g. thymus, and tissues such as skin.

The mature cells of the haemopoietic system are erythrocytes, granulocytes, lymphocytes, monocytes, macrophages, mast cells, and platelets. These all have a limited life-span, and must be replaced as they die. To achieve a balance between cell death and renewal, the bone marrow must not only continuously provide progenitor cells, but also control the commitment of these to the various lineages so that the correct proportions of mature cells are produced. The basic control mechanisms, especially of the earliest stages of haemopoiesis, are as yet poorly understood. There appears to be some compartmentalization of the marrow, and microscopic 'nests' of particular precursor cells have been identified, but these only represent the macroscopic view of proliferation and differentiation within the marrow and do not answer the question of what biochemical reactions are involved. However, the

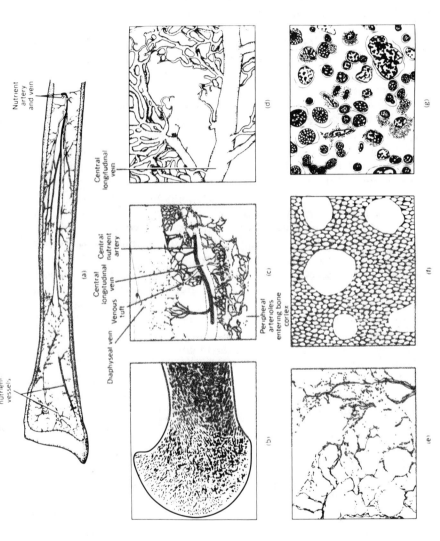

Figure 3.1 Organization of adult bone marrow. (a) Section through a long bone, showing the main blood vessels. (b) Section through head and neck of a long bone, showing sponge like trabeculae. The meshes of the sponge are occupied by bone marrow. (c) Section showing the relationship of main blood vessels. (d) The system of veins and sinuses. (e) Framework of reticular fibres. (f) Framework of reticular cells. (g) Haemopoietic cells filling the framework. (From Klein, J., 1982. *Immunology: The Science of Self-Non Self Discrimination*, John Wiley & Sons, New York; reprinted with permission from the author.)

establishment of long-term bone marrow cultures *in vitro* by Dexter and colleagues has shown that the survival and proliferation of stem and progenitor cells is dependent upon the presence of accessory cells which *in vitro* form into an adherent 'stromal' layer. In the absence of the stromal layer, stem and progenitor cells die and so presumably the stromal cells support proliferation and differentiation by intercellular interactions including production of growth factors into the extracellular milieu. In culture, stromal cells have been shown to produce GM-CSF, M-CSF, and a megakaryocyte-colony stimulating factor (or molecules functionally equivalent to these). It is widely believed that such growth factors (cytokines) are involved in haemopoiesis, but their exact role(s) in self-renewal of stem cells, differentiation of stem cells into common progenitor cells, and the proliferation and differentiation of committed progenitor cells, remains unclear. More definite roles of these cytokines in the growth stimulation and development of later-stage precursors have been evinced by the use of *in vitro* colony-forming culture systems introduced by Metcalf and colleagues in the 1970s. In these experimental systems multipotential stem cells, progenitors, or precursors are suspended in the absence of stromal cells in semi-solid agar growth medium. Without the addition of exogenous cytokines, the cells die. However, they can be stimulated to grow, multiply, and differentiate to form colonies of various blood cell lineages by adding into the growth medium dilutions of certain supernatants obtained from activated leukocytes or by addition of the now readily available purified recombinant cytokines. Experimental investigations based on these systems have led to a much greater understanding of the biological roles of cytokines, especially the haemopoietic growth factors, in the development of mature blood cells. Furthermore, injection of recombinant cytokines into experimental animals, and into patients in clinical trials to assess therapeutic potential of individual cytokine products, has shown that IL-3, GM-CSF, and G-CSF stimulate the production of white cells such as granulocytes and monocytes, thus lending support for physiological roles of such cytokines. In addition, it has also become apparent that these cytokines not only support the growth and differentiation of immature blood cells, but also in many instances are effector molecules for the functional activation of mature cells.

In summary, certain cytokines are haemopoietic growth/differentiation factors which enable the production, development, and activation of mature blood cells from bone marrow stem cells. The molecular characteristics of these cytokines will be described, together with those of their receptors where known. Their biological actions in relation to myelopoiesis (development of granulocytes, monocytes, and megakaryocytes) and erythropoiesis (generation of red blood cells, erythrocytes) is also discussed. Lymphopoiesis, the generation and development of lymphocytes, will be described in Chapter 4, since lymphocytes appear to arise from a separate pool of progenitors and are, at certain developmental stages, probably subject to growth/differentiation control by different cytokines to those discussed here.

3.3   Haemopoietic cytokines

The molecular cloning of both murine and human homologues of IL-3, GM-CSF, G-CSF, M-CSF, IL-5, and EPO has been accomplished in very recent years. For much of the investigational work carried out with these cytokines, the mouse, its tissues, or murine-derived cells have provided experimental test systems. Therefore, many of the observations and results reported in the literature are derived from mouse model systems. In many cases, such observations/results have been repeated in equivalent human cell systems. However, there are some instances where data stemming from murine systems, e.g. with IL-3, has not been reproduced in the human system and vice versa, though to a lesser extent. While the biology of these cytokines in murine systems probably reflects that in human systems, this may not always be the case and this point should be borne in mind when reading the following reviews.

Interleukin-3, a multi-colony stimulating factor

Now that its molecular identity has been established, the history of IL-3 can, in retrospect, be traced back to the 1960s. It appeared to exist in many guises and was independently named as one or other growth- or colony-stimulating factor during two decades of 'factorology' (1964–1984). Thus, it was probably one of the factors present in 'conditioned medium' from activated murine leukocytes that stimulated the growth of mast cells, granulocytes and monocytes, multipotential stem cells, megakaryocytes, erythroid precursors, etc. *in vitro*. Accordingly, it has been variously called mast cell growth factor, persisting cell-stimulating factor (PSF), haemopoietic cell growth factor (HCGF), burst-promoting activity (BPA), eosinophilic-CSF (E-CSF), multi-CSF, etc. The natural source of this pleiotropic factor was shown to be activated T-cells, and it appears not to be produced by other cell types. It is thus a lymphokine and was called 'interleukin-3' (IL-3) from the observation, now known to be erroneous, that it acted on the direct precursors of T-cells.

   For the molecular characterization of IL-3, it was fortunate that an alternative source of this cytokine had been identified. Thus, various tumour-derived cell lines, in particular a murine myelomonocytic tumour WEHI-3B, were found to secrete a factor that had many biological activities in common with the T-cell-derived IL-3. WEHI-3B constitutively produces high levels of IL-3, and tumour cell supernatants were used in early attempts to purify IL-3. It was established that erythroid burst-promoting activity and activities for granulocyte, monocyte, megakaryocyte, eosinophil, and mast cell development co-purified in a single glycoprotein (MW 25–35 000). The variable molecular weight can be attributed to the heavily glycosylated nature of IL-3; it can have oligosaccharide side chains accounting for up to 40 per cent of its mass. The WEHI-3B cell line was also used as a source of IL-3 mRNA for IL-3 cDNA cloning by rDNA technological procedures in 1984. At about the same time, a cDNA clone derived from a murine T-cell line coding for murine mast cell growth factor (MCGF) was isolated. In the event, it was shown that the coding sequences of the cDNAs for IL-3 and MCGF were identical except for a single nucleotide difference. The IL-3 cDNA encodes a polypeptide of 166 amino acids including a hydrophobic N-terminal signal sequence of 27 amino acids (Figure 3.2). The deduced amino acid sequence of IL-3 indicates that there are four potential N-linked glycosylation sites in the mature protein (MW ~15 100) and these are occupied, judging by the heavy glycosylation of natural IL-3. Comparison of the deduced sequence of IL-3 with those of other cytokines, e.g. GM-CSF, IL-2, IFNγ has revealed little sequence homology except for a striking similarity of four amino acids located at the N-terminus of IL-3, GM-CSF, G-CSF, M-CSF, IL-2, IL-1, and EPO. This sequence may serve to classify any further novel cytokines with this group of haemopoietic growth factors, but its evolutionary origin and biological significance are unknown.

Using the deduced IL-3 amino acid sequence, Schrader and colleagues chemically synthesized the entire IL-3 protein using an automated solid-phase peptide synthesizer. The IL-3 protein so produced was fully biologically active, despite being non-glycosylated, and thus provided conclusive proof that the polypeptide defined by the IL-3 cDNA possessed the pleiotropic activity attributed to it. The role of oligosaccharide side chains in the heavily glycosylated IL-3 derived from T-cells and tumour cell lines remains uncertain, but it is clear that they are not required for full biological activity. Other structure–function studies have revealed that the first seven N-terminal amino acids are also not required for biological activity, but that residues 7–16 and the cysteine residue at position 17 are required for maximum activity.

Identifying the human counterpart of murine IL-3 proved problematic because stimulated T-cells produced only low levels of this haemopoietic cytokine and no human cell lines secreting this cytokine were known. In retrospect, the fact that the primary amino acid sequence of human IL-3 is less than 30 per cent homologous to murine IL-3 made it difficult to isolate human IL-3 DNA or RNA sequences using murine IL-3 nucleic acid probes. The problem was solved by first cloning gibbon IL-3 cDNA using mRNA from the gibbon ape T-cell line, UCD-144-MLA, which produces gibbon IL-3. The deduced amino acid sequence of gibbon IL-3 is 29 per cent homologous to murine IL-3, and in contrast to the rodent factor has two cysteine residues instead of four and thus contains only one disulphide bridge. Using gibbon IL-3 DNA probes, isolation of human IL-3 cDNA then proved relatively straightforward, the human protein (Figure 3.2) turning out to be highly homologous (93 per cent) to gibbon IL-3. The nuclear genes for human and murine IL-3 are, however, similar in structure; each is composed

Figure 3.2 (opposite) Comparison of the amino acid sequences of human and mouse IL-3s. The single-letter amino acid code is used. Sequences are aligned to show maximum homology. The vertical line represents the cleavage point between signal sequences and mature polypeptides. The asterisks denote cysteine residues forming disulphide bonds. Potential N-glycosylation sites are underlined.

																				20

```
                                            20
Human (Hu)                 M  S  R  L  P  V  L  L  L  L  Q  L  L
Mouse (Mo)  M  V  L  A  S  S  T  T  S  I  H  T  M  L  L  L  L  L  M  L
                              .              .  .  .              .

                                            40
Hu          V  R  P  G  L  Q | A  P  M  T  Q  T  T  S  L  K  T  S  W  -
Mo          F  H  L  G  L  Q | A  S  I  S  G  R  D  T  H  R  L  T  R  T
               .  .  .  .

               *                            60
Hu          V  N  C  S  N  M  I  D  E  I  I  T  H  L  K  Q  P  P  L  P
Mo          L  N  C  S  S  I  V  L  E  I  I  G  K  L  -  -  -  P  E  P
               .  .  .              .        .        .           .  .

                                            80
Hu          L  L  D  F  N  N  L  N  G  E  D  Q  D  I  L  M  E  N  N  L
Mo          -  -  E  L  K  T  -  -  D  D  E  G  P  S  L  R  N  K  S  F
                                          .

                                            100
Hu          R  R  P  N  L  E  A  F  N  R  A  V  K  S  L  -  -  Q  N  A
Mo          R  R  V  N  L  S  K  F  V  E  S  Q  G  E  V  D  P  E  D  R
               .  .     .  .           .

                                 *          120
Hu          S  A  I  E  S  I  L  K  N  L  L  P  C  L  P  L  A  T  A  A
Mo          Y  V  I  K  S  N  L  Q  K  L  N  C  C  L  P  T  S  A  N  D
                  .     .     .        .     *  .  .  .

                                            140
Hu       P  T  R  H  P  I  H  I  K  D  G  D  W  N  E  F  R  R  K  L
Mo       S  A  L  P  G  V  F  I  R  -  -  D  L  D  D  F  R  K  K  L
                     .           .              .  .     .  .

                                            160
Hu       T  F  Y  L  K  T  L  E  N  A  Q  A  Q  Q  T  T  L  S  L  A
Mo       R  F  Y  M  N  H  L  N  D  L  E  T  V  L  T  S  R  P  P  Q
            .  .        .                       .

Hu       I  F
Mo       P  A  S  G  S  V  S  P  N  R  G  T  V  E  C
                                       *
```

Table 3.1   Linkage of colony stimulating factors, interleukins, growth factors, and their receptors on human chromosome 5

Cytokine/receptor	Location: long arm (q) of chromosome 5
IL-3	5q 23–q 32
IL-4	5q 23–q 32
GM-CSF	5q 23–q 31
IL-5	5q 31–q 33
FGF	5q 31–q 33
M-CSF	5q 23–q 31
M-CSF-R (c-FMS)	5q 23–q 34
PDGF-R	5q 31–q 32

of five small exons intersected by three small (first, third and fourth) and one large (second) intron. The human gene has been located to the long arm of chromosome 5 (Table 3.1) which also contains the genes of GM-CSF, M-CSF and its receptor, IL-4 and IL-5. The equivalent site in mouse is on chromosome 11.

Basically, the activities of murine, gibbon, and human IL-3 have been

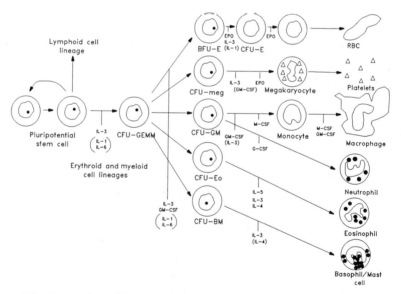

Figure 3.3   Interactions of haemopoietic growth factors with haemopoietic cells. The different progenitor cells are designated CFU-GEMM (colony-forming unit — granulocyte, erythrocyte, monocyte, megakaryocyte), CFU-Meg (CFU-megakaryocyte), CFU-GM (CFU-granulocyte, monocyte), CFU-Eo (CFU-eosinophil), CFU-BM (CFU-basophil, mast cell; it is not known if this is different from (CFU-Eo), BFU-E (burst-forming unit-erythrocyte), CFU-E (colony-forming unit-erythrocyte). The interactions of the various haemopoietic growth factors with the different lineages are as indicated.

shown to be similar, although research with the newly available human IL-3 is not as advanced or as extensive as with IL-3 from the two other species. Whereas both gibbon and human IL-3 are active in human cells, murine IL-3 shows little or no activity in heterologous human cells. Cell-surface receptors for IL-3 have been partially characterized in certain murine 'IL-3 dependent' cell lines (IL-3 dependent means that such cells require IL-3 as a mitogen to stimulate proliferation). The FDC-P1 cell line has about 5000 high-affinity receptors for IL-3, and preliminary biochemical characterization has revealed a potential receptor glycoprotein (MW 50–70000). This relatively low molecular weight distinguishes the IL-3 receptor from the high-molecular-weight receptors of other growth factors, e.g. EGF, PDGF, etc., but suggests that it may show structural similarities to the IL-2 receptor (see Chapter 4) or that of GM-CSF, a cytokine with which IL-3 has overlapping biological activities. However, there is evidence that IL-3 also binds to a 140 kDa membrane phosphoprotein, which is comparable with other receptors, and it has been speculated that the low-molecular-weight IL-3-binding protein is a proteolytic cleavage product of the 140 kDa phosphoprotein (see also p. 225).

IL-3 principally supports growth and proliferation of cells of the erythroid and myeloid lineages. In the murine system it appears to exert its effects on a larger range of erythroid/myeloid progenitors than GM-CSF, a more ubiquitous multi-CSF. IL-3 supports the proliferation and differentiation of multipotential cells in the formation of granulocyte–erythroid–macrophage–megakaryocyte colony-forming unit (GEMM-CFU)-derived colonies *in vitro* more effectively than GM-CSF (Figure 3.3). In particular, IL-3 appears more active in the stimulation of erythroid burst-forming units (BFU-E) and megakaryocyte progenitors than is GM-CSF. There is growing experimental evidence supporting the idea that IL-3 acts on early multipotential cells, thus suggesting the reason for its apparently less restricted cell specificity. It has been speculated that IL-3 acts not to stimulate the self-renewal of primitive stem cells, but to commit such cells to differentiate into the progenitors of the various haemopoietic cell lineages. Once committed in this way, these progenitors become responsive to lineage-specific cytokines, such as G-CSF and M-CSF. Alternatively, it has been proposed that IL-3 acting as a competence factor (see Chapter 2) stimulates cells to leave G_0 of the cell cycle and in doing so renders them permissive to other growth-stimulating cytokines, such as IL-1 and M-CSF, acting at later stages of the cell cycle. In this regard, it has been shown that IL-3 mediates activation of Na^+/H^+ exchange via protein kinase C causing intracellular alkanization, an early marker of signal transduction leading to the proliferative response. There is evidence for G-protein involvement in IL-3 activation, and c-*myc* proto-oncogene expression is also induced by IL-3, but these observations have been made in immortalized IL-3-dependent cell lines which may show aberrant growth control. Thus, the precise mechanism whereby IL-3 commits multipotential cells to growth and then to lineage-specific differentiation pathways remains uncertain.

While IL-3 has been clearly demonstrated to stimulate the production of erythroid and myeloid cells progenitors *in vitro*, there is no evidence that it is involved in the development of lymphoid progenitors. *In vivo*, since IL-3 is produced only by activated T-cells, the question of whether it plays a significant role in normal early haemopoiesis remains controversial. Haemopoiesis is more likely to be regulated by other cytokines and factors released by accessory cells in the bone marrow. Possibly IL-3 secreted by activated T-cells provides an additional tier of haemopoietic growth control by augmenting erythroid/myeloid cell proliferation and differentiation in times of emergency, e.g. during acute infection of the host. In support of this hypothesis, recombinant murine IL-3 injected into mice in relatively large doses increased the proliferation of erythroid/myeloid progenitors and the production of mature cell types such as granulocytes and macrophages. Perhaps as importantly, IL-3 has the potential to act as a growth factor for the production of mast cells, a heterogeneous population of mononuclear basophilic granular cells containing histamine present in connective and mucosal tissues which are involved in immune and allergic responses (Figure 3.3). Nevertheless, it has not been possible to detect natural IL-3 in the sera of normal or infected animals and possibly any IL-3 produced by activated T-cells acts locally in a paracrine fashion on responsive 'bystander' cells. In this respect, it is known that IL-3 can indirectly affect the proliferation/differentiation and function(s) of more mature cells of the myeloid lineage. For instance, IL-3 appears to regulate tissue macrophage production, probably by inducing macrophage precursors to express receptors for other cytokines, such as M-CSF. Changes in macrophage morphology and increased phagocytic activity have also been associated with IL-3 stimulation.

The genes encoding IL-3 and its receptor are not known as proto-oncogenes. Nevertheless, disruption of IL-3 gene expression may be responsible for the development of certain myeloid leukaemias (cancerous or malignant, usually immature, cells of the myeloid lineage). Although, except in T-cells, the IL-3 gene is completely repressed, it can be switched on, as for example in the WEHI-3 myelomonocytic tumour cell line, and act as an autostimulatory growth factor. The high constitutive production of IL-3 in WEHI-3 is probably caused by a retroviral DNA insertion near to the IL-3 gene located on mouse chromosome 11. The response of leukaemic cells to IL-3 or other haemopoietic cytokines is often proliferation without differentiation. Leukaemogenesis, i.e. the development of leukaemic cells, can be mimicked *in vitro* by forcing bone marrow cells to grow under certain conditions to become dependent upon the presence of exogenous IL-3 in the growth medium. In this way, several IL-3-dependent cell lines have been established which are absolutely dependent upon IL-3 for proliferation, but which are blocked at an early stage of differentiation. These 'immortalized' cell lines may be transformed to a malignant, IL-3-independent phenotype in at least two distinct ways. Infection with the Abelson murine leukaemia virus, a retrovirus containing the v-*abl* oncogene, circumvents the requirement for IL-3 or GM-CSF, probably by introducing into cells constitutive v-*abl* tyrosine kinase activity (see Chapter 2). In addition, infection with a recombinant retrovirus containing the gene for GM-CSF also leads to neoplastic transformation, this being associated with the autocrine action of GM-CSF produced by infected cells. Thus, there are clear indications that leukaemogenesis can be supported or even caused by cytokines. Interestingly, at the time of diagnosis, myeloid leukaemia cells derived from patients mostly require one or more exogenous haemopoietic cytokines to proliferate *in vitro*, strongly suggesting *in vivo* involvement of such cytokines in maintaining proliferation of leukaemia (tumour) cells. However, in some cases it has not been possible to demonstrate cytokine dependency and probably other mechanisms may be involved.

Granulocyte-macrophage colony stimulating factor

Of the four 'granulocyte-macrophage' CSFs discovered using the semi-solid agar method for growing haemopoietic cells introduced by Metcalf and colleagues, GM-CSF was the first to be isolated and characterized. GM-CSF was shown to induce the proliferation of murine bone marrow- or spleen-derived haemopoietic cells containing granulocyte and macrophage progenitors giving rise to colonies containing mainly granulocyte and macrophage precursors. In this respect, GM-CSF appears to share biological properties with the subsequently characterized IL-3 (see p. 69). However, more recent studies suggest that GM-CSF acts on 'later-stage 'multipotential cells than IL-3 (Figure 3.3). Also, GM-CSF appears to be less active than IL-3 in stimulating the proliferation of erythroid and megakaryocytic precursors. Nevertheless, like IL-3, GM-CSF can be shown to have activities in mature cells of the granulocyte and macrophage lineages.

GM-CSF can be produced by a broad range of normal cell types, including bone marrow stromal cells, fibroblasts, endothelial cells, monocytes, and T-lymphocytes. In comparison to the restricted T-cell production of IL-3, it may be considered to be ubiquitous. It may also be produced by a number of tumour cell lines grown *in vitro*. It is, however, not normally expressed in unstimulated primary cells; GM-CSF gene induction requires mitogenic, antigenic, or other stimulatory signals. *In vitro*, it is clear that the actions of other cytokines, e.g. IFNγ and IL-1, stimulate or potentiate GM-CSF production. This suggests that during episodes of microbial infection leading to activation of T-lymphocytes and macrophages, the GM-CSF produced by these cells probably augments production of both granulocytes and macrophages. As yet, as for IL-3, there is little direct evidence that GM-CSF plays a critical role in normal steady-state haemopoiesis. For instance, the identity of any indigenous inducers of the normally repressed GM-CSF gene in bone marrow stromal cells remains unknown.

Molecular cloning of murine GM-CSF cDNA followed from purification of GM-CSF from murine lung conditioned medium, and the elucidation of the N-terminal amino acid sequence of this protein. In comparison, the method of molecular cloning of human GM-CSF cDNA was similar to that of IL-3 cDNA, its isolation being dependent upon the detection of the high intrinsic activity of GM-CSF produced by monkey COS cells containing random

Table 3.2   Structure of human haemopoietic growth factors

Factor	Precursor aa	Mature protein aa	Glyco-protein MW	Disulphide bridges	Protein homology (percent) to murine factor
IL-3	152	133	15–25 kDa (N)	1	29
GM-CSF	144	127	18–24 kDa (N/O)	2	56
G-CSF	204	174	19.6 kDa (O)	2	73
M-CSF	256	(224) 149	44 kDa*	3	80
	554	189?	>50 kDa* (N)	3	
IL-5	134	114	45 kDa* (N)	1	70
EPO	193	166	36 kDa (N/O)	2	80

*dimeric
N, N-asparagine-linked carbohydrate side chains
O, O-serine/threonine-linked carbohydrate side chains

plasmid cDNAs. Human GM-CSF cDNA codes for a 144-amino-acid precursor of mature GM-CSF (Table 3.2). Cleavage of the signal sequence yields a 127-amino-acid polypeptide containing two internal disulphide bridges and with two potential sites for N-linked oligosaccharides. The deduced amino acid sequences of human and murine GM-CSF show approximately 56 per cent homology, but there is no structural homology with either human or murine IL-3 or other known cytokines. The gene for human GM-CSF is a single-copy one and is located on the long arm of chromosome 5 closely linked to the IL-3 gene. The murine GM-CSF gene is located on mouse chromosome 11. The significance of this close association of GM-CSF and IL-3 genes (Table 3.1) is, however, unclear. Both GM-CSF and IL-3 are produced by activated T-lymphocytes, suggesting that regulation of induction of their genes occurs by a common mechanism. On the other hand, only GM-CSF is expressed in cells other than T-lymphocytes; this indicates that the closely associated GM-CSF and IL-3 genes are independently regulated.

Native GM-CSF produced by T-lymphocytes or mammalian cell lines in culture is heavily glycosylated, giving rise to species with molecular weights ranging from 14 to 35 kDa, but usually in the range 18–24 kDa. In addition to N-asparagine-linked oligosaccharides, it is probable that GM-CSF is also modified by addition of O-linked oligosaccharides at several positions. Non-glycosylated GM-CSF produced by recombinant *E.coli* containing GM-CSF cDNA is, however, fully biologically active, and thus the function of the carbohydrate side chains in eukaryotic cell-derived GM-CSF remains unknown. *In vitro*, the absence or presence of carbohydrate probably does not matter much in terms of biological activity, but *in vivo* it has been demonstrated that non-glycosylated GM-CSF is more rapidly distributed among various tissues and more rapidly cleared from the body than glycosylated GM-CSF. This suggests a protective, stabilizing role for carbohydrate. As with human and murine IL-3s, there is little or no cross-reaction of human GM-CSF on murine cells and vice versa. Binding studies with radio-iodinated GM-CSF have revealed the presence of only relatively few, perhaps 100–2500, high-affinity receptors per cell in responsive cell types, the latter being restricted to erythroid and myeloid cell lineages and certain myelomonocytic tumour cell lines. The numbers of receptors appears to be highest in early haemopoietic cells and to decline as these cells differentiate into mature blood cell types such as granulocytes or macrophages. Chemical cross-linking experiments have shown that ^{125}I-GM-CSF binds to a 50–70 kDa membrane protein which in fact may be a proteolytic cleavage product of a 180 kDa receptor protein (cf. IL-3-binding 140 kDa phosphoprotein; see p. 73). There is evidence to suggest that GM-CSF and IL-3 bind to different receptors, but recent observations also suggest a third class of receptors to which they both bind. These may explain their overlapping biological activities and the fact that GM-CSF can substitute for IL-3 in IL-3-dependent cell lines in many instances. The mechanism of cell activation by GM-CSF may be similar to that of IL-3 activation, but as yet there are few details on this.

As previously mentioned, GM-CSF acts directly and selectively on granulocyte/macrophage progenitors to stimulate growth and differentiation *in vitro* of cells belonging to these lineages, e.g. neutrophils, eosinophils, macrophages (Figure 3.3). It does not appear to act on pluripotent haemopoietic stem cells, and is only active on erythroid and megakaryocytic progenitors at relatively high concentrations. These pleiotropic activities have also been demonstrated for recombinant GM-CSF. Besides regulation of the proliferation and differentiation of the progenitor/precursor cells of the myeloid lineage, GM-CSF has also been shown to activate the functions of mature myeloid cell types. For example, GM-CSF has been found to induce macrophage tumoricidal activity against the malignant melanoma cell line, A375. IFNγ can also behave as a macrophage activating factor, but in contrast to GM-CSF requires an additional secondary stimulus, e.g. bacterial LPS, to evoke tumoricidal activity. In addition, GM-CSF activates macrophages to inhibit the replication of *Trypanosoma cruzi* (a unicellular parasite that is the aetiological agent of Chagas disease, or American trypanosomiasis) and increases respiratory oxidative processes. Furthermore, the replication of HIV-1 in the human monocytic cell line U937 has been shown to be moderately inhibited by GM-CSF, and more effectively by the combination of GM-CSF and IFNγ. These *in vitro* results suggest that GM-CSF could have a potential physiological role in macrophage activation and thus possibly could be used prophylactically or therapeutically against a range of microbial agents that replicate in macrophages.

In neutrophils and eosinophils, GM-CSF stimulates a number of functions.

In particular, GM-CSF enhances phagocytosis of bacteria and yeasts by neutrophils. Purified recombinant human GM-CSF has also been shown to enhance the cytotoxic activity of neutrophils and eosinophils against anti-body-coated target cells. These observations, and others in which the anti-microbial functions of neutrophils and eosinophils are increased by GM-CSF, strongly suggest an important role for this mediator in host defence.

When mice are repeatedly injected intraperitoneally with recombinant murine GM-CSF, there is a rapid and sustained increase in the number and functional activity of peritoneal macrophages, granulocytes (neutrophils and eosinophils) as well as increased numbers of circulating monocytes. Marked increases in neutrophil, eosinophil, and monocyte numbers have also been observed following injection of recombinant human GM-CSF into AIDS patients and non-human primates. Therefore, there are strong indications that GM-CSF has the same biological activities *in vivo* as those observed *in vitro* and thus may have several potential clinical applications. (The clinical uses of haemopoietic growth factors will be dealt with in Chapter 9.) However, there may be complications associated with GM-CSF therapy and Metcalf and colleages have recently shown that transgenic mice containing a constitutively expressed murine GM-CSF gene have pathological lesions soon after birth in various tissues, including lens, retina, and striated muscle, resulting from activated-macrophage infiltration. This observation may be taken as a warning to avoid chronic macrophage activation in GM-CSF therapeutic schedules (see Chapter 9). Activated macrophages are known to produce a number of inflammatory mediators including cytokines such as TNFα and IL-1 which may induce tissue damage (see Chapter 5).

In the preceding section on IL-3, evidence for a role of IL-3 and GM-CSF in leukaemogenesis was considered. The fact that acute myeloid leukaemia cells from patients require exogenous haemopoietic growth factors such as GM-CSF for survival and proliferation in culture suggests that such cytokines act as autocrine growth stimulatory factors in maintaining tumour cell prolif-eration. Against this 'autocrine hypothesis', no evidence of myeloid or monocytic leukaemias was found in transgenic mice carrying the murine GM-CSF gene despite constitutive production of GM-CSF. The rather short life-span, less than six months, of these transgenic mice may, however, have precluded the long-term development of malignant myeloid disease, which is probably a multi-stage process. In support of the 'autocrine hypothesis', constitutive expression of GM-CSF has been found in a subset of patients with acute myeloid leukaemia (AML) (alternatively named acute non-lymphocytic leukaemia, ANLL), whereas GM-CSF production was not de-tected in patients with acute lymphocytic leukaemia (ALL) or chronic myeloid leukaemia (CML). That other mechanisms may contribute to leukaemogenesis and other myeloid disorders has been suggested by the observation that loss of part of the long arm of chromosome 5, which contains both the IL-3 and GM-CSF genes together with those of M-CSF, IL-4, IL-5, FGFs, PDGF-R, and M-CSF-R (Table 3.1) is found in some patients with AML. Loss of this part of chromosome 5, known as 5q⁻, is more frequent in patients previously treated with cytotoxic drug therapy, and the disease is more commonly referred to as therapy-induced ANLL or tANLL. The consequences of the loss of this genetic information could be either a reduction in the level of CSFs, growth factors, and receptors, or loss of the wild-type alleles resulting in expression of recessive or mutated alleles in the homologous intact chromosome. The latter consequence possibly offers a better explanation of leukaemia as in tANLL, but probably both consequences are associated with various myeloid disorders.

In contrast to its growth-stimulating effects, GM-CSF can act as a differentiation factor. Its actions on mature macrophages and neutrophils, for example, might be considered as consequences of its differentiation-inducing capacity. One way to limit the proliferation of tumour cells is to decouple growth-factor-driven self-renewal from growth-factor-induced differentiation. In other words, the more 'differentiated' tumour cells become, the less able they are to multiply. In this regard, GM-CSF has been shown in one report to induce differentiation of the myeloid leukaemic cell line HL60 and suppress its self-renewal. However, in several other studies, GM-CSF stimulated the proliferation of HL60 cells. Differentiation can be monitored by measuring expression of various plasma membrane-associated antigens, e.g. Leu-M3 (macrophage marker), Leu-7 (NK cell marker). Interestingly, these have been reported to be induced by GM-CSF in small cell lung cancer (SCLC) cell lines, suggesting that SCLC has a myeloid cell origin. This would be consistent with a proposal that SCLC arises from macrophage precursors which infiltrate damaged lung tissues, such as occur in heavy smokers. The ready availability of recombinant human GM-CSF and the limited distribution of GM-CSF receptors to cells of the myeloid and possibly erythroid lineages may thus help to define the histological origin of tumours, and suggests alternative therapeutic modalities for the treatment of cancers such as SCLC.

Granulocyte-colony stimulating factor

The third 'classic' haemopoietic growth factor is G-CSF. As its name implies, this factor acts mainly on granulocyte precursors and mature granulocytes. Haemopoietic cells grown *in vitro* in the presence of G-CSF give rise to colonies containing mostly neutrophilic granulocytes and their precursors (Figure 3.3).

The presence of a G-CSF in the serum of endotoxin-treated mice had been indicated by the observation that addition of 'endotoxin-serum' to murine leukaemic WEHI 3B (D$^+$) cells induced their differentiation to form colonies of granulocytic cells. It was also found that the conditioned medium taken from various cells and tissues cultured *in vitro* contained similar CSF activity. However, conditioned medium was shown to contain a mixture of at least two CSFs which could be separated by hydrophobic chromatography. These two CSFs were designated CSFβ, which did not bind to the chromatographic resin and which was subsequently identified as GM-CSF (see p. 75), and CSFα, a more hydrophobic factor now known to be identical to G-CSF. It is also now known that G-CSF, like GM-CSF, can be produced by a variety of cell types, principally monocytes, and certain tumour cell lines. G-CSF was first purified from mouse lung conditioned medium as a glycoprotein (MW 25 000). The purified factor was shown not only to induce the terminal differentiation of WEHI 3B (D$^+$) cells but also to stimulate the proliferation of normal granulocytic progenitor cells. The human counterpart of murine G-CSF has been purified to homogeneity from a squamous cell carcinoma (CHU-2 line), a T-leukaemia cell line (Mo), and a bladder carcinoma cell line (5637), in all cases yielding a hydrophobic 19–22 kDa glycoprotein.

The molecular cloning of G-CSF followed from amino acid sequencing of purified G-CSF derived from conditioned medium. Oligonucleotide probes constructed on the basis of amino acid sequence information were used to identify G-CSF cDNA. This cDNA was subsequently expressed to confirm that the protein it encoded had the biological properties of G-CSF. The human cDNA sequence encodes a precursor G-CSF containing 204 amino acids, which yields the 174-amino-acid mature G-CSF protein (MW 18 600) following cleavage of the signal sequence (Table 3.2). The predicted amino acid sequence suggests the formation of two intrachain disulphide bridges, but contains no sites for N-asparagine-linked carbohydrate. The slightly higher molecular weight of G-CSF produced by human cells is likely to be accounted for by some O-linked glycosylation. In contrast to IL-3, GM-CSF, and several other growth factors whose genes are located on the long arm of chromosome 5 (Table 3.1), the G-CSF gene is located on human chromosome 17. The G-CSF gene is approximately 2.5 kb and contains five exons and four introns. The murine G-CSF gene has a similar exon–intron structure. Mature mouse G-CSF consists of 178 amino acids and is approximately 73 per cent homologous to human G-CSF: there is considerable cross-species activity, i.e. human G-CSF is active in mouse cells and vice versa (cf. the non-cross-species reactivity of IL-3 or GM-CSF, which exhibit lower degrees of amino acid sequence homology between human and mouse proteins, Table 3.2). For example, recombinant human G-CSF is able to induce the terminal differentiation of murine WEHI 3B (D$^+$) cells. The G-CSF gene is normally repressed, and induction follows stimulation of primary cells by mitogens and various other activating substances, including other cytokines such as IL-1 or GM-CSF. Endotoxin (LPS) is a strong inducer of G-CSF synthesis and secretion in monocytes, for instance.

Little is so far known about the plasma membrane receptors for G-CSF. Using radio-iodinated G-CSF, receptors have been demonstrated in some murine leukaemic cell lines and on neutrophilic granulocytes with numbers of receptors apparently increasing with the degree of neutrophil maturation. The specific binding of G-CSF to its cell receptors was not competed for by other haemopoietic growth factors, indicating a unique class of G-CSF-receptors. However, murine and human G-CSF do compete for the same receptor and this is consistent with their cross-species biological effects. Chemical cross-linking experiments with ^{125}I-murine G-CSF and WEHI 3B (D$^+$) cells have identified a potential receptor protein (MW $\sim$ 150 000).

Similarly, in human circulating neutrophils, which express approximately 500 high-affinity receptors per cell, a single-subunit receptor protein (molecular weight 150 000) has been identified by ^{125}I-recombinant human G-CSF cross-linking to cells.

Besides its growth-stimulatory and differentiating activities in neutrophilic granulocyte precursors and certain leukaemic cell lines, G-CSF has also been shown to have a profound influence on the biological functions of mature neutrophils. For example, G-CSF increases the phagocytic activity of neutrophils, increases their production of superoxide anions ($O_2{}^-$) in response to the bacterial peptide f–Met–Leu–Phe, and enhances antibody-mediated cellular cytotoxicity (ADCC) against antibody-coated tumour target cells. G-CSF has also been shown to act as a chemotactic factor (this property appears to be common to GM-CSF and M-CSF as well) which induces the migration of leukocytes across polycarbonate or nitrocellulose filters. Such an activity may be important for the recruitment of neutrophils to sites of inflammation and may thus amplify resistance against certain noxious or replicating microbial agents.

Injection of G-CSF into mice, non-human primates, and man has been demonstrated to elicit marked increases in the numbers of circulating neutrophils. However, in contrast to the administration of IL-3 or GM-CSF, G-CSF often did not lead to any significant elevation in numbers of monocytes, eosinophils, or reticulocytes. Neutrophils from animals receiving G-CSF not only increase in number, but are also functionally activated. For example, neutrophil function in hamsters may be activated by *E.coli*-derived recombinant human G-CSF to give a protective effect against a lethal infection with *Staphylococcus aureus*. G-CSF may also be used in animals and patients who are neutropenic, i.e. lacking neutrophils, to restore or enhance neutrophil numbers. For instance, in cancer patients undergoing chemotherapy or ablative radiotherapy, leukocytes (white cells) are severely depressed in numbers. Therefore, G-CSF can be injected to restore leukocytes to their normal level in the circulation. In this G-CSF may be doubly beneficial in that it could also activate neutrophils to provide protection against bacterial and other microbial infections in these immunocompromised patients. In addition, it has been found that G-CSF is without the toxic side-effects of GM-CSF, presumably because it fails to stimulate macrophages to release inflammatory and pyrogenic cytokines, e.g. IL-1, TNFα (see also Chapter 9).

While most experimental evidence suggests that the actions of CSFs are largely confined to haemopoietic cells, one recent report of an enhancement of plasminogen activator activity in cultured endothelial cells by G-CSF points to the presence of G-CSF receptors in non-haemopoietic cells and extends the biological activities associated with this factor. Plasminogen activator is an enzyme that catalyses the conversion of plasminogen to plasmin, a proteolytic enzyme involved in fibrin clot lysis. The significance of this effect of G-CSF is unknown, but certainly it is one that has been associated with endothelial-cell stimulation by other cytokines, e.g. IL-1 and TNF, and thus may be consistent with a physiological role of G-CSF in inflammatory responses.

Macrophage-colony stimulating factor

Macrophage-colony stimulating factor (M-CSF), the last of the four 'classic' haemopoietic growth factors, has, in contrast to the other three factors, a seemingly complex molecular biology and a more enigmatic biology. However, unlike the receptors of the three previously described haemopoietic growth factors, for which there is as yet little information, the M-CSF receptor has been well characterized and shown to be identical to the product of the c-*fms* proto-oncogene, a rather interesting and exciting discovery. M-CSF-R (c-FMS) is an integral plasma membrane glycoprotein with an intracellular tyrosine kinase domain and thus may transduce cell-activating signals occasioned by receptor occupancy in a manner similar to that hypothesized for other growth factor receptors, e.g. PDGF-R (see Chapter 2). More details of the structure and function of M-CSF-R will be described later in this section.

Firstly, M-CSF, which is perhaps equally well known by the name CSF-1, is produced principally by monocytes and macrophages, but may also be produced by a whole variety of tumour cell lines cultured *in vitro*. For example, murine M-CSF has been purified to homogeneity from the conditioned medium obtained from the mouse L-929 'fibroblast-like' cell line. The molecular weight of M-CSF purified from various sources appears to be highly variable, ranging from 20 to over 150 kDa. Part of this heterogeneity of size is probably a reflection of a variable level of glycosylation, but it now appears that M-CSF exists naturally as dimers of glycoproteins of different subunit polypeptide lengths. Despite this molecular heterogeneity, it would appear that most or all of the dimeric species of M-CSF (but not the individual subunits) are biologically active. The main action of M-CSF is the stimulation of macrophage colony growth from haemopoietic cell precursors (colony-forming unit → monoblast → monocyte → macrophage), although M-CSF appears always to stimulate the formation of a small percentage of granulocyte-containing colonies (Figure 3.3). Human M-CSF exhibits cross-species activity and for unexplained, possibly technical, reasons is a better stimulator of the formation of murine macrophage colonies than of homologous human macrophage colonies *in vitro*. Like the other haemopoietic growth factors, M-CSF also has effects on mature monocytes and macrophages, e.g. it increases macrophage cytotoxic activity.

The strategy of the molecular cloning of M-CSF cDNA was similar to that of G-CSF. N-terminal amino acid sequences of purified human M-CSF were first determined and the oligonucleotide probes predicted on the basis of these sequences were used to 'search' cDNA libraries derived from the mRNAs of M-CSF-producing cells. For the purification of human M-CSF, conditioned medium obtained from the human pancreatic carcinoma cell line MIA PaCa, which constitutively produces M-CSF, has proved the most convenient and abundant source, and was also used to prepare a cDNA library. One cDNA isolated from this library was shown to code for a mature polypeptide of 224 amino acids and a putative signal (leader) sequence of 32 amino acids, and further shown to express M-CSF activity when inserted into monkey COS cells (Table 3.2). However, the smallest size of the M-CSF polypeptide chain appears to be more like 14–16 kDa, and not the 26 kDa indicated by the cDNA-encoded 224 amino acid sequence, strongly suggesting that some post-translational processing of the polypeptide must occur. It has been speculated that up to 80 amino acids from the C-terminal end of the 224 amino acid polypeptide are removed by proteolytic cleavage, and that in addition the resulting polypeptide is glycosylated (there are two potential sites for N-linked oligosaccharides) to form ~22 kDa subunits before associating into dimers of ~40–50 kDa.

The recent demonstration of even higher molecular weight human M-CSF precursor polypeptides translated from differently spliced M-CSF mRNAs has further complicated the pattern of molecular processing. A similar situation has been found in the cDNA cloning and expression of mouse M-CSF from L929 cells. In this case, the mature M-CSF polypeptide is

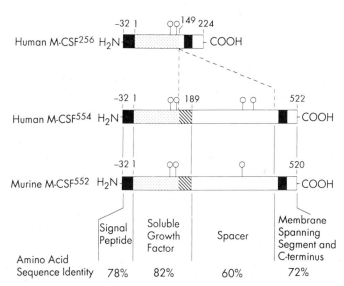

Figure 3.4 Primary translation products encoded by biologically active human and mouse M-CSF cDNAs. Each M-CSF (CSF-1) precursor consists of an amino-terminal signal peptide (black bar) and sequence for the secreted growth factor (stippled), a transmembrane segment (black bar), and a C-terminal tail. Canonical sequences for N-linked glycosylation are indicated by open circles. Human M-CSF[256] and M-CSF[554] are encoded by mRNAs derived by alternative splicing of the primary transcript. A contiguous segment of 298 amino acids present in human M-CSF[554] and absent in M-CSF[256] is delimited by the dashed lines. Polypeptide sequences from this insert, which are present in the soluble growth factor derived from M-CSF[554], are cross-hatched. Murine M-CSF[552] is similar in structure to the large human M-CSF precursor. The extent of amino acid sequence identity between the corresponding regions of the mouse and human M-CSF precursors is indicated. (Reprinted with permission from Rettenmier *et al.*, 1988; copyright The Company of Biologists Limited.)

processed from a 552 amino acid precursor (including the putative signal sequence). Both the small and large precursor human M-CSF polypeptides and the large precursor of murine origin contain a conserved hydrophobic region at their C-terminal ends which has the features of a transmembrane domain (Figure 3.4). Therefore, it has been suggested that M-CSF may exist initially as a transmembrane glycoprotein, and that the (smaller) M-CSF species detected in cell culture media and serum are the result of proteolytic cleavage of the extracellular domain (Figure 3.4). Human and mouse soluble M-CSFs are highly homologous (c. 80 per cent) at the amino acid level, which probably explains the cross-species activity of human M-CSF on mouse cells; mouse M-CSF is far less active on human cells than expected.

The gene for human M-CSF consists of many exons which are distributed over 22 kb of DNA, and is located in a cluster of genes specifying several different growth factors and receptors on the long arm of chromosome 5 (Table 3.1). The equivalent position in the mouse is on chromosome 11.

The receptor for M-CSF is coded for by the c-*fms* proto-oncogene. This discovery was made from the establishment of a link between the structure of the oncoprotein specified by a retroviral oncogene, v-*fms*, and the product of the c-*fms* gene, and the subsequent demonstration of binding of M-CSF to cells expressing v-*fms*. The v-*fms* oncogene is present in the Susan McDonough strain of feline sarcoma virus (SM-FeSV) and is therefore descended from a cellular gene of cat origin. Thus, it was found that the amino acid sequences of the feline v-FMS oncoprotein and the product of the human c-*fms* gene were highly homologous, but non-identical. Both v-*fms* and c-*fms* encode large plasma membrane glycoproteins (MW 140 000–150 000) with N-terminal extracellular domains and C-terminal tyrosine kinases (Figure 3.5). The structure of the extracellular domains shows some similarity with that of the extracellular domain of PDGF-R, in particular the spacing of cysteine residues, which therefore distinguishes M-CSF-R from the receptors of other growth factors, e.g. EGF-R and the insulin receptor. Also, unlike the large truncation of the extracellular domain of the EGF-R found in the transforming v-ERB.B oncoprotein, there is no apparent similar truncation of v-FMS oncoprotein and its binding site for M-CSF is intact. There is, however, a small deletion from the C-terminal tyrosine kinase domain of v-FMS in comparison with human c-FMS, although current evidence suggests that the missing C-terminal amino acids are not fully able to explain the oncogenicity of v-FMS. Recent work where v-FMS was compared to feline c-FMS indicates that while the C-terminal modification on v-FMS is sufficient to generate a partially transformed phenotype, at least two amino acid modifications in the N-terminal extracellular domain are required to produce full transformation. These structural modifications in v-FMS presumably lead to a constitutively activated tyrosine kinase, this activity not being found in c-FMS unless triggered by M-CSF.

As in other tyrosine kinase-containing receptors that have been previously described, e.g. EGF-R (see Section 2.5, pp. 37–40), the functioning of tyrosine kinase is probably critical for signal transduction. Tyrosine residues in the C-terminal tyrosine kinase domain of M-CSF-R are known to be autophosphorylated in the normal response to M-CSF. Further signal transduction pathways are, however, unknown. Tentative links have been established between M-CSF-R activation and a pertussis toxin-sensitive G-protein and the induction of Na^+ influx, leading to intracellular alkanization. In cell lines transformed by v-*fms* there is an increase in phosphatidylinositol turnover, but this has not been found in macrophages stimulated with M-CSF. Thus, the involvement of an activatable phospholipase C–protein kinase C pathway is uncertain. Nevertheless, in common with several other cell-activating stimuli, M-CSF triggers a rapid transient induction of a c-*fos*. In macrophage precursors this presumably leads to the induction of nuclear genes leading to a proliferative response.

When human c-*fms* DNA is transfected into the immortalized anchorage-dependent, but non-tumorigenic, mouse NIH 3T3 cell line, the resulting cells are stimulated to produce colonies in semi-solid agar in the presence of M-CSF. Moreover, when c-*fms* DNA is co-transfected with M-CSF DNA into NIH 3T3 cells they become neoplastically transformed (i.e. tumorigenic) by an autocrine mechanism. This again points to unregulated expression of a

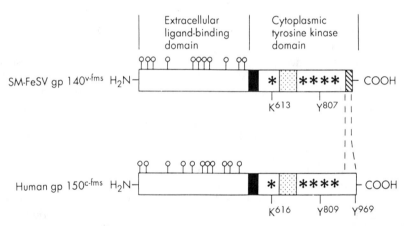

Figure 3.5 Structure of the v-*fms* and c-*fms* gene products. Schematic diagrams of the mature cell surface forms of the Susan McDonough strain of feline sarcoma virus 140 kDa glycoprotein (SM-FeSVgp140^{v-fms}) and the human 150 kDa glycoprotein (gp150^{c-fms}) are shown. A transmembrane segment of hydrophobic amino acids (black bar) divides the proteins into an extracellular domain for ligand binding and a cytoplasmic tyrosine kinase domain. Potential sites for the addition of asparagine-linked oligosaccharides in the N-terminal domain are marked by open circles. The portion of the C-terminal domain that exhibits sequences homology with other protein tyrosine kinases is indicated by asterisks. Within this region of each protein, the position of a critical lysine residue (K) at the ATP-binding site is noted. The segment of 70 fms-specific amino acids that interrupts the core kinase consensus sequence is stippled. The region of carboxyl-terminal sequence divergence between the v-*fms* and c-*fms* gene products is indicated by the cross-hatched area in gp140^{v-fms}. The location of a negative-regulatory tyrosine residue (Y^{969}) near the C-terminus of gp150^{c-fms} is noted. (Reprinted with permission from Rettenmier *et al.*, 1988; copyright The Company of Biologists Limited.)

growth factor and its receptor and the attendant autocrine stimulation being involved in oncogenesis. However, normal monocytes and macrophages both produce and respond to M-CSF in an autocrine fashion without being transformed, therefore implying that immortalized cells grown in culture may be predisposed by other mechanisms to oncogenic transformation by autocrine proliferative factors. In fact, autocrine stimulation of immortalized cell lines may not always result in neoplastic transformation as, for example, when the human M-CSF gene is transfected into the M-CSF dependent SV40-immortalized BAC1.2F5 mouse macrophage cell line. In this case, the transfected cells become factor-independent, but remain non-tumorigenic.

The significance of the *in vitro* findings on autocrine stimulation and oncogenesis to human malignancies remains uncertain, since in general it is not possible to test the relevant factors and molecular aspects of disease progression *in vivo*. However, there is growing circumstantial evidence to implicate autocrine stimulation (or autostimulation) as playing some role in the survival and proliferation of leukaemic cells. For example, c-*fms* proto-oncogene expression appears to be a molecular marker of human AMLs, although expression is not found in other types of leukaemia. Elevated levels of c-*fms* expression, as occurs in some late-stage AMLs, does not appear to result from amplification or rearrangement of the c-*fms* gene. Nevertheless, leukaemic cells from AML patients with the 5q⁻ syndrome (see p. 78) have been shown to be hemizygous for c-*fms*, raising the possibility of expression of a recessive allele encoding a structurally altered M-CSF-R. In this respect, it has been recently shown that replacement of a single amino acid in the extracellular domain of human M-CSF-R was sufficient to convert it into a transforming oncoprotein. Thus, it is tempting to speculate that some cases of AML are the result of point mutation in the c-*fms* gene and the subsequent autostimulatory effect of the structurally altered M-CSF-R. The latter in effect would be functionally equivalent to the v-*fms* product. It is also possible that some leukaemic cells produce M-CSF and respond to it. In other tumours, however, while M-CSF expression has been quite commonly found, e.g. in human ovarian, breast, and lung carcinoma cells, co-expression of M-CSF and c-*fms* genes is much rarer. That many non-haemopoietic tumour cells can produce M-CSF is in itself an interesting finding since the M-CSF released may persistently activate monocytes and macrophages with resulting inflammatory reactions and possible tissue damage.

M-CSF has been shown to be a potent activator of macrophage functions, particularly in the murine system. Thus, murine M-CSF stimulates mature macrophages to produce plasminogen activator (see p. 81), prostaglandin E, IL-1, peroxide, etc, and enhances the tumoricidal and phagocytic activities of macrophages. Since it is widely believed that such activated macrophages play an essential role in defence against cancer and infectious diseases, M-CSF has been proposed as a therapeutic agent for the treatment of these diseases. In addition, M-CSF may also find useful beneficial applications in the restoration of myeloid cell numbers in patients with natural aplastic anaemias or in cancer patients made leukopenic by chemotherapy or radiation treatment.

Interleukin-5 (eosinophil differentiating factor, EDF)

Under normal circumstances, the numbers of circulating eosinophils are relatively few compared with neutrophilic granulocytes. Their numbers can, however, increase dramatically in allergic responses and infection by parasites such as helminths. In exceptional cases of 'eosinophilia', the eosinophil can become the predominant blood leukocyte. That eosinophils are induced by parasitic infections strongly suggests that they are involved in ridding the organism of such infections. Indeed, it has been clearly shown that in the presence of antibody eosinophils *in vitro* kill parasites such the schistosomula stage of *Schistosoma mansoni*. It has also been argued that, since the eosinophil is an antibody-dependent cytotoxic cell, it may be important for host resistance in other situations of microbial infection. On the other hand, the production by activated eosinophils of inflammatory substances may be responsible for tissue damage in allergic hypersensitivity diseases such as asthma.

Eosinophils develop from multipotential stem cells committed to the myeloid cell lineage. In normal haemopoiesis, the number of eosinophils is very low and it has been shown that *in vitro* in the presence of IL-3 or GM-CSF that the number of eosinophil colonies growing out from CFU-GEMM is correspondingly small. This suggested that an additional factor(s) might be required to control eosinophil production. This has been largely confirmed, firstly by the finding that eosinophilia in rats was dependent on the presence of T-cells, and secondly by the purification of a factor from T-cell-conditioned medium which caused the proliferation and differentiation of eosinophils. However, the factor in question has a complex biology and had previously been described as a T-cell replacing factor (TRF) required for the activation of immunoglobulin-secreting B-lymphocytes (see Chapter 4). It is now known, following its molecular cloning, that the factors variously called TRF, B-cell growth factor II (BCGF-II), and eosinophil differentiating factor (EDF) are one and the same glycoprotein molecule; this has finally been designated interleukin-5 (IL-5). The cloning of mouse and human IL-5s (see below) has led to the demonstration that although they both have EDF activity *in vitro*, only recombinant mouse IL-5 appears to have the activities on B-cells formerly ascribed to TRF and BCGF-II. The reasons for this species difference in IL-5 activity are, at present, unknown, but suggests that different species may 'use' IL-5 (and perhaps other cytokines) in somewhat different ways. This emphasizes the word of caution on p. 69 that the biology of a particular cytokine in one species may not always reflect, or be relevant to, the biology of its counterpart in another species.

IL-5 is a T-lymphocyte product and was first isolated and purified from the medium conditioned by human or mouse T-cell clones. Purification yielded a heterogeneous glycoprotein in the molecular weight range 32 000–62 000, with a major species at MW~46 000. Molecular cloning of IL-5 followed the expression approach using cDNAs derived from activated T-cell clones. Mouse IL-5 cDNA was first isolated and then used to screen activated human

T-cell clone cDNA libraries to identify the corresponding human IL-5 cDNA. Fortunately, mouse and human IL-5s have turned out to be highly homologous (c. 70 per cent) at the amino acid level and so isolation of human IL-5 cDNA by this route was relatively straightforward (cf. the difficulty of this approach encountered with cytokines such as IL-3 showing low protein sequence homology, p. 71).

The mouse and human IL-5 cDNAs code for polypeptides of 133 and 134 amino acid respectively (Table 3.2). These are precursor polypeptides, and it is thought that the mature polypeptides of 113 and 114 amino acids, respectively, follow cleavage of a 20 amino acid N-terminal signal sequence, although the first N-terminal amino acid of human IL-5 remains in doubt because of a lack of sequence information on human IL-5 purified from natural sources. Both mouse and human IL-5 sequences contain two potential sites for N-linked glycosylation and two cysteines which probably form an intrachain disulphide bridge. The deduced molecular weight of these mature polypeptides is approximately 14000, but following expression in monkey COS cells, the IL-5 glycoprotein has a molecular weight of 45000–50000, suggesting that is a dimer of two heavily glycosylated subunits. The biological activity of IL-5 is relatively non-species-specific; human IL-5 is active on mouse cells, and vice versa.

The genes for human and mouse IL-5s each contain four exons and three introns, although the human gene (10 kb) is somewhat larger than the equivalent mouse gene (6 kb). The human IL-5 gene is located on the long arm of chromosome 5 together with other haemopoietic cytokine genes, e.g. IL-3, IL-4, GM-CSF (Table 3.1): the mouse IL-5 gene is on chromosome 11. Interestingly, the exon–intron organization is similar in IL-4, IL-5, and GM-CSF genes (also IL-2), but is distinct from that of IL-3, G-CSF, and M-CSF genes (Figure 3.6). Nevertheless, there are common sequence motifs in the 5' flanking regions of all of these inducible genes which are generally accepted to play a pivotal role for their regulated expression. Thus, cytokine genes are frequently co-ordinately expressed upon stimulation of T-lymphocytes with mitogen or antigen. However, the recent demonstration of functional heterogeneity of the murine T-helper lymphocyte population where one subset, T_{H1}, produces IL-2 and IFNγ but not IL-4 and IL-5 and the other, T_{H2}, produces IL-4 and IL-5 but not IL-2 and IFNγ, suggests some degree of independent regulation among cytokine genes. This qualitative difference of cytokine production between functionally distinct T_H subsets is controversial. It appears to be less marked, or not to exist at all, in humans. It should be pointed out that cytokine production following mitogenic stimulation of T-cell clones *in vitro* reflects only the capacity of such clones to produce individual cytokines, and does not necessarily correspond to either the qualitative or quantitative cytokine production by T-lymphocytes receiving physiological stimuli *in vivo*.

The plasma membrane receptors for IL-5 have not yet been well characterized. Both high- and low-affinity IL-5-binding-sites have been found in the murine chronic B-cell leukaemia, BCL_1, and chemical crosslinking experiments with ^{125}I-IL-5 have identified a 92.5 kDa IL-5–receptor complex. It is

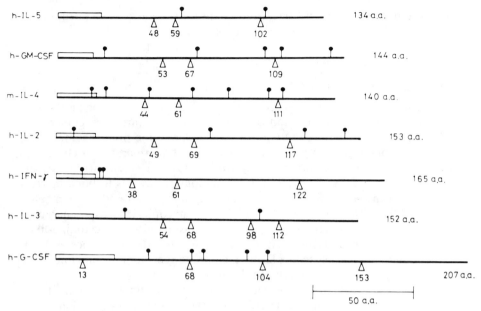

Figure 3.6 Intron–exon organization of the human IL-5 gene and comparison with the organization of human GM-CSF, murine IL-4, human IL-2, human IFNγ, human IL-3, and human G-CSF. Open boxes and thick lines represent signal sequences and mature peptides respectively. Arrowheads show the position at which an intron interrupts the gene, and the number below the arrowhead indicates the C-terminal residue number encoded by the preceding exon. Cysteine residues are shown by closed circles. (Reprinted with permission from Sideras *et al.*, 1988; copyright Munksgaard International Publishers.)

assumed that receptors are also present in eosinophils, but these have yet to be investigated and characterized (see Section 7.4, p. 225).

One of the main actions of IL-5, and probably its principal one in humans, is to stimulate the proliferation and maturation of eosinophil precursors (Figure 3.3). It does not appear to act on primitive haemopoietic stem cells, but can act on early blast cells induced by either IL-3 or GM-CSF. Neither GM-CSF nor G-CSF stimulates eosinophil colony formation to any extent, and the specific facilitation of proliferation and terminal differentiation of eosinophils has been shown to be dependent upon the presence of IL-5. Furthermore, IL-5 appears also to increase the survival of mature eosinophils in parastic infections. Recombinant human IL-5 has been shown to increase eosinophil phagocytosis of opsonized yeast particles, to enhance eosinophil killing of antibody-coated tumour cell targets, to stimulate superoxide (O_2^-) production, and to induce morphological changes. These changes were specifically induced by IL-5 in eosinophils alone, and no activity of IL-5 was found on neutrophils or macrophages. There is no evidence as yet of IL-5 acting as an autocrine stimulating factor, nor of any involvement of either IL-5 or its receptor in oncogenic mechanisms. One copy of the IL-5 gene is, however, lost in the chromosome 5_q^- syndrome, and this loss possibly contributes to myeloid cell dysfunction in these patients.

The biological activities of IL-5 relating to B-cell activation will be covered in more detail in Chapter 4.

Erythropoietin

Erythropoietin (EPO) is a glycoprotein hormone produced by the kidney that stimulates the proliferation and differentiation of erythroid precursor cells to mature erythrocytes. EPO is rather dissimilar to the other haemopoietic growth factors in that its production by kidney glomerular cells is controlled by the numbers of circulating erythrocytes and their oxygen-carrying capacity. From the kidneys, it enters the circulation and travels to bone marrow sites within the body. EPO thus acts at long range in an endocrine manner typical of 'classical' hormones. However, in terms of its molecular characteristics and biological activity, EPO may be considered to be 'cytokine-like'. For example, it is a glycoprotein of similar size to other cytokines and it is directly mitogenic via specific plasma membrane receptors for one lineage of haemopoietic cells, namely erythroid precursors.

While the activity of EPO has been known for a long time, research into the characterization of the molecule effecting erythropoiesis has been hampered by the very small amounts of EPO that could be obtained from natural sources. The steady-state production of EPO leads to circulating levels in the blood of only approximately 130 pg/ml. Sheep plasma provided one conveniently obtainable source of EPO, but the amounts of purified material that could be isolated were vanishingly small. The discovery that under conditions of anaemic or hypoxic stress large quantities of EPO were excreted into the urine, up to 10 µg/ml, led to higher yields of purified material. It became apparent that activity was contained in a glycoprotein fraction (MW 30000–40000). However, most of the details of the structure of EPO have been learnt subsequent to its molecular cloning in 1985.

The cloning strategy was based on limited amino acid sequence information, leading to synthesis of predicted oligonucleotide probes and the screening of a human genomic DNA library. In this way, EPO cDNA was isolated and sequenced, and the amino acid sequence of EPO deduced. The full-length cDNA was expressed in monkey COS cells or Chinese hamster ovary cells and the secreted glycoprotein shown to have the biological properties of EPO derived from natural sources. The mature EPO polypeptide chain contains 166 amino acids (MW 18000) and is translated from EPO mRNA as a 193 amino acid precursor including a 27 amino acid N-terminal signal sequence (Table 3.2). The polypeptide backbone of EPO contains four cysteines, at least two of which form an internal disulphide bridge, and three N-linked glycosylation sites. There is no homology of human EPO amino acid sequence with those of any other known proteins, except EPO proteins of other species (80 per cent homology with mouse EPO). The gene for human EPO is located on chromosome 7.

The EPO protein is heavily glycosylated, increasing its mass twofold or more (MW 36000). Carbohydrate analysis of human recombinant EPO produced by hamster cells has shown that there are three N-linked complex tetra-antenary oligosaccharides at amino acid positions 24, 38, and 83, and one O-linked oligosaccharide at position 126. The oligosaccharide side chains appear not be be essential for *in vitro* activity, but are required for *in vivo* activity. Their exact function remains unknown.

Recombinant human EPO is active on both human and murine erythroid precursor cells, and on certain erythroleukaemia cell lines. Binding of ^{125}I-rEPO to highly purified human and murine erythroid precursor cells of the colony-forming unit-erythroid (CFU-E) has revealed the presence of a few hundred high affinity receptors per cell. Human and murine erythro-leukaemia cells have 1600–3000 receptors per cell. In both cases, chemical cross-linking experiments with ^{125}I-rEPO have identified two putative receptor proteins of 85–95 kDa and 100–105 kDa. Further details of the structure of the EPO receptor are presented in Chapter 7, pp. 223–4.

In human bone marrow, a small proportion of erythroid progenitor and precursor cells are present, less than 1 per cent, of the total number of haemopoietic cells. EPO has no activity on pluripotential cells, but instead appears to act on commited erythroid progenitors and precursors at two distinct stages of development. Firstly, EPO stimulates an immature progeni-tor cell termed the burst-forming unit-erythroid (BFU-E) to generate large erythroid colonies which consist of clusters or 'bursts' of erythroblasts. These give rise to more mature erythroid precursor cells, CFU-E, which can be further stimulated with EPO to form small colonies of haemoglobin-synthesizing erythroblasts. The latter mature into final-stage un-nucleated erythrocytes (Figure 3.3). The oncological development of erythrocytes is strongly regulated by EPO, but may be influenced by the activities of other haemopoietic growth factors, e.g. IL-1, IL-3, with which EPO can synergize (see Section 3.4 below).

The role of EPO in the proliferation and differentiation of erythro-leukaemic cells is being intensively studied. Immature erythroid progenitor cells can be rendered leukaemic by the introduction of certain retroviral oncogenes, e.g. v-*ras*, v-*src*, v-*raf*. The action of the oncogenes is to induce erythroid cell proliferation at an early stage of differentiation. Often these leukaemic cells produce a factor (or factors) that stimulates their proliferation *in vitro* (cf. myeloid leukaemias, see pp. 74, 78). However, in the presence of EPO erythroleukaemia cells differentiate into more mature, frequently haemoglobin-producing, erythroid cells. As the erythroleukaemia cells be-come more transformed with serial passage in culture and lose their growth-factor dependence, they become progressively unresponsive to the dif-ferentiating effect of EPO while normally maintaining expression of high-affinity EPO receptors. The progression from factor-dependent erythroid progenitor proliferation to autonomous erythroleukaemia cell proliferation is widely considered to be a model system for the study of oncogenesis. Moreover, it clearly suggests that transformation to the malignant cell phe-notype is a multi-stage process.

Patients with deficiences in EPO production, such as those with chronic renal (kidney) failure, often suffer severe anaemia. Since EPO has been demonstrated both *in vitro* and *in vivo* to increase production of erythrocytes, a clear clinical application is indicated. Prior to the development of human recombinant EPO (hrEPO), it was not possible to treat kidney disease patients because there simply was insufficient EPO available from natural sources. In the late 1980s that situation has been dramatically reversed with the increasing availability of hrEPO. Clinical trials in progress in 1989 indicate that hrEPO is very effective in correcting the anaemia of advanced renal disease. Analysis of bone marrow progenitors in patients receiving hrEPO has indicated that CFU-E and BFU-E are significantly increased and that in addition there is some increase in myeloid and megakaryocytic progenitors. This suggests that hrEPO in therapeutic doses synergizes with endogenous haemopoietic growth factors in the bone marrow.

3.4   Other cytokines regulating haemopoiesis

To a large extent, although not completely, the actions of the haemopoietic growth factors, IL-3, GM-CSF, G-CSF, M-CSF, IL-5, and EPO, are restricted to haemopoietic cells (summarized in Table 3.3). This appears to be solely due to the limited distribution of specific receptors for individual haemopoietic growth factors on haemopoietic progenitor/precursor cells and their mature counterparts. From the multipotential stem cell through to mature blood cells there is, as expected, a progressive restriction with regards

Table 3.3   Sources and *in vitro* actions of haemopoietic growth factors

Factor	*Sources*	In vitro *effects*
IL-3	T-lymphocytes	Stimulates proliferation of early granulocyte, macrophage, erythrocyte and megakaryocyte progenitors. Activates monocytes and macrophages
GM-CSF	T-lymphocytes, monocytes/macrophages, fibroblasts, endothelial cells	Stimulates proliferation of granulocyte, macrophage (erythrocyte and megakaryocyte) precursors. Activates macrophages, neutrophils, and eosinophils
G-CSF	Monocytes/macrophages, fibroblasts, endothelial cells	Stimulates proliferation of granulocyte colonies. Activates mature granulocytes
M-CSF	Monocytes/macrophages, fibroblasts	Weakly stimulates growth of monocyte/macrophage colonies. Activates mature monocytes
IL-5	T-lymphocytes	Stimulates growth of eosinophil colonies. Activates mature eosinophils
EPO	Kidney	Stimulates growth of erythroid and megakaryocytic colonies

expression of receptors, and thus of cell responsiveness to haemopoietic growth factors. Early haemopoietic cells have receptors for pleiotropic IL-3 and GM-CSF molecules, whereas once these differentiate into cells of particular types they express lineage-restricted receptors for the largely monotropic G-CSF, M-CSF, IL-5, and EPO molecules. All of the haemopoietic growth factors have inducible expression and except for EPO and possibly M-CSF are not normally present in the circulation or bone marrow. Again, with the notable exception of EPO, the haemopoietic growth factors are produced mainly by activated T-lymphocytes and activated monocytes/macrophages during episodes of antigenic- and endotoxic-stimulation, respectively (Table 3.3). No mRNAs for IL-3, GM-CSF, or G-CSF have been detected in unstimulated bone marrow stromal cells, and so it remains controversial as to whether these haemopoietic growth factors produced as a result of peripheral immune responses have any bearing on normal steady-state haemopoiesis.

There are two possibilities that may account for steady-state haemopoiesis. Either there is a separate group of growth factors that mediates haemopoietic cell development, or the currently described haemopoietic growth factors are present at very low, undetectable, levels but are able to maintain haemopoietic cell proliferation/differentiation by synergizing among themselves or with the activities of other cytokines. The second alternative looks more attractive because, as yet, no other growth factors/cytokines have been described that have the capacity to cause haemopoietic progenitor/precursor cells to develop into mature blood cells, and in vitro synergistic effects between or among individual haemopoietic growth factors or other particular cytokines have been readily demonstrable. For example, EPO and IL-3 have been shown to synergize in the induction of erythroid burst colony formation (Figure 3.3). In addition, it has been shown that only low levels (5–10 per cent) of haemopoietic growth factor-receptor occupancy is necessary to trigger cell activation and most progenitor/precursor cells express relatively few (100–1000) high-affinity receptors. Thus, these cells probably respond to extremely low amounts of haemopoietic growth factors. However, the problem remains of identifying the indigenous stimuli of haemopoietic growth factor expression in the bone marrow and the cell types involved in their production.

If it is assumed that other cytokines play a role in steady-state haemopoiesis, there appears to be several 'candidates', the principal being interleukin-1 (IL-1), which on the basis of in vitro studies could be critically involved. IL-1 is a cytokine that has a broad spectrum of in vitro and in vivo biological actions. There are two distinct molecular forms of IL-1, known as IL-1α and IL-1β, which act through the same receptor. They are non-glycosylated proteins (MW 17 500). (More details of the molecular characteristics of IL-1 will be found in Chapter 4.) They are produced by monocytes/macrophages, endothelial cells, and fibroblasts, and thus are quite ubiquitous. Originally, it was found that a factor present in conditioned medium from certain tissues or a human bladder carcinoma cell line (5637), facilitated the development of haemopoietic multipotential stem cells to the stage at which they could respond to particular haemopoietic growth factors. This factor was first called haemopoietin-1 (H-1), but it was subsequently discovered with the availability of human recombinant IL-1 (rIL-1) that the activity of II-1 is also present in purified rIL-1α. H-1 and rIL-1α are not mitogenic by themselves and in the presence of H-1 alone stem cells eventually die out. However, if other specific haemopoietic growth factors, e.g. IL-3, GM-CSF, M-CSF are added then the proliferation of multipotential stem cells and formation of myeloid colonies is stimulated at much lower concentrations of these factors than if each was used alone. For example, H-1 plus IL-3 increased the number of colonies formed by primitive multipotential cells by 30-fold *in vitro*, whereas H-1 plus EPO had no effect. Further, H-1 has also been shown to act synergistically with M-CSF in the generation of monocyte precursor cells. These observations indicate that H-1 permits IL-3 or M-CSF to act on cells more primitive than those acted on by either growth factor alone. It has been speculated that H-1 induces 'commitment' of primitive haemopoietic cells to respond to secondary stimulation by particular colony stimulating factors. This commitment would involved transcriptional activation of nuclear genes, probably including expression of receptor genes. Thus, H-1 (IL-1α) may be considered to be acting as a 'competence' factor (see Chapter 2) in haemopoietic cell development, with the secondarily acting colony stimulating factors as 'progression' factors.

In the *in vitro* long-term model system of bone marrow haemopoiesis, it is known that direct contact of haemopoietic cells with stromal cells, which comprise a heterogeneous collection of cell types, is required for haemopoietic cell proliferation and differentiation. IL-1 is probably a poorly secreted cytokine and there is some evidence that it, and particularly the IL-1α form, may exist as an integral plasma membrane protein. Therefore, cells which produce IL-1 probably contain IL-1 molecules facing out from the cell surface which on contact with IL-1 receptors on other cells induce commitment to respond to subsequent signals. Thus, it may be reasonably conjectured that stromal cells expressing cell surface-IL-1 could by cell contact alone induce the commitment of haemopoietic cells. Moreover, IL-1 has been demonstrated to induce synthesis of colony stimulating factors, e.g. GM-CSF and M-CSF, and other strongly mitogenic growth factors such as PDGF. In this respect, it is also widely believed that several cytokines besides IL-1, e.g. M-CSF, TNFα, EGF, etc., exist as transmembrane proteins before being released from cytokine-producing cells by proteolytic cleavage, and could thus trigger other cells from the cell surface. Therefore, normal steady-state haemopoiesis could possibly be regulated by cell-to-cell contacts of inducer (stromal) cells expressing plasma membrane forms of cytokines and responder (haemopoietic) cells expressing the appropriate receptors (Figure 3.7). Low-level constitutive production of appropriate plasma-membrane-bound cytokines may be all that is required for normal steady-state haemopoietic cell development. Amplification of this haemopoietic process could, however, readily occur when CSFs released into the circulation by activated macrophages and T-lymphocytes reached the bone marrow (see Figure 3.7).

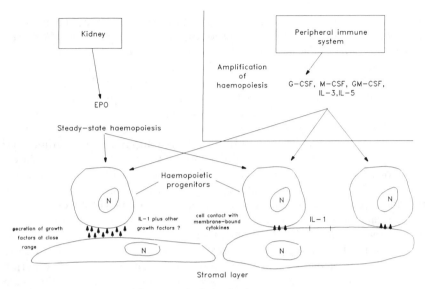

Figure 3.7   Regulation of haemopoiesis in the bone marrow.

The speculative model of the haemopoietic system proposed above may have attractive features, but regrettably several of these are extremely difficult to test experimentally even *in vitro*. However, there is preliminary evidence that the synergistic effects among the haemopoietic growth factors and other cytokines observed *in vitro* may also occur *in vivo*. For instance, intravenous injection of IL-1 into rats produced neutrophilia in much the same way as GM-CSF or G-CSF. This observation may, however, have as much to do with IL-1-induced colony stimulating factor-production as any direct effect of IL-1 on haemopoietic cells, although as previously discussed IL-1 potentiates the growth stimulatory effects of GM-CSF and M-CSF *in vitro*. Combinations of haemopoietic growth factors have been demonstrated to have synergistic actions *in vivo*. For example, injection of low-dose combinations of murine IL-3, GM-CSF, and M-CSF into mice produced synergistic myelopoietic actions.

In addition to IL-1, several other cytokines either individually or in combination with particular haemopoietic growth factors have been demonstrated to affect the proliferation and differentiation of haemopoietic cells and their leukaemic cell counterparts *in vitro*. Such cytokines may stimulate or inhibit proliferation or induce differentiation depending on cell phenotype and stage of development. Growth factors such as TGFβ whose expression has been located in sites of haemopoietic cell development *in vivo*, e.g. fetal liver, spleen, bone marrow, are almost certainly involved in the regulation of haemopoiesis (see p. 55). TNFα appears to increase early haemopoietic cell proliferation while inhibiting that of later-stage myeloid precursors. In particular, there are a growing number of cytokines, including TNFα, IFNs, and ILs, which have been shown to affect the growth and differentiation of myeloid cells. It is not possible to describe all of these in the space available and instead attention will be focused on just two cytokines: IL-6 and leukaemia inhibitory factor (LIF). The actions of TNF and IFNs on myeloid cell growth and differentiation will be described in subsequent chapters.

IL-6, like IL-1, is a broad-acting cytokine with multiple biological activities. It is an inducible glycoprotein (MW~22 000), produced by monocytes, lymphocytes, and fibroblasts. (The molecular characterization of IL-6 will be given in Chapter 4.) Although IL-6 is molecularly very different to IL-1, it has been shown to act very similarly to IL-1 in the potentiation of IL-3-stimulated multipotential haemopoietic cell proliferation *in vitro*. It has also been shown to enhance GM-CSF- or IL-3-stimulated proliferation of factor-dependent blast cells of AML. Most interestingly, IL-6 has been demonstrated to be an autocrine growth factor for human multiple myeloma (MM) cells: these constitutively produce IL-6 and express the IL-6 receptor. In this regard, neutralizing antibody to IL-6 has been shown to inhibit the growth of MM cells indicating that unregulated expression of IL-6 and/or its receptors are involved in the oncogenesis of MM, thus lending support to the 'autocrine hypothesis'. However, myeloma cells whilst being produced in the bone marrow are antibody-producing tumour cells derived from B-lymphocyte precursors, i.e. are non-myeloid, and the autocrine stimulatory effect of IL-6 relates to its known B-cell stimulating action (IL-6 is alternatively known as B-cell stimulatory factor-2 (BSF-2)).

In marked contrast to the growth stimulating effect of IL-6 in MM cells, IL-6 appears to act as a differentiation-inducing factor for certain myeloid leukaemia cells. For example, IL-6 has been shown to cause the differentiation of murine myeloleukaemic M1 cells and human 'monocyte-like' histiocytic lymphoma U937 cells. In other words, such IL-6-treated cells become less responsive to proliferation signals and adopt the morphology and other characteristics of mature macrophages. These observations are, however, less remarkable given that G-CSF and GM-CSF are able to induce the differentiation of myelomonocytic WEHI-3B (D^+) leukaemic cells (p. 80), G-CSF, the differentiation of M1 cells (see above) and TNFα, the differentiation of both HL-60 (promyelocytic) and ML-1 leukaemic cells. In fact, the differentiation of M1 cells has been used to isolate a further novel cytokine, LIF.

Both murine and human LIF have been molecularly cloned and their respective cDNAs encode mature polypeptides of 179 amino acids (MW ~20 000) which show 78 per cent overall sequence homology. The LIF gene has two exons and one intron. In the LIF polypeptide chain there are seven potential N-linked and four potential O-linked-glycosylation sites. Purified recombinant LIF derived from medium conditioned by monkey COS cells transfected with LIF cDNA has a molecular weight of 43 000, indicating heavy glycosylation. Subsequent to the initial cloning of LIF, it has been shown that the polypeptide factors previously known as differentiation inhibitory activity (DIA) which suppresses the differentiation of murine embryonic stem (ES) cells *in vitro* and human interleukin for DA cells (HILDA) which supports the proliferation of murine IL-3-dependent leukaemic cell line,

DA-la, are identical to LIF. Therefore, LIF is not only an inducer of myeloid cell differentiation but, like other cytokines, such as IL-6 and TNFα, has growth-promoting and differentiating actions in other cell types. For example, LIF stimulates the proliferation of murine ES cells, thus maintaining their multipotency, by inhibiting their differentiation in culture. This suggests, together with other similar observations mentioned elsewhere in this chapter, that the mechanisms controlling proliferation and differentiation are interrelated and that individual cytokines exert profoundly different effects on these two processes depending upon the phenotype of target cells. In other words, it is very difficult to generalize about the biological effects of different individual cytokines and to place them with any certainty into playing specific regulatory roles in physiological processes such as haemopoiesis. For the haemopoietic growth factors as a group it is possible to have some confidence in presuming their involvement in haemopoiesis, but the role (or roles) of cytokines such as IL-6 and LIF are uncertain and controversial.

Further reading

General

Clark, S.C. and Kamen, R. (1987) The human hematopoietic colony-stimulating factors. *Science* **236**, 1229.

Devereux, S. and Linch, D.C. (1989). Clinical significance of the haemopoietic growth factors. *British Journal of Cancer* **59**, 2.

Dexter, T.M. and Spooner, E. (1987) Growth and differentiation in the hemopoietic system. *Annual Review of Cell Biology* **3**, 423.

Dexter, T.M., Whetton, A.D., Spooncer, E., et al. (1985) The role of stromal cells and growth factors in haemopoiesis and modulation of their effects by the src oncogene. *Journal of Cell Science, Supplement* **3**, 83.

Garland, J.M. (1987) Cell stimulation by haemopoietic lymphokines. *Immunology Letters* **16**, 233.

Kanz, L., Löhr, G.W. and Fauser, A.A. (1986) Lymphokine(s) from isolated T lymphocyte subpopulations support multilineage hematopoietic colony and megakaryocytic colony formation. *Blood* **68**, 991.

Metcalf, D. (1984) *The Hemopoietic Colony Stimulating Factors*. Elsevier, Amsterdam.

Metcalf, D. (1985) The granulocyte-macrophage colony-stimulating factors. *Science* **229**, 16.

Metcalf, D. (1986) The molecular biology and functions of the granulocyte-macrophage colony-stimulating factors. *Blood* **67**, 257.

Morstyn, G. and Burgess, A.W. (1988) Haemopoietic growth factors: a review. *Cancer Research* **48**, 5624.

Platzer, E. (1989) Human haemopoietic growth factors. *European Journal of Haematology* **42**, 1.

Sachs, L. (1987) The molecular control of blood cell development. *Science* **238**, 1374.

Schrader, J.W., Ziltener, H.J. and Leslie, K.B. (1986) Structural homologies among the hemopoietins. *Proceedings of the National Academy of Sciences USA* **83**, 2458.

Interleukin-3

Chen, B., D-M., Mueller, M., and Olenki, T. (1988) Interleukin-3 (IL-3) stimulates the cloned growth of pulmonary alveolar macrophage of the mouse: role of IL-3 in the regulation of macrophage production outside the bone marrow. *Blood* **72**, 685.

Clark-Lewis, I., Aebersold, R., Ziltener, H., *et al.* (1986) Automated chemical synthesis of a protein growth factor for hemopoietic cells, interleukin-3. *Science* **231**, 134.

Emerson, S.G., Yang, Y-C., Clark, S.C., and Long, M.W. (1988) Human recombinant granulocyte-macrophage colony stimulating factor and interleukin 3 have overlapping but distinct hematopoietic activities. *Journal of Clinical Investigation* **82**, 1282.

Isfort, R.J., Stevens, D., May, W.S. and Ihle, J.N. (1988) Interleukin 3 binds to a 140-kDa phosphotyrosine-containing cell surface protein. *Proceedings of the National Academy of Sciences USA* **85**, 7982.

Lang, R.A., Metcalf, D., Gough, N.M., *et al.* (1985) Expression of a hemopoietic growth factor cDNA in a factor-dependent cell line results in autonomous growth and tumorigenicity. *Cell* **43**, 531.

Lopez, A.F., Dyson, P.G., To, L.B., *et al.* (1988) Recombinant human interleukin-3 stimulation of hematopoiesis in humans: loss of responsiveness with differentiation in the neutrophilic myeloid series. *Blood* **72**, 1797.

Migliaccio, A.R., Migliaccio, G., and Adamson, J.W., (1988) Effect of recombinant hematopoietic growth factors on proliferation of human marrow progenitor cells in serum-deprived liquid culture. *Blood* **72**, 1387.

Miyatake, S., Yokota, T., Lee, F., and Arai, K-I. (1985) Structure of the chromosomal gene for murine interleukin 3. *Proceedings of the National Academy of Sciences USA* **82**, 316.

Schrader, J.W. (ed.) (1988) *Interleukin 3: The Panspecific Hemopoietin. Lymphokines* **15**, Academic Press, New York.

Whetton, A.D., Vallance, S.J., Monk, P.N., *et al.* (1988) Interleukin-3 stimulated haemopoietic stem cell proliferation. *Biochemical Journal* **256**, 585.

Yang, Y-C., Ciarletta, A.B., Temple, P.A., *et al.* (1986) Human IL-3 (multi-CSF): identification by expression of a novel hematopoietic growth factor related to murine IL-3. *Cell* **47**, 3.

Yang, Y-C., Kovacic, S., Kriz, R., *et al.* (1988) The human genes for GM-CSF and IL-3 are closely linked in tandem on chromosome 5. *Blood* **71**, 958.

Ziltener, H.J., Fazekas de St Groth, B., Leslie, K.B., and Schrader, J.W. (1988) Multiple glycosylated forms of T-cell-derived interleukin-3 (IL-3). *Journal of Biological Chemistry* **263**, 14511.

Granulocyte-macrophage colony stimulating factor

Cantrell, M.A., Anderson, D., Cerretti, D.P., *et al.* (1985) Cloning, sequence and expression of a human granulocyte/macrophage colony-stimulating factor. *Proceedings of the National Academy of Sciences USA* **82**, 6250.

Chung, S.W., Wong, P.M.C., Shen-Ong, G., *et al.* (1986) Production of granulocyte-macrophage colony-stimulating factor by Abelson virus-induced tumorigenic mast cell lines. *Blood* **68**, 1074.

Fibbe, W.E., Van Damme, J., Billiau, A., *et al.* (1988) Human fibroblasts produce granulocyte-CSF, macrophage-CSF and granulocyte-macrophage-CSF following stimulation by interleukin-1 and poly(rI), poly(rC). *Blood* **72**, 860.

Fleischmann, J., Golde, D.W., Weisbart, R.H., and Gasson, J.C. (1986) Granulocyte-macrophage colony-stimulating factor enhances phagocytosis of bacteria by human neutrophils. *Blood* **68**, 708.

Grabstein, K.H., Urdal, D.L., Tushinski, R.J., *et al.* (1986) Induction of macrophage tumoricidal activity by granulocyte-macrophage colony-stimulating factor. *Science* **232**, 506.

Kelso, A. and Owens, T. (1988) Production of two hemopoietic growth factors is differentially regulated in single T lymphocytes activated with an anti-T cell receptor antibody. *Journal of Immunology* **140**, 1159.

Lang, R.A., Metcalf, D., Cuthbertson, R.A., *et al.* (1987) Transgenic mice expressing a hemopoietic growth factor gene (GM-CSF) develop accumulations of macrophages, blindness and a fatal syndrome of tissue damage. *Cell* **51**, 675.

Le Beau, M.M., Westbrook, C.A., Diaz, M.O., *et al.* (1986) Evidence for the involvement of GM-CSF and FMS in the deletion (5q) in myeloid disorders. *Science* **231**, 984.

Lee, F., Yokota, T., Otsuka, T., *et al.* (1985) Isolation of cDNA for a human granulocyte-macrophage colony-stimulating factor by functional expression in mammalian cells. *Proceedings of the National Academy of Sciences USA* **82**, 4360.

Lopez, A.F., Williamson, D.J., Gamble, J.R., *et al.* (1986) Recombinant human granulocyte-macrophage colony-stimulating factor stimulates *in vitro* mature human neutrophil and eosinophil function, surface receptor expression, and survival. *Journal of Clinical Investigation* **78**, 1220.

Metcalf, D. and Moore, J.G. (1988) Divergent disease patterns in granulocyte-macrophage colony-stimulating factor transgenic mice associated with different transgene insertion sites. *Proceedings of the National Academy of Sciences USA* **85**, 7767.

Metcalf, D., Burgess, A.W., Johnson, G.R., *et al.* (1986) *In vitro* actions of hemopoietic cells of recombinant murine GM-CSF purified after production in *Escherichia coli:* comparison with purified native GM-CSF. *Journal of Cellular Physiology* **128**, 421.

Park, L.S., Friend, D., Gillis, S., and Urdal, D.L. (1986) Characterization of the cell surface receptor for human granulocyte/macrophage colony stimulating factor. *Journal of Experimental Medicine* **164**, 251.

Reed, S.G., Nathan, C.F., Pihl, D.L., *et al.* (1987) Recombinant granulocyte/macrophage colony-stimulating factor activates macrophages to inhibit *Trypanosoma cruzi* and release hydrogen peroxide. *Journal of Experimental Medicine* **166**, 1734.

Ruff, M.R., Farrar, W.L., and Pert, C.B. (1986) Interferon gamma and granulocyte/macrophage colony-stimulating factor inhibit growth and induce antigens characteristic of myeloid differentiation in small-cell lung cancer cell lines. *Proceedings of the National Academy of Sciences USA* **83**, 6613.

Sisson, S.D. and Dinarello, C.A. (1988) Production of interleukin-1α and interleukin-1β and tumour necrosis factor by human mononuclear cells stimulated with granulocyte-macrophage colony-stimulating factor. *Blood* **72**, 1368.

Steward, W.P., Scarffe, J.H., Austin, R., *et al.* (1989) Recombinant human granulocyte macrophage colony stimulating factor (rhGM-CSF) given as daily short infusions — a phase I dose-toxicity study. *British Journal of Cancer* **59**, 142.

Williams, D.E., Bicknell, D.C., Park, L.S., *et al.* (1988) Purified murine granulocyte/macrophage progenitor cells express a high-affinity receptor for recombinant murine granulocyte/macrophage colony-stimulating factor. *Proceedings of the National Academy of Sciences USA* **85**, 487.

Young, D.C., Wagner, K., and Griffin, J.D. (1987) Constitutive expression of the granulocyte-macrophage colony-stimulating factor gene in acute myeloblastic leukaemia. *Journal of Clinical Investigation* **79**, 100.

Granulocyte-colony stimulating factor

Begley, C.G., Metcalf, D., and Nicola, N.A. (1987) Purified colony stimulating factors (G-CSF and GM-CSF) induce differentiation in human HL60 leukemic cells with suppression of clonogenicity. *International Journal of Cancer* **39**, 99.

Dührsen, U., Villeval, J-L., Boyd, J., *et al.* (1988) Effects of recombinant human granulocyte colony-stimulating factor on hematopoietic progenitor cells in cancer patients. *Blood* **72**, 2074.

Kitagawa, S., Yuo, A., Souza, L.M., *et al.* (1987) Recombinant human granulocyte colony-stimulating factor enhances superoxide release in human granulocytes stimulated by the chemotactic peptide. *Biochemical and Biophysical Research Communications* **144**, 1143.

Kojima, S., Tadenuma, H., Inada, Y., and Saito, Y. (1989) Enhancement of plasminogen activator activity in cultured endothelial cells by granulocyte colony-stimulating factor. *Journal of Cellular Physiology* **138**, 192.

Morstyn, G., Souza, L.M., Keech, J. *et al.* (1988) Effect of granulocyte colony stimulating factor on neutropenia induced by cytotoxic chemotherapy. *The Lancet*, **i**, 667.

Nagata, S., Tsuchiya, M., Asano, S., *et al.* (1986) The chromosomal gene structure and two mRNAs for human granulocyte colony-stimulating factor. *The EMBO Journal* **5**, 575.

Nicola, N.A. and Peterson, L. (1986) Identification of distinct receptors for two hemopoietic growth factors (granulocyte colony-stimulating factor and multipotential colony-stimulating factor) by chemical cross-linking. *Journal of Biological Chemistry* **261**, 12384.

Nomura, H., Imazeki, I., Oheda, M., *et al.* (1986) Purification and characterization of human granulocyte colony-stimulating factor (G-CSF). *The EMBO Journal* **5**, 871.

Souza, L.M., Boone, T.C., Gabrilove, J., *et al.* (1986) Recombinant human granulocyte colony-stimulating factor: effects on normal and leukemic myeloid cells. *Science* **232**, 61.

Tsuchiya, M., Kaziro, Y., and Nagata, S. (1987) The chromosomal gene structure for murine granulocyte colony-stimulating factor. *European Journal of Biochemistry* **165**, 7.

Tsuchiya, M., Asano, S., Kaziro, Y., and Nagata, S. (1986) Isolation and characterization of the cDNA for murine granulocyte colony-stimulating factor. *Proceedings of the National Academy of Sciences USA* **83**, 7633.

Uzumaki, H., Okabe, T., Sasaki, N., *et al.* (1988) Characterization of receptor for granulocyte colony-stimulating factor on human circulating neutrophils. *Biochemical and Biophysical Research Communications* **156**, 1026.

Wang, J.M., Chen, Z.G., Colella, S., *et al.* (1988) Chemotactic activity of recombinant human granulocyte colony-stimulating factor. *Blood* **72**, 1456.

Watson, J.D., Crosier, P.S., March, C.J., *et al.* (1986) Purification to homogeneity of a human hematopoietic growth factor that stimulates the growth of a murine interleukin-3-dependent cell line. *Journal of Immunology* **137**, 854.

Macrophage-colony stimulating factor

Ampel, N.M., Wing, E.J., Waheed, A., and Shadduck, R.K. (1988) Stimulatory effects of purified macrophage colony-stimulating factor on murine resident peritoneal macrophages. *Cellular Immunology* **97**, 344.

Csejtey, J. and Boosman, A. (1986) Purification of human macrophage colony stimulating factor (CSF-1) from medium conditioned by pancreatic carcinoma cells. *Biochemical and Biophysical Research Communications* **138**, 238.

Dubreuil, P., Torrès, H., Courcoul, M-A., *et al.* (1988) c-*fms* expression is a molecular marker of human acute myeloid leukaemias. *Blood* **72**, 1081.

Guilbert, L.J. and Stanley, R.E. (1986) The interaction of ^{125}I-colony-stimulating factor-1 with bone marrow-derived macrophages. *Journal of Biological Chemistry* **261**, 4024.

Horiguchi, J., Sherman, M.L., Sampson-Johannes, A., *et al.* (1988) CSF-1 and c-*fms* gene expression in human carcinoma cell lines. *Biochemical and Biophysical Research Communications* **157**, 395.

Imamura, K. and Kufe, D. (1988) Colony-stimulating factor 1 induced Na^+ influx into human monocytes involves activation of a pertussis toxin-sensitive GTP-binding protein. *Journal of Biological Chemistry* **263**, 14093.

Kawasaki, E.S., Ladner, M.B., Wang, A.M., *et al.* (1985) Molecular cloning of a complementary DNA encoding human macrophage-specific colony-stimulating factor (CSF-1). *Science* **230**, 291.

Ladner, M.B., Martin, G.A., Noble, J.A., *et al.* (1988) cDNA cloning and expression of murine macrophage colony-stimulating factor from L929 cells. *Proceedings of the National Academy of Sciences USA* **85**, 6706.

Nakoinz, I. and Ralph, P. (1988) Stimulation of macrophage antibody-dependent killing of tumor targets by recombinant lymphokine factors and M-CSF. *Cellular Immunology* **116**, 331.

Ralph, P. and Nakoinz, I. (1987) Stimulation of macrophage tumoricidal activity by the growth and differentiation factor CSF-1. *Cellular Immunology* **105**, 270.

Rettenmier, C.W., Roussel, M.F., and Sherr, C.J. (1988) The colony-stimulating factor 1 (CSF-1) receptor (c-*fms* proto-oncogene product) and its ligand. *Journal of Cell Science Supplement* **9**, 27.

Roussel, M.F., Downing J.R., Rettenmier, C.W., and Sherr, C.J. (1988) A point mutation in the extracellular domain of the human CSF-1 receptor (c-*fms* proto-oncogene product) activates its transforming potential. *Cell* **55**, 979.

Sacca, R., Stanley, E.R., Sherr, C.J., and Rettenmier, C.W. (1986) Specific binding of the mononuclear phagocyte colony-stimulating factor CSF-1 to the product of the v-*fms* oncogene. *Proceedings of the National Academy of Sciences USA* **83**, 3331.

Sengupta, A., Liu, W-K., Yeung, Y.G., *et al.* (1988) Identification and subcellular localization of proteins that are rapidly phosphorylated in tyrosine in response to colony-stimulating factor 1. *Proceedings of the National Academy of Sciences* **85**, 8062.

Woolford, J., McAuliffe, A., and Rohrschneider, L.R. (1988) Activation of the feline c-*fms* proto-oncogene: multiple alterations are required to generate a fully transformed phenotype. *Cell* **55**, 965.

Interleukin-5

Butterworth, A.E., Sturrock, R.I., Houba, V., *et al.* (1975) Eosinophils as mediators of antibody dependent damage to schistosomula. *Nature* **256**, 727.

Campbell, H.D., Tucker, W.Q.J., Hort, Y., *et al.* (1987) Molecular cloning, nucleotide sequence and expression of the gene encoding human eosinophil differentiation factor (interleukin 5). *Proceedings of the National Academy of Sciences USA* **84**, 6629.

Cherwinski, H.M., Schumacher, J.H., Brown, K.D., and Mosmann, T.R. (1987) Two types of mouse helper T cell clone. III. Further differences in lymphokine synthesis between T_h1 and T_h2 clones revealed by RNA hybridization, functionally monospecific bioassays, and monoclonal antibodies. *Journal of Experimental Medicine* **166**, 1229.

Clutterbuck, E., Shields, J.G., Gordon, J., *et al.* (1987) Recombinant human interleukin 5 is an eosinophil differentiation factor but has no activity in standard human B cell growth factor assays. *European Journal of Immunology* **17**, 1743.

Gleich, G.J. and Adolphson, C.R. (1986) The eosinophilic leukocyte: structure and function. *Advances in Immunology* **39**, 177.

Kinashi, T., Harada, N., Severinson, E., *et al.* (1986) Cloning of a complementary DNA encoding T-cell replacing factor and identity with B-cell growth factor II. *Nature* **324**, 70.

Lopez, A.F., Sanderson, C.J., Gamble, J.R., *et al.* (1987) Recombinant human interleukin-5 (IL-5) is a selective activator of human eosinophil function. *Journal of Experimental Medicine* **167**, 219.

Sanderson, C.J., Campbell, H.D., and Young, I.G. (1988) Molecular and cellular biology of eosinophil differentiation factor (IL-5) and its effects on human and mouse B cells. *Immunological Reviews* **102** (Möller, G., ed.) p. 29.

Sideras, P., Noma, T. and Honjo, T.,(1988) Structure and function of interleukins 4 and 5'. *Immunological Reviews*, **102** (Möller, G. ed.), p. 189.

Strath, M. and Sanderson, C.J. (1985) The production and functional properties of eosinophils from bone marrow cultures. *Journal of Cell Science* **74**, 207.

Takatsu, K., Tominaga, A., Harada, N., *et al.* (1988) T-cell-replacing factor (TRF)/interleukin 5 (IL-5): molecular and functional properties. *Immunological Reviews*, **102** (Möller, G. ed.), p. 107.

Yokota, T., Aai, N., De Vries, J., *et al.* (1988) Molecular biology of interleukin-4 and interleukin-5 genes and biology of their products that stimulate B cells, T cells and hemopoietic cells. *Immunological Reviews*, **102**, (Möller, G. ed.) p. 137.

Erythropoietin

Broudy, V.C., Lin, N., Egrie, J., *et al.* (1988) Identification of the receptor for erythropoietin on human and murine erythroleukaemia cells and modulation by phorbolester and dimethyl sulfoxide. *Proceedings of the National Academy of Sciences USA* **85**, 6513.

Dessypris, E.N., Graber, S.E., Krantz, S.B., and Stone, W.J. (1988) Effects of recombinant erythropoietin on the concentration and cycling status of human marrow hematopoietic progenitor cells *in vivo*. *Blood* **72**, 2060.

Dubé, S., Fisher, J.W., and Powell, J.S. (1988) Glycosylation at specific sites of erythropoietin is essential for biosynthesis, secretion and biological function. *Journal of Biological Chemistry* **263**, 17516.

Graber, S.E. and Krantz, S.B. (1978) Erythropoietin and the control of red cell production. *Annual Review of Medicine* **29**, 51.

Jacobs, K., Shoemaker, C., Rudersdorf, R., *et al.* (1985) Isolation and characterization of genomic and cDNA clones of human erythropoietin. *Nature* **313**, 806.

Klinken, S.P., Nicola, N.A., and Johnson, G.R. (1988) *In vitro*-derived leukaemia erythroid cell lines induced by a *raf*- and *myc*-containing retrovirus differentiate in response to erythropoietin. *Proceedings of the National Academy of Sciences USA* **85**, 8506.

Krantz, S.B., Sawyer, S.T., and Sawada, K-I. (1988) Purification of erythroid progenitor cells and characterization of erythropoietin receptors. *British Journal of Cancer* **58** Supplement IX, 31.

Lin, F-K., Suggs, S., Lin, C-H., *et al.* (1985) Cloning and expression of the human erythropoietin gene. *Proceedings of the National Academy of Sciences USA* **82**, 7580.

Powell, J.S., Berkner, K.L., Lebo, R.V., and Adamson, J.W. (1986) Human erythropoietin gene: high level expression in stably transfected mammalian cells and chromosome location. *Proceedings of the National Academy of Sciences USA* **83**, 6465.

Sasaki, H., Ochi, N., Dell, A., and Fukuda, M. (1988) Site-specific glycosylation of human recombinant erythropoietin: analysis of glycopeptides or peptides at each glycosylation site by fast atom bombardment mass spectrometry. *Biochemistry* **27**, 8618.

Sherwood, J.B. (1984) The chemistry and physiology of erythropoietin, in *Vitamins and Hormones* **41** (McCormick, D.B. ed.) Academic Press, New York, p. 161.

Weiss, T.L., Barker, M.E., Selleck, S.E., and Wintroub, B.U. (1989) Erythropoietin binding and induced differentiation of Rauscher erythroleukaemia cell line Red 5-1.5. *Journal of Biological Chemistry* **264**, 1804.

Other cytokines regulating haemopoiesis

Asaoku, H., Kaurano, M., Iurato, K., *et al.* (1988) Decrease in BSF-2/IL-6 response in advanced cases of multiple myeloma. *Blood* **72**, 429.

Broxmeyer, H.E., Williams, D.E., Hangoc, G., *et al.* (1987) Synergistic myelopoietic actions *in vivo* after administration to mice of combinations of purified natural murine colony-stimulating factor 1, recombinant murine interleukin-3 and recombinant murine granulocyte/macrophage colony-stimulating factor. *Proceedings of the National Academy of Sciences USA* **84**, 3871.

Chen, L., Novick, D., Rubinstein, M., and Revel, M. (1988) Recombinant interferon-beta 2 (interleukin 6) induces myeloid differentiation. *FEBS Letters* **239**, 299.

Fibbe, W.E., Goselink, J.M., Van Eden, G., *et al.* (1988) Proliferation of myeloid progenitor cells in human long-term bone marrow cultures is stimulated by interleukin-1 beta. *Blood* **72**, 1242.

Gearing, D.P., Gough, N.M., King, J.A. *et al.* (1987) Molecular cloning and expression of cNDA encoding a murine myeloid leukaemia inhibitory factor (LIF). *The EMBO Journal* **6**, 3995.

Gough, N.M., Gearing, D.P., King, J.A., *et al.* (1988) Molecular cloning and expression of the human homologue of the murine gene encoding myeloid leukaemia-inhibitory factor. *Proceedings of the National Academy of Sciences USA* **85**, 2623.

Hoang, T., Haman, A., Goncalves, O., *et al.* (1988) Interleukin-1 enhances growth factor-dependent proliferation of the clonogenic cells in acute myeloblastic leukaemia and of normal human primitive hemopoietic precursors. *Journal of Experimental Medicine* **168**, 463.

Hoang, T., Haman, A., Goncalves, O., *et al.* (1988) Interleukin-6 enhances growth factor-dependent proliferation of the blast cells of acute myeloblastic leukaemia. *Blood* **72**, 823.

Johnson, C.S., Chang, M-J., and Furmanski, P. (1988) *In vivo* hematopoietic effects of tumour necrosis factor-α in normal and erythroleukemic mice: characterization and therapeutic applications. *Blood* **72**, 1875.

Koike, K., Nakahata, T., Takagi, M., *et al.* (1988) Synergism of BSF-2/interleukin 6 and interleukin 3 on development of multi-potential hemopoietic progenitors in serum-free culture. *Journal of Experimental Medicine* **168**, 879.

Lotem, J. and Sachs, L. (1988) *In vivo* control of differentiation of myeloid leukaemic cells by cyclosporine A and recombinant interleukin-1. *Blood* **72**, 1595.

Migliaccio, G., Migliaccio, A.R. and Visser, J.W.M. (1988) Synergism between erythropoietin and interleukin-3 in the induction of hematopoietic stem cell proliferation and erythroid burst colony formation. *Blood* **72**, 944.

Moreau, J-F., Donaldson, D.D., Bennett, F., *et al.* (1988) Leukaemia inhibitory factor is identical to the myeloid growth factor human interleukin for DA cells. *Nature* **336**, 690.

Segal, G.M., McCall, E. and Bagby, Jr. G.C. (1988) Erythroid burst-promoting activity produced by interleukin-1 stimulated endothelial cells is granulocyte-macrophage colony-stimulating factor. *Blood* **72**, 1364.

Shabo, Y., Lotem, J., Rubinstein, M., *et al.* (1988) The myeloid blood cell differentiation-inducing protein MGI-2A is interleukin-6. *Blood* **72**, 2070.

Smith, A.G., Heath, J.K., Donaldson, D.D., *et al.* (1988) Inhibition of pluripotential embryonic stem cell differentiation by purified polypeptides. *Nature* **336**, 688.

Stanley, E.R., Bartocci, A., Patinkin, D., *et al.* (1986) Regulation of very primitive, multipotent, hemopoietic cells by hemopoietin-1. *Cell* **45**, 667.

Troutt, A.B. and Lee, F. (1989) Tissue distribution of murine hemopoietic growth factor mRNA production. *Journal of Cellular Physiology* **138**, 38.

Ulich, T.R., Del Castillo, J., Guo, K., and Souza, L. (1989) The hematologic effects of chronic administration of the monokines tumor necrosis factor, interleukin-1 and granulocyte-colony stimulating factor on bone marrow and circulation. *American Journal of Pathology* **134**, 149.

Williams, D.E. and Broxmeyer, H.E. (1988) Interleukin-1α enhances the *in vitro* survival of purified murine granulocyte-macrophage progenitor cells in the absence of colony-stimulating factors. *Blood* **72**, 1608.

4

Lymphocyte activation

4.1 Introduction

The process of lymphopoiesis, the generation of B- and T-lymphocytes, may be subdivided into three distinct stages. As in the initial stage of granulopoiesis and erythropoiesis, lymphocyte progenitors are produced in the fetal liver and subsequently in the bone marrow. Very little is known about the commitment of multipotential stem cells to the lymphoid lineage or the development of very early lymphocyte progenitors in terms of the proliferative and differentiating stimuli they respond to. From the fetal liver and bone marrow, lymphocyte precursors enter the circulation and colonize the primary lymphoid organs, the thymus (T-lymphocyte precursors) and, in birds only, the bursa of Fabricius (B-lymphocyte precursors). In these organs they undergo secondary development. In mammals, which have no bursa, B-lymphocyte precursors differentiate in the bone marrow.

Both B- and T-lymphocyte precursors contain immunoglobulin or 'immunoglobulin-like' genes which, as these cells mature, undergo a series of rearrangements to produce antigen-recognition molecules or receptors that are expressed at the cell surface. In B-lymphocytes, this results in the expression of a plasma-membrane-bound form of immunoglobulin which serves to recognize particular antigens. In contrast, in T-lymphocytes, this results in the expression of the so-called T-cell receptor, a complex glycoprotein containing two subunits, α and β (Figure 4.1) which can recognize certain antigenic epitopes of protein molecules when they are presented in association with the self-distinguishing major histocompatibility (MHC) antigens. It is beyond the scope of this chapter to describe the series of gene rearrangements leading to immunoglobulin (antibody) expression and to T-cell recep-

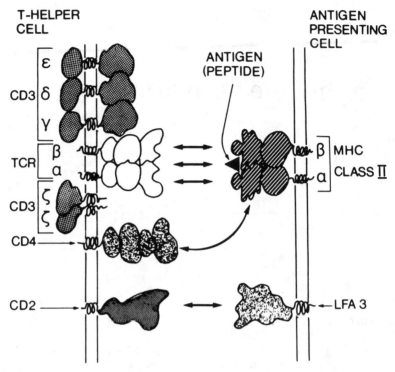

Figure 4.1 A simplified view of the interface between a helper T-cell and an antigen-presenting cell. TCR, T-cell receptor; CD, cell-surface cellular differentiation antigens; LFA, leukocyte function antigen; MHC, major histocompatibility complex; Greek letters denote the molecular subunits of the various cell surface antigens. (Reprinted with permission from Traunecker *et al.* (1989), *Immunology Today* **10**, 29; copyright 1989 Elsevier Science Publishers Ltd, UK.)

tor formation, or the intricacies of the MHC system; any reader who requires more information should refer to basic immunology textbooks.

In the thymus, T-lymphocyte precursors or thymocytes undergo a further maturation step in which they are 'educated' to discriminate between self and non-self antigens. The thymic epithelium expresses self-MHC molecules and this either determines non-self antigen/self-MHC reactivity in thymocytes or leads to the elimination of self antigen/self-MHC- or self-reactive-thymocytes. From recent studies, it is clear that some self-reactive T-cell clones are present in the circulation and that, while the thymus may limit their number, their elimination is not absolute. This problem of 'tolerance' to self antigens is currently the subject of some controversy as to how positive selection of thymocytes occurs in the presence of MHC, but no apparent self antigen. For this reason, it will not be further pursued here.

The secondary development of T-lymphocyte precursors is also associated

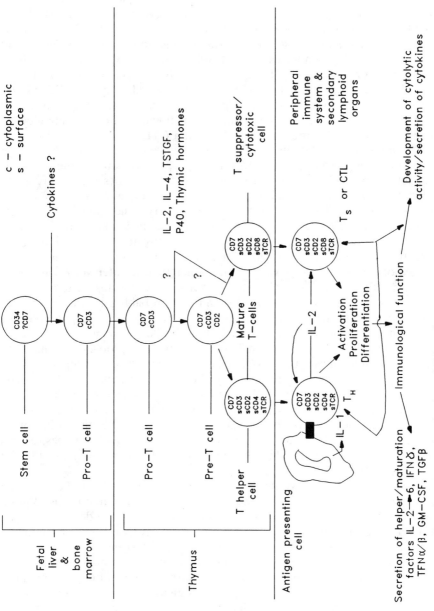

Figure 4.2 Development and activation of T-lymphocytes.

with the expression of particular cell-surface antigens or markers that are recognized by monoclonal antibodies. These markers serve to identify certain functionally distinct lymphocyte subsets and/or particular stages of their ontological development. It is clear, for example, that T lymphocytes may be subdivided into at least two functionally distinct subsets: the T-helper (T_H) cells, so-called because they provide helper factors for the maturation and activation of B-lymphocytes, are identified by the expression of cellular differentiation antigen-4 (CD4), while cytotoxic T-lymphocytes (CTL), so called because they kill antigen-expressing target cells, express CD8 (Figure 4.2). There are several other CD antigens which are either unique to certain lymphocyte subsets or are shared among functionally different lymphocytes. For example, CD3 is present on both T_H and CTL.

It is not clear whether any cytokines are involved in the thymic maturation stage of T-lymphocytes (Figure 4.2). However, it is known that the thymus is capable of producing a number of polypeptide hormones which may affect both the intra-thymic differentation of thymocytes and the proliferation/ differentiation of T-lymphocytes in the periphery. The 'thymic hormones' comprise a heterogeneous collection of molecules including thymosin (more than 30 peptides), thymopoietin (two peptides), thymulin (nine amino acids), and thymic humoral factor (30 amino acids) which appear to act at early stages of T-lymphocyte development, rather than at later stages involving antigen activation of T-lymphocytes. Nevertheless, they appear to mimic the actions of certain cytokines, e.g. ILs, and thus probably play important roles in T-lymphocyte maturation. In addition, they may possibly potentiate or augment T-lymphocyte responses to antigen and/or cytokines.

The classification of the thymic hormones poses a problem. Should they also be considered as cytokines? Thymopoietin and some polypeptides in the heterogeneous thymosin are certainly above the molecular weight of 5000 which would include them in the cytokine definition (see p. 3, Chapter 1). However, because in general they are less well characterized than most of the cytokines included in this book, and for reasons of space, they will not be discussed further. This was a difficult decision, and the author hopes readers will not be too disappointed by the omission (see Further reading, p. 137, for reviews on thymic hormones).

Once lymphocytes have matured to a certain stage, they leave the bone marrow (or bursa of Fabricius) and thymus, enter the circulation and migrate to secondary lymphoid organs such as the spleen, lymph nodes, and tonsils. At this stage B- and T-lymphocytes are able to respond to many non-self antigens such as would be carried by invasive pathogens, e.g. viruses and bacteria. In fact, each individual clone of B- or T-lymphocytes recognizes only one antigen. Further activation is therefore dependent upon stimulation of clonal B- and T-lymphocytes by their cognate antigen, usually a defined epitope of a foreign protein. As has been mentioned, activation occurs only when antigen is presented in combination with appropriate MHC antigens, class I in the case of CTL and class II in the cases of T_H (Figure 4.1) and B-lymphocytes. It should however be pointed out that there is a population of large granular lymphocytes (LGL), known as null cells, which do not appear to require MHC antigen co-expression, i.e. are not MHC-restricted. Included in the LGL are cytotoxic cells such as the so-called NK cells and lymphokine activated killer (LAK) cells. As the name of the latter implies, such lymphocytes can be activated by stimulation with certain lymphokines, e.g. IL-2, without apparent involvement of antigen or MHC. This 'non-specific' activation leads to the development of lymphocytes capable of killing certain tumour cell- or virus-infected cell-targets *in vitro*.

Thus, summarizing at this stage, there are antigen-requiring, MHC-restricted lymphocytes and antigen-non-requiring, MHC-non-restricted lymphocytes. Both categories, however, require stimulation with cytokines to become fully functional. The actions of particular interleukins in relation to lymphocyte proliferation and differentiation will be the main concern of this chapter.

The rest of the chapter provides descriptions of the molecular and biological characteristics of IL-1, IL-2, IL-4, IL-6, IL-7, and other relevant lymphocyte-activating cytokines.

4.2   Interleukins-1 and -2

Interleukin-1

The origins of our knowledge of IL-1 go back to the late 1940s, when it was isolated as a fever-inducing substance from neutrophils and thus called granulocyte pyrogen (GP). Subsequently, a factor with similar properties known as endogenous pyrogen (EP) was isolated from the blood of rabbits made febrile by injection of bacteria. In the 1960s, leukocyte endogenous mediator (LEM), a substance thought to induce the acute phase response, was also described. Then in the 1970s, immunologists working with mitogen-stimulated thymocytes discovered a factor derived from mononuclear phagocytes that enhanced mitogen-driven thymocyte proliferation; this they called lymphocyte activating factor (LAF). The molecular characterization of EP did not proceed quickly until it was found, in the late 1970s, that LPS-stimulated monocytes, rather than neutrophils, are the major cellular source of this factor. By that time, it was beginning to be realized that EP and LAF had similar characteristics. The agents that stimulated EP release also stimulated LAF production, the kinetics of EP and LAF release were similar, and the molecular weight and isoelectric points (pI) of EP and LAF were broadly the same. However, purification of EP/LAF from the supernatants of LPS-stimulated monocytes initially yielded active protein products of heterogeneous molecular weight with a broad spectrum of isoelectric points. These proteins had molecular weights ranging from 12 000 to 17 000 with pI from 5 to 7. In 1979, at the Second International Lymphokine Workshop in Ermatingen, Switzerland, the term 'interleukin' was coined. This terminology was devised primarily to name the soluble mediators produced by activated

T-lymphocytes that acted at short-range on 'responder' lymphocytes. However, it was proposed and accepted that the 'monokine' variously referred to as EP, LEM, and LAF should thenceforward be known as interleukin-1 (IL-1).

Although IL-1 could be resolved into two principal molecular species with pI 5 (α) and pI 7 (β), the precise structure of these proteins and their molecular relatedness was not revealed until their molecular cloning was accomplished in about 1984. IL-1 cDNAs were isolated by screening a cDNA library prepared from LPS-stimulated monocyte poly(A)$^+$ RNA (essentially mRNA enriched) with ^{32}P-labelled cDNA probes prepared from stimulated- and unstimulated-monocyte poly(A)$^+$RNA and subsequently identified by *in vitro* translation systems, e.g. rabbit reticulocyte lysate. In this way, two separate cDNAs coding for the precursor polypeptides of murine IL-1α and human IL-1β were cloned. Subsequently, the corresponding cDNAs for human IL-1α and murine IL-1β have been isolated. The precursor polypeptides of human IL-1α and IL-1β are 271 and 269 amino acids long, respectively (MW ~31 000). Active IL-1s are produced following cleavage of 159 carboxy-terminal amino acid residues (IL-1α) and 153 carboxy-terminal residues (IL-1β), from their respective precursors. The unusually long N-terminal 'leader' sequences do not appear to contain the usual signal sequence that characterizes most secreted proteins. In fact, the leader sequence is predominantly hydrophilic in nature and this therefore poses the problem of how IL-1 leaves the cell (see below). The active 17.5 kDa IL-1s appear to be functionally similar despite there being only about 25 per cent amino acid sequence identity between IL-1α and IL-1β. The murine IL-1s are approximately 63 per cent homologous to their respective human IL-1 counterparts. The amino acid sequences of mature IL-1α and IL-1β deduced from the cDNA sequences have subsequently been confirmed by chemical sequencing of human IL-1α and IL-1β purified from monocytes.

As far as is known, neither IL-1α nor IL-1β is glycosylated. There is one potential N-linked glycosylation site in IL-1α, which contains one cysteine residue. IL-1β contains two cysteine residues which probably form an intra-chain disulphide bridge, although the integrity of this does not appear to be necessary for biological activity. Both IL-1α and IL-1β are readily produced by *E.coli* containing plasmids with inserted IL-1 cDNAs. Circular dichroism measurements of the purified recombinant human (rh) IL-1β product have suggested that is is a non-helical protein with approximately 60 per cent of its residues in β-sheets or β-strands. A recent preliminary crystallographic study of rhIL-1β at the 3.0 Å resolution level further indicates that the structure is probably tetrahedral and is composed of 12 β-strands forming a complex of hydrogen bonds (Figure 4.3). The overall folding suggests a threefold internal structural pseudosymmetry which strongly resembles that of soybean trypsin inhibitor, a completely unrelated protein.

The nuclear gene for human IL-1β is located on the long arm of chromosome 2. The structure of the gene is complex, and there are seven exons. A comparative analysis of the structures of human IL-1α and murine IL-1β genes has shown extremely high conservation of the exon–intron junctions.

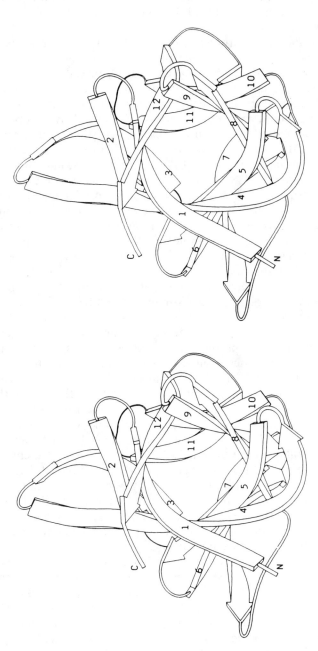

Figure 4.3 Stereo cartoon of IL-1β. The twisted arrows represent β-strands and they are numbered sequentially from the N-terminal. The view is down the axis of the barrel formed by six of the β-strands. (Reprinted with permission from Priestle *et al.*, 1988; copyright EMBO/IRL Press Ltd, UK.)

This observation, together with similarities in the number and size of the exons between the two species, has suggested that these genes have diverged from a common ancestral gene.

Monocytes are the major producers of IL-1, but it has been found that virtually every type of nucleated cell may produce IL-1 under the appropriate conditions. Thus, fibroblasts, endothelial cells, dendritic cells, keratinocytes, neutrophils, astrocytes, and cells in the stromal layer of bone marrow and in the thymic epithelium have all been demonstrated to produce IL-1. In addition, several cultured cell lines including monocytoid, lymphoblastoid, melanoma, glioma, and other tumour cell lines can be stimulated to produce IL-1. Generally, IL-1 is not produced without stimulation, but it is clear that a whole variety of substances including LPS, phorbol esters, muramyl dipeptide, calcium ionophore A 23187, immune complexes, bacteria, etc. can act as stimulants. Furthermore, IL-1 may stimulate its own production and that of other cytokines such as CSFs, and IFNγ may either induce or prime cells for IL-1 production. In most instances, cells produce a mixture of IL-1α and IL-1β following stimulation, although not usually in equal proportions. For example, LPS-stimulated monocytes produce approximately ten times more IL-1β than IL-1α. In the apparent absence of exogenous stimuli, there appears to be a low 'spontaneous' expression of both IL-1α and IL-1β mRNA in monocytes. However, following LPS-stimulation, IL-1β mRNA expression increases up to 40-fold greater than the basal level whereas IL-1α mRNA expression increases only two- to threefold. This observation strongly suggests that regulation of the production of the two IL-1 species is mainly controlled at the level of transcription. The difference in levels of the two IL-1 proteins accumulating in the cell medium may also reflect differential release from monocytes. It is clear that, following stimulation, IL-1α and IL-1β, probably as 31 kDa precursors, steadily accumulate intracellularly and that release into the medium, unlike most secreted proteins with a signal sequence, is relatively slow. The means of exit from the cell is not known, but there is controversial evidence that IL-1, and in particular IL-1α, enters the plasma membrance as a 23 kDa processed molecule. The recent demonstration that IL-1 precursors are post-translationally acylated with the fatty acid myristate suggests a means whereby they may be localized in hydrophobic cell membranes. However, the presence of active IL-1 in plasma membranes has not been universally confirmed and while the expression of plasma membrane IL-1 in relation to cell contact interactions (see Section 3.4) remains an attractive mechanism for cell activation, further evidence of its existence in membranes is required to substantiate this hypothesis. The alternative, continuous slow release of 17.5 kDa IL-1α and IL-1β from producer cells would presumably have the same effects, and so it may not be necessary to formulate a plasma membrane-bound IL-1 mechanism of cell activation at all.

Despite their apparent structural dissimilarity, both IL-1α and IL-1β bind to a common cell surface receptor. This implies that the structural element of IL-1 that binds to the receptor must be sufficiently conserved between IL-1α and IL-1β to permit specific receptor binding. The situation may be analogous to that of TNFα and TNFβ where, despite a seemingly wide divergence of primary amino acid sequences, the two polypeptides probably fold up into similarly shaped molecules (see Chapter 5). The production of IL-1 precursors and several subpeptides by recombinant DNA technology has suggested that these, besides the mature 17.5 kDa proteins, bind to receptors and are in many instances biologically active. The so-called 'active site' of IL-1β appears to be present in the N-terminal domain of the 17.5 kDa mature protein. More specifically, it has been shown that a nonapeptide, produced by chemical synthesis, whose amino acid sequence is homologous to residues 163–171 of the IL-1β precursor sequence, mimics the immunostimulatory activity of IL-1. However, the latter could not be shown to produce the inflammatory responses, such as prostaglandin synthesis, characteristic of intact IL-1 activity (see Chapter 5), nor is the nonapeptide sequence conserved in IL-1α, and it remains to be determined whether the nonapeptide acts through binding to the IL-1 receptor or by another means.

Just as the production of IL-1 is widespread among different cell types, the presence of IL-1 receptors (IL-1R) on cells is ubiquitous. Its widespread distribution should, however, be qualified by saying that in many cell types it is not very abundant, with numbers of receptors ranging from tens up to a few hundred per cell. For example, resting or quiescent T-lymphocytes express only about 40 receptors per cell, but this number increases approximately 10-fold in two days following antigenic stimulation. Thus, in normal cells IL-1R expression is probably an inducible phenomenon which itself may depend upon stimulation by other cytokines such as PDGF or the action of IL-1-induced prostaglandins. However, in certain tumour cells, for example the murine thymoma cell line EL4 clone 6.1, IL-1R expression appears to be unregulated. These cells express up to 20000 receptors per cell. For this reason, the murine IL-1R from EL4 cells has been most intensively investigated. Chemical cross-linking experiments with ^{125}I-IL-1α to EL4 cells have revealed the presence of an 80 kDa receptor protein. Putative receptor proteins of a similar size have also been demonstrated in human fibroblasts, keratinocytes, endothelial cells, and B-lymphoblastoid cells. Solubilization of EL4 cell membranes has also yielded an 80 kDa glycoprotein capable of binding IL-1 in solution (see below). There have been reports of other membrane proteins of a different size to the IL-1-binding glycoprotein, which may be part of a complex IL-1R or form low-affinity binding sites. Following binding of IL-1 to its receptor, the receptor–ligand complex is internalized, probably by endocytosis, and is either degraded or possibly recycled. There is also evidence of a nuclear 'receptor' for IL-1, presumably similar to that proposed for NGF and other growth factors (see p. 57).

The murine 80 kDa IL-1R glycoprotein from EL4 cells has recently been cloned. This was carried out by preparing cDNA from EL4 cells, linking cDNA to a highly efficient expression vector and transfecting into monkey COS cells, following which IL-1R bearing cells were identified by binding of ^{125}I-IL-1α and autoradiographical techniques. This led to the isolation of a cDNA coding for the 80 kDa protein and the deduction of its amino acid sequence from the nucleotide sequence of this cDNA. The polypeptide sequence predicts a 19 amino acid signal sequence followed by a putative mature receptor sequence of 557 amino acids. The latter may be subdivided up into the three-domain structure typical of growth factor plasma membrane receptors (see Figure 7.2, p. 222). Thus, the N-terminal domain of 319 amino acids is probably the glycosylated extracellular segment which contains the IL-1 binding site. The C-terminal domain of 217 amino acids, which is presumably intracellular, is linked by a hydrophobic stretch of 21 amino acids which is the presumed transmembrane domain. Comparison of the sequence of the extracellular domain with the sequences of other growth factor receptors and cell-surface members of the immunoglobulin (Ig) superfamily such as CD8 and T-cell receptor chains has revealed significant similarities between the IL-1R and PDGF-R, M-CSF-R (c-FMS), rat CD8 chain II, and human T-cell receptor Cβ. This analysis therefore strongly suggests that the IL-1R is also a member of the Ig superfamily. In contrast, the C-terminal domain sequence does not show homology with any tyrosine kinase sequences and thus distinguishes the IL-1R from the receptor-tyrosine kinase class of receptors such as EGF-R, PDGF-R, and the insulin receptor.

The lack of a tyrosine kinase in the IL-1R suggests a different mechanism of receptor activation to that of tyrosine phosphorylation envisaged for tyrosine kinase receptors. However, whatever the initial biochemical reactions, the 'downstream' signalling pathways may be similar. For example, IL-1 has been shown to rapidly induce inositol phospholipid breakdown in murine macrophages and synthesis of cAMP in a variety of IL-1-responsive target cells, steps which have previously been implicated in signal transduction. Alternatively, and in apparent contradiction to the above, in human T-lymphoblastoid Jurkat cells IL-1 fails to modify inositol phospholipid and cAMP levels, but induces synthesis of phosphatidylserine. This compound is a necessary co-factor of protein kinase C, another enzyme widely believed to play a role in signal transmission to the nucleus. IL-1 also appears to activate the cyclo-oxygenase–arachidonic acid metabolic pathway which acts on the breakdown product of membrane-associated phospholipases A and C to yield a variety of products including thromboxanes, prostacyclins, and several species of prostaglandins, and this too has been suggested to be involved in signal transmission. Clearly there is still some confusion about the means of IL-1-induced signal transmission, and further investigations are required to clarify this situation. There may be different routes of transmission in different cell types, which may account for the various cellular responses accorded to IL-1-mediated cell activation (see also Chapter 5). Nevertheless, in common with growth factor stimulation in general, IL-1-induced signal transmission leads to early expression of c-*fos* proto-oncogene followed sequentially by c-*myc* induction. This suggests that either IL-1R and other growth factor receptors are linked to a common response pathway, or they may be linked to different signalling pathways which converge in the nucleus to elicit a response which is a common feature of cell activation processes.

The possible involvement of IL-1 in the activation of T-lymphocytes is described in Section 4.3 pp. 119–25 following the description of the molecular characteristics of interleukin-2 (IL-2) and its receptor (pp. 116–19). Some knowledge of the structure of these molecules is necessary to aid perception of the sequential events of T-lymphocyte activation. The inflammatory properties of IL-1 will be dealt with separately in Chapter 5.

Interleukin-2

The first step along the road to the isolation of a factor that stimulated the proliferation of T-lymphocytes was the discovery by Nowell in 1960 that certain plant lectins are mitogenic for lymphocytes. Soon afterwards, it was found that the medium conditioned by cultured lymphocytes contained soluble mitogenic factors. In particular, medium conditioned by lymphocytes stimulated by phytohaemagglutinin (PHA), a plant lectin, could be used to support the long-term survival and proliferation of normal T-lymphocytes. This finding was of great importance to cellular immunology, as it led on directly to the isolation and culture of physiological relevant antigen-specific T-lymphocyte or T-cell clones. It has subsequently proved possible to characterize T-cell differentiation markers and the T-cell antigen receptor, and to investigate the molecular mechanisms underlying T-cell cytolytic behaviour.

The means for purification and further molecular characterization of this as yet undefined T-cell growth factor (TCGF) was instigated by using a cloned murine T-cell line, which was dependent on conditioned-medium factors for proliferation. The principal source of TCGF was identified as T-lymphocytes themselves, and tonsillar lymphocytes, which could be obtained in large numbers, were used to generate large quantities of conditioned medium for TCGF purification. All this was taking place in the early 1980s, by which time the Second International Lymphokine Workshop (Switzerland, 1979) had already designated TCGF as interleukin-2 (IL-2). From 100 litres of conditioned medium, IL-2 was purified to virtual homogeneity as a single glycoprotein moiety (MW 15 500). The IL-2 glycoprotein is remarkably hydrophobic, a characteristic that was exploited for its purification. Murine IL-2 was purified from medium conditioned by lectin-stimulated mouse splenocytes and shown not only to be molecularly similar to human IL-2 but also to exhibit a nearly equivalent specific biological activity to human IL-2 as determined in a murine IL-2-dependent T-cell line (CTLL).

Molecular cloning of human IL-2 followed quite quickly from these purification studies, but the cloning strategy was based upon the preparation of cDNA from either human splenocytes or a T-lymphoblastoid cell line, Jurkat, hybridization with mRNA derived from PHA-stimulated cells, and translation of IL-2 mRNA in *Xenopus* oocytes rather than on knowledge of N-terminal amino acid sequences of IL-2 that were becoming available at the same time (1982–83). The IL-2 cDNAs so isolated encoded a polypeptide of 153 amino acids of which the 20 N-terminal amino acids formed a signal sequence. The mature IL-2 polypeptide of 133 amino acids (MW 15 420) has three cysteines, two of which form an intrachain disulphide bond, and an

O-linked glycosylation site on threonine residue position 3 from the N-terminus. Human recombinant (rh) IL-2 synthesized by *E.coli* transformed by plasmids containing IL-2 cDNA inserts lacks the variable O-linked oligosaccharides present in IL-2 derived from human T-cells, but is fully biologically active. Interestingly, substitution with alanine of the cysteine residue at position 125, which is not involved in disulphide bond formation, improves the yield of active IL-2 from *E.coli*, probably by preventing mis-matching of cysteines and the formation of interchain dimers. The primary sequence of human IL-2 shows little if any homology with the amino acid sequences of other known cytokines. However, the gibbon IL-2 sequence is identical to human, but bovine and murine IL-2s are much less homologous (60–70 per cent homology to human). The gene for human IL-2 is located on the long arm of chromosome 4 and contains four exons and three introns. A similar exon–intron organization has been subsequently found in the genes coding for IL-4, IL-5, GM-CSF, and IFNγ (see also p. 89). In addition, perhaps rather coincidentally, the human IL-3 gene has been shown to code for a polypeptide of exactly the same length, 133 amino acids, as that of IL-2, although molecularly they are unrelated.

The complete three-dimensional structure of IL-2 has been elucidated from X-ray crystallographic studies at the 3Å resolution level. The IL-2 molecule has been shown to be composed mainly of α-helical segments, similar in some respects to α-helix-containing unrelated proteins such as human growth hormone and IFNα, but in contrast to the β-strand structure predicted for IL-1β (see p. 111). It has a short α-helix (A) near to the N-terminus (residues 11–19), which joins a more extensive helical region (BB′) via a bent loop, followed by Cys-58, which is involved in the intrachain disulphide bond (Cys58-Cys105) and four further α-helical segments (C, D, E, F) to form an apparent antiparallel antihelical bundle (Figure 4.4). Studies involving neutralizing monoclonal α-bodies and site-specific or deletion-mutant IL-2 molecules have suggested that amino acid residues in the N-terminal region are necessary for receptor binding, e.g. deletion of residues 1–20 abolishes the activity of human IL-2. On the basis of the three-dimensional structure this would suggest that the N-terminal α-helix or part of the ensuing loop structure, which are presumably on the surface of the IL-2 molecule, can fit into the receptor binding site. It also appears possible that the E-helix, based on the stereogeography of the molecule, makes contact with the receptor.

The investigators attempting to characterize the IL-2 receptor (IL-2R) started out in the early 1980s with one great advantage, namely the availability of a monoclonal antibody, anti-Tac, that bound to a component of IL-2R and blocked T-cell proliferation. Firstly, it was shown that anti-Tac immunoprecipitated a cell surface protein present in T-lymphocyte plasma membranes. This protein, the Tac antigen, had a molecular weight of 50 000–55 000. Although it appeared likely at that time that Tac was a receptor protein, inconsistent data on the numbers and affinities of IL-2R suggested that the latter was a complex of two or more closely associated proteins, of which the 55 kDa Tac protein was a subunit. In human T-cell lines, e.g. the

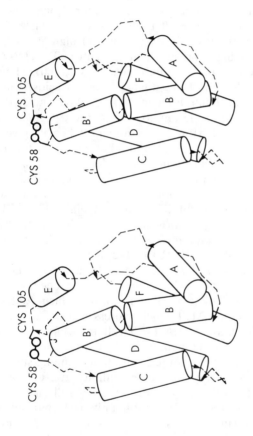

Figure 4.4 Schematic stereo drawing of IL-2; helices are represented as cylinders and are lettered sequentially from the N-terminus. (Reprinted with permission from Brandhuber *et al.*, 1987; copyright American Association for the Advancement of Science 1987.)

adult T-cell leukaemia line HUT102, both high- and low-affinity binding sites for IL-2 were demonstrated, with the high-affinity sites comprising only 1–2 per cent of the total sites. However, anti-Tac was shown to bind to both classes of binding sites, whereas IL-2 itself bound preferentially to the high affinity binding sites. This difference in binding between anti-Tac and IL-2 provided the means for the demonstration in 1987 of a second component of the high-affinity IL-2R (see below).

In parallel to these studies to characterize IL-2R, two research groups worked towards the molecular cloning of this receptor. Complementary (c) DNA libraries were prepared from adult T-cell leukaemia cell lines (HUT102 and MT1), which express the low-affinity receptor at high levels, and both groups using the same cloning strategy, isolated identical Tac cDNAs which encoded a mature polypeptide of 251 amino acids (MW 28 400). The deduced amino acid sequence of Tac predicted that 219 amino acids from the N-terminus formed the extracellular domain with a 19-residue hydrophobic transmembrane domain and only 13 amino acids at the C-terminus likely to be intracellular. Although the extracellular domain is heavily glycosylated, in keeping with the features of this domain in other growth factor receptors, the apparent lack of a C-terminal domain and thus of any enzymic signal transduction device suggested that Tac was not the complete IL-2R. In addition, when expressed in mouse fibroblasts, the Tac cDNA exclusively directed the synthesis and expression of low-affinity binding sites. The gene coding for Tac has subsequently been located on the short arm of chromosome 10 and characterized as containing eight exons spanning 25 kb.

The second component of the IL-2R isolated as a result of IL-2 binding to high-affinity binding sites has been shown to be a 70–75 kDa protein, subsequently referred to as p70. This component has been found to be present in the adult T-cell leukaemia line HUT-102 which contains high-affinity binding sites, but not in MT1 which expresses only Tac. In addition, p70 has been found in the gibbon MLA-144 T-cell line which, however, does not express Tac. Fusion of plasma membranes from MT1 and MLA-144 has been subsequently shown to reconstitute high-affinity binding sites for IL-2. Despite this, actual rigorous proof that the high-affinity IL-2R is composed of a complex of p70 and Tac, e.g. as a heterodimer, is still lacking, and the primary amino acid sequence of p70 is still unknown (but see p. 224). Nevertheless, there is growing circumstantial evidence that p70 and Tac are linked and that the inducible expression of Tac regulates the formation of high affinity IL-2R. First, in addition to the MLA-144 T-cell line, p70 has also been demonstrated in other T-cell lines, in resting or quiescent T-lymphocytes and in NK cells without the simultaneous presence of Tac. Second, p70 has been shown to bind IL-2 at an affinity intermediate between that of the low-affinity Tac antigen and the high-affinity IL-2R and to be able itself to transduce activating signals into cells. In this regard, site-specific mutants of the IL-2 molecule again suggest that amino acids in the N- and C-terminal segments are required for binding to p70. Third, Tac expression which is induced upon T-cell activation (see below) correlates well with the appearance of high-affinity IL-2R, and the latter contains both p70 and Tac on the evidence of chemical cross-linking experiments with ^{125}I-IL-2. Fourth, the IL-2-to-IL-2R complex is rapidly internalized, probably by an endocytic mechanism, and this is normally associated with the presence of an intracellular receptor domain. Since Tac lacks, or has very little of, an intracellular domain, this suggests that p70, or yet another putative receptor subunit, contains this domain. Recent investigations in which evidence has been obtained of the association of Tac with a 95 kDa antigen designated T27, or another membrane protein of 100 kDa, has tended to suggest an even more complex structure for the IL-2R than the proposed p70.Tac heterodimer. It should be pointed out that Tac is now often referred to as the α-chain of IL-2R and p70 as the β-chain, hence IL-2Rα and IL-2Rβ, but rather confusingly one group reverses this nomenclature. Thus Tac is β and p70 is α! It is hoped that future developments will not only resolve the structure of IL-2R, but also remove such nomenclature problems (see also p. 223).

4.3   T-lymphocyte activation, proliferation, and differentiation

The wish to support the growth of T-lymphocytes in culture has over several years generated a great quest to understand the processes of T-lymphocyte activation, proliferation, and differentiation. These three processes are probably interrelated, proliferation and/or differentiation following on autonomously from the activation step. This latter is now known to require the combination, through cell-to-cell contact, of the T-cell antigen receptor (a heterodimer of two immunoglobulin-like chains associated with CD3 antigens) and antigen presented in combination with MHC on accessory cells, such as macrophages or dendritic cells (Figure 4.1). Following this trigger, there are changes in cell metabolism, in ion fluxes, and in cell size that are similar to those occasioned by growth factors occupying their cognate receptors. For example, antigen binding to the T-cell receptor increases inositol phospholipid turnover, intracellular Ca^{2+} levels, and protein kinase C (PKC) activity, these changes being associated with putative signal transmission pathways for several different growth factors or cytokines. The antigen-mediated activation step has been found to mimicked by a combination of Ca^{2+}-ionophore, which allows increased Ca^{2+} uptake into the T-cell, and phorbolesters, e.g. phorbol myristate acetate (PMA), which substitute for diacylglycerol in the activation of PKC. Antibodies to the T-cell receptor or other cell surface antigens, such as CD2 and CD3, and certain plant lectins, such as PHA and concanavalin A (ConA), also appear to produce the same effect. However, while the activation step is necessary, it is possibly not sufficient, for the proliferative response.

It has been known for some time that accessory cells such as macrophages or monocytes appear to be necessary for lectin-stimulated T-cell proliferation. Thus, it is widely believed that accessory cells produce a factor (or factors) that is essential, or at least enhances, T-cell proliferation. The prime candidate for this role is IL-1, a macrophage/monocyte cytokine that has already been implicated as a co-factor in the proliferation of early haemopoietic progenitor cells (see Section 3.4). On its own, IL-1 is a poor stimulator of T-cell proliferation, but in combination with lectin or antigen produces a synergistic effect on the proliferative response (Figure 4.2). Probably, therefore, IL-1 is not an obligatory factor for T-cell proliferation, but acts more as an enhancer, much in the same way as it has been shown to synergize in IL-3-driven proliferation of haemopoietic cells. Indeed, the addition of neutralizing anti-IL-1 antibodies to unfractionated lymphocytes and mononuclear cells was shown to have no effect on antigen- or lectin-stimulated T-cell proliferation, suggesting that endogenously produced IL-1 is not an absolute requirement for this process. This has led to speculation that another factor or cytokine is involved, and there are already several papers in the literature reporting the preliminary characterization of such a factor or factors.

Alternatively, as has been previously hypothesized, IL-1 may be active in an unreleased form present in the plasma membrane of accessory cells. While there remain doubts about the existence of plasma-membrane-bound IL-1 and the source of endogenous inducers of its synthesis, the increased numbers of IL-1R in activated T-lymphocytes (see p. 113), together with the proven capacity of IL-1 to induce the production of IL-2 and other cytokines, strongly suggests that it could have a functional role in T-cell proliferation.

Following the initial activation step, the T-cell may be considered to be committed to respond to further or contingent regulatory events. Under the microscope, the activated T-cell appears to progress autonomously through a number of morphologic changes; from early cell swelling to blastogenesis at about 12 hours post-activation, and to cell division occurring at between 24 and 48 hours. Obviously, underlying metabolic and structural changes occur throughout this period, but is has become apparent that molecular events happening during only the first two hours after activation are sufficient for the mitogenic response leading to DNA synthesis and cell division. On the basis of the cell cycle, it is thought that antigen-mediated activation commits resting T-cells in G_0 to proceed into G_1 when possibly they become responsive to IL-1 or to other regulatory factors which lead to the induction of synthesis of IL-2 and IL-2R. The autocrine action of IL-2 (Figure 4.2) on the newly formed high-affinity IL-2R is thought to lead to the expression of transferrin receptors (all proliferating cells require iron) and the progression from G_1 to the S-phase, in which DNA synthesis commences. Since the entry of cells into the S-phase has been found to be dependent upon the IL-2 concentration in the extracellular milieu and on the number of IL-2R expressed, the regulation of the induction and expression of the IL-2 and the IL-2R-genes, which occurs during the first two-hour activation period, is of central importance to the proliferative response.

The initiation of IL-2 gene expression has been tentatively linked to the prior 'early' inositol phospholipid hydrolysis, Ca^{2+} mobilization, and phosphorylation of membrane and cytoplasmic proteins occurring within 5 minutes of the activation signal. For instance, T-cells normally require PKC activation for IL-2 production. Nevertheless, the actual control of transcription of the IL-2 gene appears to be regulated by a transcription enhancer in the 5′ flanking region of the IL-2 gene, proximal to the IL-2 protein-coding sequence. There are at least two and possibly three defined regions within this 5′ flanking region to which particular nuclear factors may bind in order to activate transcription. These factors, designated NFAT-1, AP-1, and NFIL-2A, may themselves be regulated by separate signal pathways emanating from the cell surface, for example from the antigen receptor or from PKC. In this context, since IL-1 has been shown to enhance IL-2 production, the signal generated from IL-1R might be to amplify the cooperation of nuclear transcription factors at the level of the responsive IL-2 gene. Alternatively, IL-1 may act by inducing c-*fos* (see p. 114), the product of which complexes with AP-1 (c-*jun* product) to form a transcriptional promoter responsive to other signals. Further, IL-1 induces c-*myc* which, although the function of c-MYC is not known, appears also to be an obligatory step of the proliferative response.

Thus, summarizing so far, the molecular events involved in T-cell activation in temporal order appear to be as follows:

1   inositol phospholipid hydrolysis, intracellular Ca^{2+} mobilization, PKC activation (5 min);
2   induction of c-*fos* and other nuclear transcriptional factors, e.g. NFAT-1, NFIL-2A required for IL-2 gene activation (15 min);
3   induction of c-*myc* (30 min);
4   induction of IL-2 gene (45 min).

Further events are then apparently contingent on the secretion of IL-2 and its action on IL-2R-bearing lymphocytes. This can lead both to the autocrine stimulation of IL-2 producing T-lymphocytes and the paracrine stimulation of other lymphocytes bearing receptors. It is widely believed that IL-2 mediated effects are first transmitted inside lymphocytes by p70 (IL-2Rβ), the medium-affinity receptor and that the signals so generated lead to IL-2Rα (Tac) gene expression and ultimately to the formation of the heterodimeric, high-affinity IL-2Rα/β. In contrast to the т-cell antigen receptor, neither IL-2Rβ or IL2Rα/β signal transduction leads to hydrolysis of phosphatidylinositols or increase of intracellular Ca^{2+}, and PKC activation does not appear to be required for IL-2-induced cell proliferation. On the other hand, IL-2R occupancy has been shown to lead to:

1   intracellular alkanization via activation of the Na^+/H^+ antiport
2   increased Ca^{2+} association with cells
3   increased proto-oncogene expression and
4   perhaps activation of a receptor-associated protein kinase.

In this respect, the activating mechanism whereby the IL-2R operates may possibly be similar to that of the insulin receptor which also does not appear to use the inositol phospholipid-Ca^{2+}-PKC pathway, but which does activate the Na^+/H^+ antiport. With regard to proto-oncogene expression, IL-2 binding to its receptor induces c-*myc*, but not c-*fos*. In addition, IL-2 induces the expression of c-*myb*, the product of which appears to be essential for progression from the G_1 to the S-phase of the cell cycle. The expression of the IL-2Rα (Tac)-gene appears to be regulated by similar, but probably non-identical, nuclear transcription factors to those controlling IL-2-gene expression and presumably these are also induced by IL-2. IL-2Rα synthesis takes place approximately 2 hours after the initial activation step and increases up to 8 hours; the peak of c-MYB synthesis also occurs at 8 hours, the midpoint of G_1. Transferrin receptor synthesis then ensues and the cell progresses to DNA synthesis in the S-phase. It should be pointed out that the times indicated are only very approximate and that the length of G_1 may vary considerably in T-lymphocytes and in different T-cell clones.

The T-lymphocyte has provided a unique mammalian cell type in which to study cell activation and proliferation. In many ways the proliferative response in T-lymphocytes is similar to that in fibroblasts triggered by PDGF. In both cases, cells are 'committed' to enter the cell cycle by an early activation step; such cells become competent to respond to other stimuli necessary for proliferation. Activated T-lymphocytes are able themselves to produce the requisite progression factors, IL-2, IL-2R, c-MYB, etc., in a strict temporal sequence to enable the cell to proceed to blastogenesis (DNA synthesis) and cell division; in fibroblasts it is presumed that similar progression factors operate, but in most cases their identity remains unknown. Thus, T-lymphocyte activation and proliferation appears to fit nicely into the model advanced in Chapter 2 where it was proposed that for each stimulus there would be a corresponding wave of specific gene modulation and competence/progression protein synthesis. It is, however, unwise to take this simplistic version of activation/proliferation at face value. It may well be that some of the 'main players' involved in T-lymphocyte-activation/proliferation have been identified and characterized, but that certainly is not the end of the story. For instance, it is known that at least 15 plasma membrane proteins may modulate T-cell activation and that during the G_0–G_1 transition T-cells are expressing 8000–10 000 genes. In only four of the latter, c-*myc* and the genes coding for IL-2, IL-2Rα, and IFNγ, has the pattern of expression been well characterized! Furthermore, following T-cell activation more than 50 different gene products have been identified, some not being expressed until days after the initial stimulation. This raises questions about the nature of signals required to maintain the necessary series of contingent gene activations for the long-term development of immunological function. Part of the answer to these questions may be provided by the secretion by T-cells of various cytokines with differentiation-inducing activities.

The production of cytokines by activated T-lymphocytes may be considered both to be part of the proliferation response and part of their differentiation or maturation pathway (Figure 4.2). As has been seen, T-lymphocyte secretion of IL-2 is important in initiating and sustaining proliferation. On the other hand, IL-2, which is essentially only produced by T-lymphocytes, and in particular by a subset of T_H cells, may be considered to be a product of a cell at a specific stage of differentiation. IL-2 then enables responsive cells to proceed to a further stage of differentiation at which other differentiation-inducing cytokines are produced. One of these is IFNγ, a pleiotropic cytokine produced by activated T_H, CTL, and NK cells which has profound effects relating to immunological and cytolytic functions in many cell types (see Chapter 5). In addition, there are several other cytokines, IL-3, IL-4, IL-5, IL-6, IL-7, GM-CSF, TNFα and β, and TGFβ which may be produced by activated T-lymphocytes and which, although their principal role appears to be as 'helper factors' for the growth and differentiation of leukocytes other than T-lymphocytes, could be also involved in the differentiation of the latter. For instance, the receptors for certain of these cytokines, e.g. TNFα/β, are not present in resting T-cells, but are induced following activation suggesting that such cytokines could have functional roles in T-cell differentiation. For example, TNFα may be a necessary factor for the maturation of CTL to express cytolytic activity, an effect that is inhibited by TGFβ. Thus, the autostimulatory effects of cytokines probably are important for the late-stage differentiation/maturation events in activated T-lymphocytes.

The autocrine actions of IL-1 and IL-2 suggest that they may be involved in oncogenesis and, specifically, in leukaemogenesis. *In vitro*, the establishment of both IL-1- and IL-2-dependent cell lines has been described. In many cases, these cell lines do not produce the cytokine they are dependent upon for proliferation, e.g. the murine CTLL which are absolutely dependent upon the addition of exogenous IL-2. On the other hand, there are many cell lines which appear to have lost their cytokine dependence, but which produce IL-2 following appropriate stimulation. For example, the Jurkat T-cell line produces high titres of human IL-2 when stimulated with PHA and PMA, and the EL4 thymoma line produces murine IL-2 following stimulation with IL-1. The EL4 cell line expresses high levels of IL-1R, as previously discussed (see p. 113), but shows no apparent dependence on IL-1 for proliferation. A similar situation exists in several established T_H-cell lines which are chronically infected by the adult T-cell leukaemia (ATL) virus, a human retrovirus called HTLV-1, where there is aberrantly high constitutive expression of (usually) low-affinity IL-2R without apparent stimulation by IL-2. It has been speculated that HTLV-1 may initially cause polyclonal T_H-cell proliferation by inducing constitutive expression of IL-2R and thus rendering T-cells permanently responsive to autocrine or paracrine stimulation by IL-2. Then following unknown genetic changes, the autostimulatory loop breaks down with the loss of IL-2 dependence, resulting in the uncontrollable, proliferation of a particular monoclonal T_H cell and leading to ATL (Figure 4.5). The loss of IL-2 dependence may reflect the presence of an abnormal or mutated IL-2R component and/or its unregulated expression and/or the breakdown of growth control mechanisms associated with IL-2R or elsewhere inside these tumour cells. The pattern of events involved in leukaemogenesis in this case may thus be similar to that occurring in AML (see Chapter 3), although the latter have no apparent viral cause.

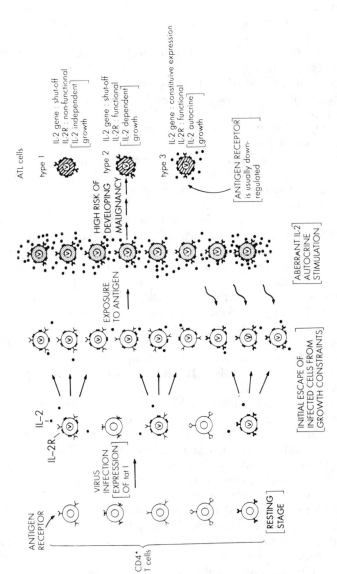

Figure 4.5 The two-step activation model of adult T-cell leukaemia (ATL). Possible involvement of the operation of an aberrant IL-2 autocrine loop in the ATL development at an early stage. An intriguing possibility is that some if not all of the ATL cells become responsive to other cytokines in acquisition of the malignant phenotype as a consequence of dysregulation of the IL-2 system. (Reproduced, with permission, from *Annual Review of Immunology* **6**; copyright 1988 by Annual Reviews Inc.)

Several recent observations and studies have lent support to the autocrine self-stimulation hypothesis, as suggested above, and its possible operation in the development of other types of leukaemia, besides those of T_H-cell origin. For example, there is suggestive evidence in at least one T-cell line, the gibbon T-cell line MLA 144, which constitutively produces IL-2, that its proliferation is dependent upon this IL-2. In addition, IL-2 autocrine stimulation has been demonstrated for the *in vitro* growth of a human T-cell line isolated from a patient with non-Hodgkin's T-cell leukaemia. Furthermore, IL-2 cDNA has been transfected into murine CTLL cells, which express IL-2R but which are normally dependent on the addition of exogenous IL-2 for proliferation, and shown to give rise to autonomously growing cell lines. In fact, the cell lines producing the most IL-2 were more tumorigenic than lines producing low IL-2 levels. Thus, *in vitro* at least, the dysregulation of the IL-2/IL-2R system of growth control leads to neoplastic transformation and suggests that similar aberrant autostimulatory mechanisms are involved in leukaemogenesis (*in vivo*).

4.4   Interleukins-4, -6, and -7

In the preceding sections, the molecular characteristics of IL-1 and IL-2 together with their biological activities in relation to T-cell activation, proliferation, and differentiation were described and discussed. As previously mentioned, these two cytokines are pleiotropic, i.e. they act on several cell types, besides T-lymphocytes. Receptors for IL-1 are to be found on virtually all cell types. IL-2R are also not limited to T-cells, being present also on NK cells, B-cells, and monocytes/macrophages. Thus, IL-1 and IL-2 potentially could have roles in the proliferation and maturation of non-T-cells. For example, B-lymphocyte or B-cell development is probably influenced by the activities of these two cytokines. However, for simplicity, B-cell development will be related to a separate set of cytokines, including a subset of interleukins, i.e. IL-4, IL-5, IL-6, and IL-7. However, many if not all of these display the same lack of cell-type specificity as IL-1 and IL-2, and therefore, conversely, they may also affect the growth and differentiation of non-B-cells. IL-4, for example, may be important for the maturation of thymocytes.

In the following sections, the molecular characterization of IL-4, IL-6, and IL-7 will precede an account of B-cell development. Descriptions of the structure and functions of IL-3 and IL-5 have been previously given in Chapter 3.

Interleukin-4

The cytokine now known as interleukin-4 (IL-4) was originally discovered through its action on B-lymphocytes. The latter, which express surface immunoglobulin (Ig), were found to proliferate in response to anti-Ig only if the medium they were cultured in was supplemented by particular T-cell-derived supernatants. These supernatants were subsequently shown (*circa* 1982) to contain a novel cytokine which, because of its mitogenic activity was called B-cell growth factor-I (BCGF-I). Further studies revealed pleiotypic effects of this cytokine in B-cells and consequently it was renamed B-cell stimulating factor-1 (BSF-1). Then, in 1985, there arose a dispute as to whether BSF-1 or eosinophil differentiating factor (EDF; BCGF-II in the mouse) should be designated IL-4; in the event, agreement was reached that BSF-1 would be IL-4 and EDF/BCGF-II, IL-5.

IL-4 is probably exclusively produced by cells of T-lymphocyte origin, e.g. activated T_H-cells. In the mouse, Mosmann's group have delineated two kinds of T_H-lymphocytes, a suppressor–inducer (cytotoxic) T_H1 subset and a helper–inducer (non-cytotoxic) T_H2 subset. These functionally distinct subsets have been shown to produce different 'packages' of cytokines: the production of IL-2 and IFNγ (T_H1) and that of IL-4 and IL-5 (T_H2) was found to be mutually exclusive. Thus, only the T_H2 subset could provide 'helper factors' for B-cell development. However, there are differences of opinion as to whether the distinction in terms of cytokine production between T_H1 and T_H2 is truly watertight, and certainly in most human CD4$^+$ T_H-cell clones IL-2, IL-4, and IFNγ are produced simultaneously. Qualitative and quantitative differences in cytokine production by different T_H-cell clones may reflect differences in methods of culture and stimulation as much as any phenotypic distinctions. Besides activated T_H-cells, IL-4 is produced by certain 'T-cell-like' cell lines, e.g. the murine EL4 thymoma cell line, by some T-cell hybridomas and by some HTLV-I infected/transformed human T_H cells. With respect to the latter, it has recently been demonstrated that the leukaemic cells from some ATL patients proliferate in responses to exogenously added IL-4. This suggests that a dysregulation of the IL-4/IL-4R system, similar to that discussed for IL-2/IL-2R, may be involved in leukaemogenesis in certain cases of ATL.

The molecular cloning of IL-4 was achieved virtually simultaneously in 1986 by two research groups who, however, cloned this cytokine under two different names, murine mast cell growth factor-2 (MCGF-2) and murine T-cell growth factor-2 (TCGF-2). This illustrates the pleiotropic nature of IL-4; besides having the activities implied by the names above, IL-4 also has effects in resting and differentiated B-cells, in macrophages, and in NK cells. Complementary DNAs were prepared from mRNAs derived from activated murine T-cell clones and IL-4 (MCGF-2, TCGF-2)-cDNA identified by expression vector systems. The IL-4 cDNAs so isolated contained an open reading frame sufficient to code for 140 amino acids. The first 20 N-terminal amino acids are mainly hydrophobic and probably comprise a signal sequence. The deduced amino acid sequence of mature IL-4 (MW 14 137) contains six cysteines, which are believed to be all involved in the formation of three intrachain disulphide bridges, and three potential N-linked glycosylation sites. Since the molecular weight of murine IL-4 derived from transfected monkey COS cells appears to be *c.* 20 000, substantial glycosylation is likely to be a feature of IL-4 produced by activated T-lymphocytes. More recently, human IL-4 has been cloned and the deduced amino acid sequence shown to be ~50 per cent homologous to murine IL-4. However, the human IL-4 precursor polypeptide chain is longer at 153 amino acids than that of the murine homologue; it is thought that this precursor contains a 24 amino acid N-terminal signal sequence and a 129 residue mature IL-4 protein sequence. The latter has three disulphide bridges, in approximately the same positions as in murine IL-4, and two potential N-linked glycosylation sites. While human IL-4 is likely therefore to be highly glycosylated (MW 25 000), non-glycosylated IL-4 produced in *E.coli* is also biologically active. Nevertheless, human and murine IL-4 are sufficiently molecularly distinct for them to be essentially species-specific, i.e. human IL-4 is not active in mouse cells and vice versa. Comparison of the IL-4 amino acid sequence with those of known proteins has indicated that IL-4 shares some significant but rather limited homology with GM-CSF and IFNγ, suggesting a remote phylogenetic relationship of these cytokines. Rather interestingly, the genes coding for IL-4, GM-CSF, and IFNγ share a similar four exon–three intron organization and IL-4- and GM-CSF-genes are closely linked on human chromosome 5 (murine chromosome 11).

As expected, receptors for the pleiotropic IL-4 molecule are widely distributed among lymphoid and myeloid cells such as B-cells, T-cells, macrophages, mast cells, etc. The number of receptors present in resting B- or T-cells has been estimated to be of the order of a few hundred per cell. However, following polyclonal stimulation, e.g. with anti-IgM or ConA, the number of IL-4R increases four- to eightfold. IL-4R are also expressed in several lymphoblastoid, e.g. Burkitt's lymphomas, and leukaemic cell lines with an average of around 1000 receptors per cell. IL-4R has been shown to be totally specific for IL-4, i.e. no other cytokines bind to it. Further, murine IL-4 competes very poorly with human IL-4 for binding to human IL-4R, which is in line with the lack of cross-species biological activity between human and murine IL-4. Only high-affinity binding sites (dissociation constant, $K_d = 5 \times 10^{-11}$M) have been demonstrated and chemical cross-linking experiments with ^{125}I-IL-4 have revealed the presence of a single putative 55–60 kDa receptor (glyco-) protein. The details of the structure of IL-4R have just become available, but the mechanism of signal transduction remains obscure. However, it has been shown that murine IL-4 binding to its receptor does not cause phosphoinositol breakdown, intracellular Ca^{2+} mobilization, PKC activation, or plasma membrane depolarization. In contrast, there is some suggestive evidence that human IL-4 induces transient phosphoinositol breakdown, Ca^{2+} mobilization and cyclic AMP formation. Phosphorylation of plasma membrane proteins, in particular an unidentified 42 kDa protein, has been demonstrated in IL-4 stimulated mouse B-cells. Rather interesting, IFNγ has been shown to inhibit IL-4 mediated B-cell-activation and production of IgE, although IFNγ does not interfere with IL-4 binding to its receptors. In contrast, IL-4 appears to block the stimulatory effects of IL-2 in LAK cells, although in other circumstances IL-4 may synergize with the actions of IL-2. Such observations possibly suggest interactions between IL-4R and the receptors of other cytokines, e.g. cross-modulation in receptor functionality or numbers.

Interleukin-6

Originally, the molecule that was eventually to become IL-6 was discovered and characterized in completely different circumstances to those when it was 're-discovered' to be a B-cell stimulating factor. In the early 1980s, a cytokine secreted by polyinosinic polycytidylic acid (poly I:C)-induced human diploid fibroblasts was first described as an interferon. Messenger RNA for this cytokine coded for a 26 kDa protein which came to be known as interferon beta-2 (IFNβ2). The latter had very low to non-existent antiviral activity in comparison to other cloned IFNs and thus has since been the subject of a debate as to whether it should be designated an IFN at all. It has subsequently been molecularly cloned and shown to have very little sequence homology with any of the known IFN types.

At about the same time, in a completely different setting where the biological characteristics of T-cell replacing factors (TRF), i.e. factors that would replace the presence of T-cells for the proliferation and differentiation of B-cells, was being investigated, it was found that medium conditioned by PHA-activated T cells contained a B-cell differentiation factor (BCDF). In the presence of this BCDF, the human B-lymphoblastoid cell line, CESS, was induced to secrete Ig at a high rate, characteristic of terminally differentiated B-cells (also known as plasma cells). The BCDF was produced in small quantities by activated T-cells, but subsequently it was shown that T-cell hybridomas and an HTLV-1-transformed T-cell line also produced this cytokine in relatively large amounts. Therefore, BCDF was purified from the supernatant culture fluids of the HTLV-1-transformed T-cell line and, following its purification to homogeneity, the N-terminal amino acid sequence determined. Since the purified cytokine had potent IgG and IgM secretion-inducing activity, a nomenclature committee in 1983 renamed it BSF-2. Further amino acid sequence determinations and the construction of the oligonucleotide probes corresponding to BSF-2 subpeptides led to its molecular cloning in 1986. At first it was thought that the BSF-2 cDNA encoded a novel cytokine, but it was quickly realized from comparing its amino acid sequence with other known proteins that it was identical to IFNβ2. The subsequent demonstration that BSF-2/IFNβ2 is a pleiotropic cytokine and can mediate different responses in different cell types, e.g. it induces the production of acute-phase proteins in liver hepatocytes, led to it being called IL-6 by some researchers. This designation has now been generally accepted.

Human IL-6 cDNA from both the IFNβ2 and BSF-2 cloning studies codes for a precursor polypeptide of 212 amino acids which is processed by cleavage of a 28 amino acid N-terminal signal sequence into a mature form of 184 amino acids (see Figure 6.1, Chapter 6). The amino acid sequence of mature

IL-6 predicts two potential N-linked glycosylation sites and two potential intrachain disulphide bridges. IL-6 shows no significant homology with other known proteins except G-CSF where, in particular, the positions of the four cysteine residues are conserved between the two cytokines, suggesting that their tertiary structures may be similar. Additionally, it has been shown that the structure of the IL-6 gene, on the basis of exon–intron organization, is extraordinarily similar to that of the G-CSF gene, suggesting that these two genes arose from a common ancestral gene. Both genes consist of five exons and four introns, but the IL-6 gene is located on human chromosome 7 whereas the G-CSF gene is on chromosome 17. Murine IL-6, which has only been cloned more recently, has 187 amino acids (MW = 21 710) which are preceded by a 24 amino acid N-terminal signal sequence in the precursor form, and shows 42 per cent overall homology with human IL-6. The murine IL-6 sequence predicts no N-linked glycosylation sites, but there are several possible O-linked glycosylation sites. The murine IL-6 gene has been located to mouse chromosome 5.

Both human and mouse IL-6 have been shown to be produced by several cell types, including T-lymphocytes, monocytes, macrophages, fibroblasts, and endothelial cells, either constitutively or in response to many different stimuli. The latter include viruses, bacterial components such as LPS, double-stranded RNA such as poly I:C, mitogens, other cytokines such as IL-1, and second-messenger agonists such as phorbolesters, cAMP analogues, etc. As has been mentioned it is not simply a B-cell stimulating factor, but has

Table 4.1   Biological activities of IL-6

Terminal B-cell differentiation and stimulation of IgG production

Hybridoma/plastocytoma growth factor

Growth factor for:
  B-cells transformed with EBV (low cell density only)
  Myeloma cells
  Lennert's lymphoma-derived T-cell line

Co-stimulant (second signal) for:
  IL-2 production by mature T-cells
  Proliferation of thymocytes
  IL-3-dependent proliferation of multipotential haemopoietic cells
  Proliferation of myeloid leukaemic blast cells

Hepatocyte stimulating factor; inducer of acute-phase protein production

Inducer of ACTH secretion

Mediator of fever in rabbits

Differentiation factor for CTL

wide-ranging activities in many different cell types and is probably a mediator of inflammatory responses (Table 4.1, see also Chapter 5). Besides acting as a differentiation inducer, one of its main activities appears to be as a growth factor for many B-cell hybridomas cultured *in vitro*. It may also be involved in the autocrine stimulation of proliferation of myelomas (see Chapter 3, Section 3.4, p. 96) and possibly of B-cell lymphomas. Thus again there is evidence of a particular cytokine being involved in the leukaemogenic process: IL-1, IL-2, IL-3, IL-4, GM-CSF, and M-CSF have all been implicated in contributing to autostimulatory mechanisms leading to particular leukaemias.

The wide variety of cell types acted on by IL-6 indicates that receptors for this cytokine are widely distributed. In common with the receptors for other ILs which are expressed only at low levels in resting lymphocytes, IL-6R were not found to be present in resting, normal B-lymphocytes. However, activated B-cells have been demonstrated to express IL-6R with a K_d of 3–5 $\times$ 10^{-10}M. The highest number of IL-6R have been found in human myeloma cell lines, e.g. U266, which have around 10 000 high-affinity receptors per cell. B-lymphoblastoid cell lines also express high numbers of IL-6R whereas, in marked contrast, Burkitt's lymphomas, which express IL-4R, do not generally express IL-6R. Both glycosylated (MW $\sim$ 26 000) and non-glycosylated (MW 21 000) human IL-6 bind to IL-6R and stimulate cell responses, and thus the function of oligosaccharide side chains remains obscure. Possibly the latter increase the stability of IL-6, although it has been recently shown that IL-6 binds to α_2-macroglobulin which, acting as a carrier protein, may also serve to protect IL-6 from degradative proteases present in plasma.

The structure of IL-6R was until recently unknown. Chemical cross-linking experiments with ^{125}I-IL-6 had suggested the presence of a two-subunit receptor, perhaps similar to the probably heterodimeric IL-2R (a similar two-chain model has also been suggested for NGF-R and IL-3R). However, such is the power of modern rDNA cloning techniques that it has been possible to isolate a cDNA encoding IL-6R, or a major component thereof. In this case, a cDNA library was prepared from a human NK-like cell line, YT, which contains high levels of IL-6R and IL-6R mRNA, and plasmid-linked cDNA expressed in monkey COS cells. Clones of transfected cells expressing IL-6R were identified with biotinylated-rhIL-6 and fluorescein-conjugated avidin (FITC-A) and subsequently IL-6R cDNA isolated. A full-length IL-6R cDNA has been shown to encode a polypeptide chain of 467 amino acids of which, on the basis of a hydropathy plot, the first 19 hydrophobic amino acids probably form a signal sequence and the 28 hydrophobic amino acids between residues 359 and 386 form a transmembrane segment (see Figure 7.2, Chapter 7). There are five potential N-linked glycosylation sites in the N-terminal extracellular domain and, by comparison of the predicted amino acid sequence of this domain with those of other known proteins, there is significant homology with several members of the Ig superfamily, including the Ig light-chain variable region, the CD4 molecule, and alpha-1-β-glycoprotein. It is likely that IL-6R belongs to a subset of the Ig superfamily which includes several adhesion molecules, PDGF-R, M-CSF-R (c-FMS), and IL-1R. Unlike PDGF-R and M-CSF-R, but like IL-1R, it does not contain an intracellular tyrosine kinase domain. Other cytokine and hormone receptors in different structural categories, e.g. IL-2Rα (Tac), NGF-R, and growth hormone receptor, also lack a tyrosine kinase domain. (It is not known if other components of these receptors have tyrosine kinase domains.) The mechanism of signal transduction by IL-6R remains unknown, but probably will be different to that of tyrosine kinase receptors. Similar to IL-4, IL-6 stimulation did not increase

1 inositol phospholipid turnover,
2 intracellular Ca^{2+} mobilization or
3 PKC activity,

indicating that IL-6 mediates growth and differentiation responses by an alternative, but as yet unknown, biochemical pathway.

Interleukin-7

In addition to cytokines that mediate activation and differentiation of mature B-cells, it is clear that there must be some that mediate the proliferation and differentiation of B-cell progenitors and precursors. The earliest identified cells in the B-cell lineage are those which contain the immunoglobulin heavy- and light-chain genes in the germline configuration. These committed B-cell progenitors, also known as pro-B-cells, are present in the bone marrow and appear to respond to stimuli elaborated by bone marrow stromal cells. Indeed, murine bone marrow stromal cells have been shown to support the proliferation of pro-B-cells *in vitro*. Recently (1988), by transforming murine bone marrow stromal cells with viral (SV40) DNA, a transformed stromal cell line (IXN/A6) was isolated that constitutively produced a factor capable of supporting pro-B-cells in culture. Subsequently, a cDNA library was prepared from the mRNA derived from IXN/A6 and transfected into monkey COS cells to yield factor-expressing cells. This enabled the molecular cloning of cDNA encoding this factor, now designated IL-7, to take place and the determination of its primary amino acid sequence.

Murine IL-7 cDNA encodes a 25 amino acid signal sequence, followed by a 129 amino acid mature IL-7 protein (MW 14900). The predicted amino acid sequence contains two potential N-linked glycosylation sites, the glycosylation of which accounts for the higher molecular weight of 25000 found for IL-7 produced by IXN/A6 cells. There are also six cysteine residues, some or all of which may be involved in disulphide bridge formation.

Using the murine IL-7 cDNA as a hybridization probe, a cDNA encoding biological active human IL-7 has recently been isolated. Comparison of the predicted amino acid sequence of human IL-7 with that of murine IL-7 indicates that, although the signal sequence lengths are identical (25 amino acids), the mature form of human IL-7 is longer at 152 amino acids than murine IL7 (129 amino acids) and this is mainly due to an insertion of 19

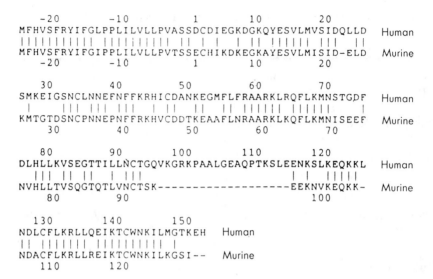

Figure 4.6 Alignment of amino acid sequences (single-letter code) encoded by human and murine IL-7 cDNAs. Reprinted from Goodwin *et al.*, 1989, with permission of the authors.

amino acids (residues 96–114) in human IL-7 (Figure 4.6). However, human and murine IL-7 show a strong degree of homology (*c.* 60 per cent) and the six cysteine residues are all conserved. Human IL-7 is active in both human and mouse pro-B-cells, being apparently more active in the murine assay system. On the other hand, murine IL-7 appears only to be active in mouse pro-B-cells.

The full spectrum of biological activities of IL-7 has yet to be elucidated. However, it is already apparent that, in common with the majority of cytokines, it is pleiotropic. For instance, recombinant IL-7 has very recently been demonstrated to have co-stimulatory activity on purified mature T-cells. IL-7 was found to synergize with conA stimulation of purified murine T-cells to increase IL-2/IL-2R production and proliferation, and thus may be similar to IL-1 and IL-6 in this respect. Clearly, receptors for IL-7 are not limited to the B-cell lineage and it will be interesting to learn whether non-lymphoid cells bear receptors and respond to this novel cytokine.

A summary of the molecular properties of the cytokines and receptors covered in this chapter is given in Table 4.2.

4.5   B-cell development

The initial stages of commitment from pluripotential haemopoietic stem cells to the B-cell lineage takes place in the bone marrow. The nature of these events and the molecular mechanisms underlying them are as yet unknown. The first identifiable cells of the B-cell lineage are progenitor B-cells (pro-B-

Table 4.2 Molecular characteristics of human interleukins and their receptors

Cytokine	Precursor (aa)	Mature protein (aa)	Glycosylation	Disulphide bonds	Chromosome assignment of gene	Receptors
IL-1α	271	159 (17.5 kDa)	—	0	unknown	80 kDa glycoprotein, non-tyrosine kinase
IL-1β	269	153 (17.5 kDa)	—	1	2	Ig-superfamily member (cloned)
IL-2	153	133 (15.5 kDa)	O-linked	1	4	55 kDa Tac antigen: p70 heterodimer (see Section 7.4.3) (both subunits cloned)
IL-4	154	129 (25 kDa)	N-linked	3	5	55–60 kDa glycoprotein (no details)
IL-6	212	184 (26 kDa)	N-linked	2	7	80 kDa glycoprotein, non-tyrosine kinase, Ig-superfamily member (cloned)
IL-7	177	152	N-linked	3	8	unknown

Development and activation of B-lymphocytes

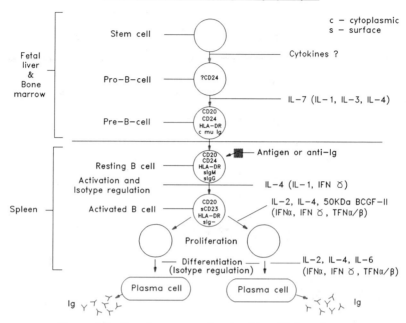

Figure 4.7   Development and activation of B-lymphocytes.

cells) in which the immunoglobulin genes are in the germ line configuration. In the mouse, pro-B-cells are recognized by the expression of a surface marker known as B220. The equivalent marker in human pro-B-cells may be the CD24 antigen, but this has not been clearly defined. Nevertheless, similar to T-cell ontological development, B-cell development progresses through a series of stages characterized by the expression of specific cell surface antigenic determinants and the appearance of different Ig isotypes. Thus, pro-B-cells proliferate and differentiate into precursor-B-cells (pre-B-cells) which are identified by the coexpression of MHC class II antigens and B220/CD24 and the presence of cytoplasmic μ Ig chain. Pre-B-cells then progress to the so-called immature B-cell stage in which cells express surface IgM and synthesize ϰ and λ Ig light chains. The latter may also express other recognizable cell surface molecules such as IgD and CD20 antigen. Subsequently, immature B-cells migrate from the bone marrow to secondary lymphoid organs such as the spleen where they undergo further Ig isotype switching, giving rise to B-cell subsets expressing surface IgM and another class, or either IgG, IgA, or IgE alone. Once this stage has been reached, B-cell clones may be activated by their specific cognate antigens to proliferate and differentiate into mature Ig-secreting B-cells known as plasma cells (Figure 4.7). This is necessarily a rather simplistic account of B-cell development and readers should refer to standard immunology textbooks for more details.

The involvement of cytokines in B-cell differentiation is a complex one, with each cytokine performing different functions depending on the stage of development of their 'target' B-cell. However, teleologically there should be some order in the 'use' of cytokines to effect normal B-cell development. For instance, although the full range of activities of IL-7 is yet to be delineated, IL-7, a bone marrow stromal cell product, appears to be a prime candidate for stimulating the proliferation and differentiation of pro-B-cells. It is tempting to speculate that IL-7 may perform this function in normal steady-state haemopoietic processes, while other T-cell- and monocyte-derived cytokines such as IL-1, IL-3, and IL-4 augment proliferative and differentiating responses during episodes of host infection with micro-organisms. It is clear that any of the above cytokines can act on pro- and pre-B-cells. For example, IL-4 has been demonstrated to induce human pro-B-cells to synthesize cytoplasmic μ Ig chains and induce cytoplasmic μ chain-positive pre-B-cells to express surface Ig. (In contrast, IL-4 has been shown to antagonize the proliferative effects of haemopoietic growth factors, e.g. M-CSF, on myeloid cell precursors.) In most investigations reported, cytokines such as IL-4 act as co-stimulants or competence factors, and do not as a rule individually trigger proliferation. For early B-cell proliferation, the nature of the proliferation-inducing stimuli remains obscure. However, once B-cells acquire surface Ig they are then able to respond to antigenic stimulation or molecules that cross-link surface Ig or other cell-surface antigens.

Rather more is known about activation, proliferation, and differentiation of resting, surface-Ig positive, B-cells regarding the actions of particular cytokines, although it should be remembered that this information is largely derived from *in vitro* studies with isolated, purified B-cells, which may or may not be relevant to the situation *in vivo*. The first step in B-cell activation is occasioned by the binding of antigen to surface 'receptor' Ig, or by molecules which mimic this, which trigger increased

1   inositol phospholipid turnover,
2   intracellular Ca^{2+} mobilization and
3   PKC activity,

leading, by unknown signalling pathways and response elements, to early nuclear gene induction events. IL-4 may also independently activate resting B-cells by an alternative pathway probably involving protein phosphorylation, which may involve the phosphoinositide – Ca^{2+} – PKC activation system. IL-4 stimulation results in increased expression of a number of cell-surface molecules, e.g. MHC class II, CD23, and surface IgM. In murine but not in human-B-cells, IL-5 (see Chapter 3 for details of molecular characterization) may also provide an activation signal leading in this case to induction of the expression of IL-2R. The function of murine IL-5 in this respect may in human B-cells be the property of an as yet not fully characterized 50 kDa human B-cell growth factor-II (BCGF-II). It should be noted that activation by antigen or IL-4, or murine IL-5/human 50 kDa BCGF-II, results in transition of resting B-cells from G_0 to G_1, but without further stimulation does not lead to proliferation.

In order to obtain a proliferative response two separate signals are necessary. This may be achieved, at least *in vitro*, by combining antigenic (or mitogenic) stimulation with either IL-4 or murine IL-5/human 50 kDa BCGF-II. Other cytokines such as IL-1, TNF, IFNγ, and a recently cloned human low-molecular-weight BCGF may also act as co-stimulants for proliferation (Figure 4.7). It appears possible that proliferation induced by co-stimulation with IL-4 on the one hand and by co-stimulation with murine IL-5/human 50 kDa BCGF-II on the other might lead B-cells to differentiate along separate pathways, perhaps involving isotype switching. Murine IL-5/human 50 kDa BCGF-II induce IL-2R (Tac) and responsiveness to IL-2, whereas IL-4 co-stimulation does not. IL-4 also antagonizes IL-2-mediated B-cell proliferation. While it is widely believed that T-cells and monocytes provide the major stimulatory cytokines for B-cells, it is becoming apparent that B-cells themselves are also capable of producing some mediators to which they also respond. For instance, CD23 antigen, a B-cell plasma membrane 45 kDa glycoprotein with low-affinity receptor activity for IgE, can be proteolytically released from the B-cell surface to yield a soluble 25 kDa CD23 and this has been claimed to be a progression factor or BCGF for B-cell proliferation.

Apart from acting as co-stimulants for B-cell proliferation, a major role of several cytokines is in B-cell differentiation (Figure 4.7). One of the facets of B-cell maturation is Ig isotype switching and at least three cytokines, IL-4, IL-5, and IFNγ have been implicated as 'switch factors' for murine B-cells. For example, IL-4 stimulation causes B-cells to undergo an Ig class switch from IgM to IgG in the absence of proliferation and enhances IgG production. Following a period of proliferation and differentiation, mature B-cells, responding to high doses of IL-4, switch on IgE synthesis. In human B-cells cultured *in vitro*, IL-4 appears to be directly responsible for inducing IgE synthesis. Both IgG and IgE production stimulated by IL-4 was repressed in the presence of IFNγ. Terminal differentiation of B-cells into Ig-secreting plasma cells appears also to be up-regulated by IL-6.

The precise details of the autocrine and paracrine stimulatory actions of cytokines on B-cells are yet to be fully elucidated. 'Fine-tuning' within such a regulatory network probably will depend in part upon a temporally ordered sequence of cytokine-mediated events, involving autocrine and paracrine mechanisms, and their interactions with one another. *In vivo*, particular tissues and organs probably provide unique micro-environments, which could also control B-cell development, and which would be difficult or impossible to reproduce *in vitro*. Thus, understanding in this area may be restricted to knowledge evinced from B-cells 'dissected' from their natural environment and the actions and interactions of various cytokines in artificially maintained cultures. Nevertheless, it is to be hoped such knowledge on the selective regulation of B-cell responses by cytokines will be of relevance and value to clinical practice, where the therapeutic application of cytokines in diseases of B-cell dysfunction, such as allergy and autoimmunity, is already indicated.

Further reading

General

Adkins, B., Mueller, C., Okada, C.Y., *et al.* (1987) Early events in T-cell maturation. *Annual Reviews of Immunology* **5**, 325.

Fowlkes, B.J. and Pardoll, D.M. (1989) Molecular and cellular events in T cell development, in *Advances in Immunology* **44** (Dixon, F.J. ed.) Academic Press, San Diego, p. 207.

Hamblin, A.S. (1988) *Lymphokines.* In Focus Series (Male, D. ed.). IRL Press, Oxford.

Male, D., Champion, B. and Cooke, A. (1987) *Advanced Immunology.* Gower Medical Publishing, London. Chapters 4 and 11.

Roitt, I., Brostoff, J., and Male, D. (1985) *Immunology.* Gower Medical Publishing, London.

Schulof, R.S. (1985) Thymic peptide hormones: basic properties and clinical application in cancer. *CRC Critical Reviews on Oncology and Haematology* **3**, 309.

Von Boehmer, H. (1988) The developmental biology of T-lymphocytes. *Annual Reviews of Immunology* **6**, 309.

Interleukin-1

Akahoshi, T., Oppenheim, J.J., and Matsushima, K. (1988) Interleukin-1 stimulates its own receptor expression on human fibroblasts through the endogenous production of prostaglandins. *Journal of Clinical Investigation* **82**, 1219.

Antoni, G., Presentini, R., Perin, F., *et al.* (1986) Short synthetic peptide fragment of human interleukin-1 with immunostimulatory but not inflammatory activity. *Journal of Immunology* **137**, 3201.

Bensi, G., Raugei, G., Palla, E., *et al.* (1987) Human interleukin-1 beta gene. *Gene* **52**, 95.

Beuscher, H.U. and Colten, H.R. (1988) Structure and function of membrane IL-1. *Molecular Immunology* **25**, 1189.

Bird, T.A., Gearing, A.J.H., and Saklatvala, J. (1988) Murine interleukin-1 receptor: direct identification by ligand blotting and purification to homogeneity of an interleukin-1 binding glycoprotein. *Journal of Biological Chemistry* **263**, 12063.

Bonin, P.D. and Singh, J.P. (1988) Modulation of interleukin-1 receptor expression and interleukin-1 response in fibroblasts by platelet-derived growth factor. *Journal of Biological Chemistry* **263**, 11052.

Bron, C. and MacDonald, H.R. (1987) Identification of the plasma membrane receptor for interleukin-1 on mouse thymoma cells. *FEBS Letters* **219**, 365.

Bursten, S.L., Locksley, R.M., Ryan, J.L., and Lovett, D.H. (1988) Acylation of monocyte and glomerular mesangial cell proteins; myristyl acylation of the interleukin-1 precursors. *Journal of Clinical Investigation* **82**, 1479.

Cameron, P.M., Guadalupe, A., Limjuco, J.C., *et al.* (1986) Purification to homogeneity and amino acid sequence analysis of two anionic species of human interleukin-1. *Journal of Experimental Medicine* **164**, 237.

Colotta, F., Lampugnani, M.G., Polentarutti, N., *et al.* (1988) Interleukin-1 induces c-*fos* protooncogene expression in cultured human endothelial cells. *Biochemical and Biophysical Research Communications* **152**, 1104.

Craig, S., Schmeissner, U., Wingfield, P., and Pain, R.H. (1987) Conformation, stability and folding of interleukin-1β. *Biochemistry* **26**, 3570.

Didier, M., Aussel, C., Pelassy, C., and Fehlmann, M. (1988) IL-1 signalling for IL-2 production in T-cells involves a rise in phosphatidylserine synthesis. *Journal of*

Immunology **141**, 3078.
Dinarello, C.A. (1984) Interleukin-1. *Reviews of Infectious Diseases* **6**, 51.
Dinarello, C.A. (1989) Interleukin-1 and its biologically related cytokines. In *Advances in Immunology* **44** (Dixon, F.J. cd.) Academic Press, San Diego, p. 153.
Dinarello, C.A., Clark, B.D., Puren, A.J., *et al.* (1989) The interleukin-1 receptor. *Immunology Today* **10**, 49.
Forni, G., Musso, T., Jemma, C., *et al.* (1988) Lymphokine-activated tumour inhibition in mice: ability of a nonapeptide of the human IL-1β to recruit anti-tumour reactivity in recipient mice. *Journal of Immunology* **142**, 712.
Fuhlbrigge, R.C., Fine, S.M., Unane, E.R. and Chaplin, D.D. (1988) Expression of membrane interleukin 1 by fibroblasts transfected pro-interleukin-1α cDNA. *Proceedings of the National Academy of Sciences USA* **85**, 5649.
Humes, J.L. and Farrar, W.L. (1985) The role of arachidonic acid metabolism in the activities of interleukin-1 and 2. *Journal of Immunology* **135**, 1153.
Hunkapiller, T. and Hood, L. (1989) Diversity of the immunoglobulin gene superfamily. *Advances in Immunology* **44** (Dixon, F.J. ed.) Academic Press, San Diego, p. 1.
Kovacs, E.J., Oppenheim, J.J., and Young, H.A. (1986) Induction of c-*fos* and c-*myc* expression in T-lymphocytes after treatment with recombinant interleukin-1α. *Journal of Immunology* **137**, 3649.
Martin, M. and Resch, K. (1988) Interleukin-1: more than a mediator between leukocytes. *Trends in Pharmacological Sciences* **9**, 171.
Minnich-Carruth, L.L., Suttles, J. and Mizel, S.B. (1989) Evidence against the existence of a membrane form of murine IL-1. *Journal of Immunology* **142**, 526.
Mizel, S.B. (1987) Interleukin-1 and T-cell activation. *Immunology Today* **8**, 330.
Oppenheim, J.J., Kovacs, E.J., Matsushima, K., and Durum, S.K. (1986) There is more than one interleukin-1. *Immunology Today* **7**, 45.
Priestle, J.P., Schär, H.P., and Grütter, M.G. (1988) Crystal structure of the cytokine interleukin-1β. *The EMBO Journal* **7**, 339.
Shirakawa, F., Yamashita, U., Chedid, M., and Mizel, S.B. (1988) Cyclic AMP — an intracellular second messenger for interleukin-1. *Proceedings of the National Academy of Sciences USA* **85**, 8201.
Sims, J.E., March, C.J., Cosman, D., *et al.* (1988) cDNA expression cloning of the IL-1 receptor, a membrane of the immunoglobulin superfamily. *Science* **241**, 585.
Wijelath, E.S., Kardasz, A.M., Drummond, R., and Watson, J. (1988) Interleukin-one induced inositol phospholipid breakdown in murine macrophages: possible mechanism of receptor activation. *Biochemical and Biophysical Research Communications* **152**, 392.
Williams, A.F. (1987) A year in the life of the immunoglobin superfamily. *Immunology Today* **8**, 298.
Williams, A.F. and Barclay, A.N. (1988) The immunoglobulin superfamily — domains for cell surface recognition. *Annual Reviews of Immunology* **6**, 381.

Interleukin-2

Brandhuber, B.J., Boone, T., Kenney, W.C., and McKay, D.B. (1987) Three-dimensional structure of interleukin-2. *Science* **238**, 1707.
Cohen, F.E., Kosen, P.A., Kuntz, I.D., *et al.* (1986) Structure-activity studies of interleukin-2. *Science* **234**, 349.
Colamonici, O.R., Rosolen, A., Cole, D., *et al.* (1988) Stimulation of the β-subunit of the IL-2 receptor induces MHC-unrestricted cytotoxicity in T acute lymphoblastic leukaemia cells and normal thymocytes. *Journal of Immunology* **141**, 1202.

Collins, L., Tsien, W.H., Seals, C., *et al.* (1988) Identification of specific residues of human interluekin 2 that affect binding to the 70 kDa subunit (p70) of the interleukin 2 receptor. *Proceedings of the National Academy of Sciences USA* **85**, 7709.

Degrave, W., Tavernier, J., Derinck, F., *et al.* (1983) Cloning and structure of the human interleukin-2 chromosomal gene. *The EMBO Journal* **2**, 2349.

Edidin, M., Aszalos, A., Danyanovich, S., and Waldmann, T.A. (1988) Lateral diffusion measurements give evidence for association of the Tac peptide of the IL-2 receptor with the T27 peptide in the plasma membrane of HUT-102-B2 T cells. *Journal of Immunology* **141**, 1206.

Fujita, T., Takaoka, C., Matsui, H. and Taniguchi, T. (1983) Structure of the human interleukin-2 gene. *Proceedings of the National Academy of Sciences USA* **80**, 7437.

Greene, W.C., Wano, Y., and Dukovich, M. (1988) New insights into the structure of high-affinity interleukin-2 receptors. *Recent Progress in Hormone Research* **44** (Clark J.H., ed.) Academic Press, New York.

Hermann, T. and Diamantstein, T. (1988) The high affinity interleukin 2 receptor: evidence for three distinct polypeptides chains comprising the high affinity interleukin 2 receptor. *Molecular Immunology* **25**, 1201.

Leonard, W.J., Depper, J.M., Kanehisa, M., *et al.* (1985) Structure of the human interleukin-2 receptor gene. *Science* **230**, 633.

Möller, G. (ed.) (1986) *IL-2: Receptors and Genes. Immunological Reviews* **92**. Munksgaard, Copenhagen.

Robb, R.J. (1984) Interleukin 2: the molecule and its function. *Immunology Today* **5**, 203.

Siegel, J.P., Sharon, M., Smith, P.L., and Leonard, W.J. (1987) The IL-2 receptor beta chain (p70): role in mediating signals for LAK, NK and proliferative activities. *Science* **238**, 75.

Smith, K.A. (ed.) (1988) *Interleukin-2*. Academic Press, San Diego. Chapters 1, 2, and 3.

Takemoto, J., Murai, Y., and Ide, M. (1988) Monoclonal antibodies which differentiate high- and low-affinity binding sites of interleukin-2. *FEBS Letters* **242**, 53.

T-cell activation, proliferation, and differentiation

Bird, P.R., Freeman, G.J., Wilson, S.D., *et al.* (1987) Cloning and characterization of a novel T cell activation gene. *Journal of Immunology* **139**, 3126.

Cantrell, D.A., Collins, M.K.L., and Crumpton, M.J. (1986) Autocrine regulation of T-lymphocyte proliferation: differential induction of IL-2 and IL-2 receptor. *Immunology* **65**, 343.

Chaudhri, G., Hunt, N.H., Clark, I.A., and Ceredig, R. (1988) Antioxidants inhibit proliferation and cell surface expression of receptors for interleukin-2 and transferrin in T-lymphocytes stimulated with phorbol myristate acetate and ionomycin. *Cellular Immunology* **115**, 204.

Crabtree, G.R. (1989) Contingent genetic regulatory events in T lymphocyte activation. *Science* **243**, 355.

Everson, M.P., Spalding, D.M., and Koopman, W.J. (1989) Enhancement of IL-2-induced T-cell proliferation by a novel factor(s) present in murine spleen dendritic cell-T-cell culture supernatants. *Journal of Immunology* **142**, 1183.

Karasuyama, H., Tohyama, N., and Tada, T. (1989) Autocrine growth and tumorigenicity of interleukin-2-dependent helper T cells transfected with IL-2 gene. *Journal of Experimental Medicine* **169**, 13.

Maizel, A.L. and Lachman, L.B. (1984) Control of human lymphocyte proliferation by soluble factors. *Laboratory Investigation* **50**, 369.

Mizel, S.B. (1987) Interleukin 1 and T-cell activation. *Immunology Today* **8**, 330.

Mizushima, Y., Saitoh, M., Ogata, M., *et al.* (1989) Thymic stroma-derived T cell growth factor (TSTGF). *Journal of Immunology* **142**, 1195.

Shaw, S. (1989) Lymphocyte differentiation: not all in a name. *Nature* **338**, 539.

Shirakawa, F., Tanaka, Y., Oda, S., *et al.* (1989) Autocrine stimulation of interleukin 1 alpha in the growth of adult human T-cell leukaemic cells. *Cancer Research* **49**, 1143.

Smith, K.A. (ed.) (1988) *Interleukin-2*. Academic Press, San Diego. Chapters 1, 6, 7, 9 and 10.

Taniguchi, T. (1988) Regulation of cytokine gene expression. *Annual Reviews of Immunology* **6**, 439.

Thompson, C.B., Lindsten, T., Ledbetter, J.A., *et al.* (1989) CD28 activation pathway regulates the production of multiple T-cell derived lymphokines/cytokines. *Proceedings of the National Academy of Sciences USA* **86**, 1333.

Van Snick, J., Goethals, A., Renauld, J.-C., *et al.* (1989) Cloning and characterization of a cDNA for a new mouse T cell growth factor (p40). *Journal of Experimental Medicine* **169**, 363.

Interleukin-4

Brooks, B. and Rees, R.C. (1988) Human recombinant IL-4 suppresses the induction of human IL-2 induced lymphokine activated killer (LAK) activity. *Clinical and Experimental Immunology* **74**, 162.

Cabrillat, H., Galizzi, J.-P., Djossou, O., *et al.* (1987) High affinity binding of human interleukin-4 to cell lines. *Biochemical and Biophysical Research Communications* **149**, 995.

Fernandez-Botran, R., Sanders, V.M. and Vitelta, E.S. (1989) Interactions between receptors for interleukin-2 and interleukin-4 on lines of helper T-cells (HT-2) and B-lymphoma cells (BCL$_1$). *Journal of Experimental Medicine* **169**, 379.

Gallagher, G., Wilcox, F. and Al-Azzauri, F. (1988) Interleukin-3 and interleukin-4 each strongly inhibit the induction and function of human LAK cells. *Clinical and Experimental Immunology* **74**, 166.

Kishimoto, T. and Hirano, T. (1988) Molecular regulation of B-lymphocyte response. *Annual Reviews of Immunology* **6**, 485.

Möller, G. (ed.) (1988) *IL-4 and IL-5: Biology and Genetics. Immunological Reviews* **102**. Chapters beginning pp. 5, 77, 137, 189.

Mosley, B., Beckmann, M.P., March, C.J. *et al.* (1989) The murine interleukin-4 receptor: molecular cloning and characterisation of secreted and membrane bound forms. *Cell* **59**, 335.

Ohara, J. and Paul, W.E. (1988) Up-regulation of interleukin-4/B-cell stimulatory factor 1 receptor expression. *Proceedings of the National Academy of Sciences USA* **85**, 8221.

Paul, W.E. and Ohara, J. (1987) B-cell stimulatory factor-1/interleukin-4. *Annual Reviews of Immunology* **5**, 429.

Uchiyama, T., Kamio, M., Kodaka, T., *et al.* (1988) Leukemic cells from some adult-T-cell leukemia patients proliferate in response to interleukin-4. *Blood* **72**, 1182.

Umadome, H., Uchiyama, T., Onishi. R., *et al.* (1988) Leukemic cells from a chronic T-lymphocytic leukaemia patient proliferated in response to both interleukin-2 and interleukin-4 without prior stimulation and produced interleukin-2 mRNA with stimulation. *Blood* **72**, 1177.

Interleukin-6

Billiau, A. (1987) Interferon β2 as a promoter of growth and differentiation of B-cells. *Immunology Today* **8**, 84.

Brakenheff, J.P.J., De Groot, E.R., Evers, R.F., *et al.* (1987) Molecular cloning and expression of hybridoma growth factor. *Journal of Immunology* **139**, 4116.

Content, J., De Wit, L., Pierard, D., *et al.* (1982) Secretory proteins induced in human fibroblasts under conditions used for the production of interferon β. *Proceedings of the National Academy of Sciences USA* **79**, 2768.

Gauldie, J., Richards, C., Harnish, D., *et al.* (1987) Interferon β2/B cell stimulatory factor type 2 shares identity with monocyte-derived hepatocyte-stimulating factor and regulates the major acute phase protein response in liver cells. *Proceedings of the National Academy of Sciences USA* **84**, 7251.

Haegeman, G., Content, J., Volekaert, G., *et al.* (1986) Structural analysis of the sequence coding for an inducible 26 kDa protein in human fibroblasts. *European Journal of Biochemistry* **159**, 625.

Hirano, T., Yasukawa, K., Harada, H., *et al.* (1986) Complementary DNA for a novel interleukin (BSF-2) that induces B lymphocytes to produce immunoglobulin. *Nature* **324**, 73.

Hirano, T., Matsuda, T., Hosoi, K., *et al.* (1988) Absence of antiviral activity in recombinant B cell stimulatory factor 2 (BSF-2). *Immunology Letters* **17**, 41.

Ikebuchi, K., Wong, G.G., Clark, S.C., *et al.* (1987) Interleukin 6 enhancement of interleukin-3 dependent proliferation of multi-potential hemopoietic progenitors. *Proceedings of the National Academy of Sciences USA* **84**, 9035.

Kishimoto, T. and Hirano, T. (1988) Molecular regulation of B lymphocyte response. *Annual Reviews of Immunology* **6**, 485.

Lotz, M., Jirik, F., Kabouridis, P., *et al.* (1988) B-cell stimulating factor 2/interleukin-6 is a costimulant for human thymocytes and T lymphocytes. *Journal of Experimental Medicine* **167**, 1253.

Matsuda, T., Hirano, T., Nagasawa, S., *et al.* (1989) Identification of α2-macroglobulin as a carrier for IL-6. *Journal of Immunology* **142**, 148.

Mock, B.A., Nordan, R.P., Justice, M.J., *et al.* (1989) The murine IL-6 gene maps to the proximal region of chromosome 5. *Journal of Immunology* **142**, 1372.

Muraguchi, A., Hirano, T., Tang, B., *et al.* (1988) The essential role of B-cell stimulatory factor 2 (BSF-2/IL-6) for the terminal differentiation of B-cells. *Journal of Experimental Medicine* **167**, 332.

Ray, A., Tatter, S.B., May, L.T., and Sehgal, P.B. (1988) Activation of the human β2-interferon/hepatocyte stimulating factor/interleukin 6 promoter by cytokines, viruses and second messenger agonists. *Proceedings of the National Academy of Sciences USA* **85**, 6701.

Sehgal, P.B., May, L.T., Tamm, I., and Vilcek, J. (1987) Human β2 interferon and B-cell differentiation factor BSF-2 are identical. *Science* **235**, 731.

Shimizu, S., Hirano, T., Yoshioka, R., *et al.* (1988) Interleukin-6 (B-cell stimulatory factor 2) dependent growth of a Lennerts lymphoma-derived T-cell line (KT-3). *Blood* **72**, 1826.

Takai, Y., Wong, G.G., Clark, S.C., *et al.* (1988) B cell stimulatory factor-2 is involved in the differentiation of cytotoxic T lymphocytes. *Journal of Immunology* **140**, 508.

Van Snick, J., Cayphas, S., Szikora, J.-P., *et al.* (1988) cDNA cloning of murine interleukin-HP1: homology with human interleukin-6. *European Journal of Immunology* **18**, 193.

Weissenbach, J., Chernajovsky, Y., Zeevi, M, *et al.* (1980) Two interferon mRNAs in human fibroblasts: *in vitro* translation and *Escherichia coli* cloning studies.

Proceedings of the National Academy of Sciences USA **79**, 2768.

Wong, G.C. and Clark, S.C. (1988) Multiple actions of interleukin-6 within a cytokine network. *Immunology Today* **9**, 137.

Yamasaki, K., Taga, T., Hirata, Y., *et al.* (1988) Cloning and expression of the human interleukin-6 (BSF-2/IFNβ2) receptor. *Science* **241**, 825.

Zilberstein, A., Ruggieri, R., Korn, J.H., and Revel, M. (1986) Structure and expression of cDNA and genes for human interferon-beta-2, a distinct species inducible by growth stimulatory cytokines. *The EMBO Journal* **5**, 2529.

Interleukin-7

Goodwin, R.G., Lupton, S., Schmierer, A., *et al.* (1989) Human interleukin-7: molecular cloning and growth factor activity on human and murine B-lineage cells. *Proceedings of the National Academy of Sciences USA* **86**, 302.

Morrissey, P.J., Goodwin, R.G., Nordan, R.P., *et al.* (1989) Recombinant interleukin-7, pre-B cell growth factor, has costimulatory activity on purified mature T-cells. *Journal of Experimental Medicine* **169**, 707.

Namen, A.E., Lupton, S., Hjerrild, K., *et al.* (1988) Stimulation of B-cell progenitors by cloned murine interleukin-7. *Nature* **333**, 571.

Namen, A.E., Schmierer, A.E., March, C.J., *et al.* (1988) B-cell precursor growth-promoting activity: purification and characterization of a growth factor active on lymphocyte precursors. *Journal of Experimental Medicine* **167**, 988.

B-cell development

Callard, R.E. (1989) Cytokine regulation of B-cell growth and differentiation, in *Growth Factors: British Medical Bulletin* **45**(2) (Waterfield, M.D., ed.). Churchill Livingstone, New York p. 371.

Cambier, J.C. and Ransom, J.T. (1987) Molecular mechanisms of transmembrane signalling in B lymphocytes. *Annual Reviews of Immunology* **5**, 175.

Defrance, T., Vandervliet, B., Aubrey, J.-P., and Banchereau, J. (1988) Interleukin 4 inhibits the proliferation but not the differentiation of activated human B cells in response to interleukin-2. *Journal of Experimental Medicine* **168**, 1321.

Defrance, T., Vandervliet, B., Pène, J., and Banchereau, J. (1988) Human recombinant IL-4 induces activated B lymphocytes to produce IgG and IgM. *Journal of Immunology* **141**, 2000.

Delespesse, G., Sarfati, M., and Peleman, R. (1988) Influence of recombinant IL-4, IFN-α and IFN-γ on the production of human IgE-binding factor (soluble CD23). *Journal of Immunology* **142**, 134.

Gordon, J., Cairns, J.A., Millsum, M.J., *et al.* (1988) Interleukin 4 and soluble CD23 as progression factors for human B lymphocytes: analysis of their interactions with agonists of the phosphoinositide 'dual pathway' of signalling. *European Journal of Immunology* **18**, 1561.

Hofman, F.M., Brock, M., Taylor, C.R., and Lyons, B. (1988) IL-4 regulates differentiation and proliferation of human precursor B cells. *Journal of Immunology* **141**, 1185.

Kawano, M., Matsushima, K., Masuda, A., and Oppenheim, J.J. (1988) A major 50-kDa human B-cell growth factor-II induces both Tac antigen expression and proliferation by several types of lymphocytes. *Cellular Immunology* **111**, 273–286.

Kincade, P.W. (1987) Experimental models for understanding B lymphocyte formation. *Advances in Immunology* **41** (Dixon, F.J., ed.) Academic Press, San Diego, p. 181.

Kincade, P.W., Lee, G., Pietrangeli, C.E., *et al.* (1989) Cells and molecules that regulate B lymphopoiesis in bone marrow. *Annual Review of Immunology* **7**, 111–143.

Lebman, D.A. and Coffman, R.L. (1988) Interleukin-4 causes isotype switching to IgE in T-cell-stimulated clonal B cell cultures. *Journal of Experimental Medicine* **168**, 853.

Möller, G. (ed.) (1988) *IL-4 and IL-5: Biology and Genetics. Immunological Reviews* **102**. Munksgaard, Copenhagen.

Pène, J., Rousset, F., Brière, F., *et al.* (1988) IgE production by normal human lymphocytes is induced by interleukin 4 and suppressed by interferons γ and α and prostaglandin E_2. *Proceedings of the National Academy of Sciences USA* **85**, 6880.

Romagnani, S., Giudizi, M.G., Biaglotti, R., *et al.* (1986) B cell growth factor activity of interferon-γ: recombinant interferon-γ promotes proliferation of anti-μ-activated human B lymphocytes. *Journal of Immunology* **136**, 3513.

Roth, C., Moreau, J.-L., Korner, M., *et al.* (1988) Biochemical characterization and biological effects of partially purified B cell-activating factor (BCAF). *European Journal of Immunology* **18**, 577.

Sharma, S., Mehta, S., Morgan, J. and Maizel, A. (1987) Molecular cloning and expression of a human B-cell growth factor gene in *Escherichia coli. Science* **235**, 1489.

Vazquez, A., Mills, S., and Maizel, A. (1989) Modulation of IL-2 induced human B-cell proliferation in the presence of human 50 kDa B-cell growth factor and IL-4. *Journal of Immunology* **142**, 94.

5

Mediators of immune responses and inflammatory reactions

5.1 Introduction

From the previous chapter, it is clear that there are a number of cytokines, principally interleukins, which are probably involved in lymphocyte activation, proliferation and differentiation. Obviously, the up-regulation of the immunological functions of lymphocytes and their clonal expansion in response to antigen are central to the immune response. Therefore, while 'new' cytokines will be included in this chapter, it is inevitable that discussion of immune responses will have to include some of these cytokines, for instance IL-1, IL-2, and IL-6, previously cited as being involved in lymphocyte regulation. Moreover, cytokines such as IL-1 and IL-6 are known to have, or are linked to, several different biological effects and importantly are implicated as mediators of inflammatory reactions, the second topic of this chapter. Thus, the following cytokines are considered here: IL-1, IL-6, IL-8, IFNγ, TNFα/β. What these all have in common is that besides having activities in myeloid and lymphoid cells, they are active in many, if not all, cell types outside of the immune system. In addition, the immunosuppressive activity of TGFβ will be discussed.

5.2 Immunoregulatory and inflammatory cytokines

Interferons: origins and nomenclature

The name interferon (IFN) was given to a substance, isolated by Isaacs and Lindemann in 1957, that protected cells against viral infection. IFN was produced in very small quantities by virus-infected cells, and early research

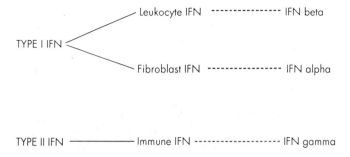

Figure 5.1   Classification of interferons.

was hampered by the low availability of purified IFN. It was not until the late 1970s, when genetic manipulation methods led to the expression in large quantities of human proteins in bacteria, that intensive research into the biological actions of IFN and their clinical application was possible. Even 30 years or more after its discovery, the complexity of the IFN system is still being unravelled.

Before the advent of gene cloning, it had long been recognized from physico-chemical and antigenic studies that there was more than one type of IFN. From the early 1960s, different types of IFN were named according to their cell source, e.g. fibroblast IFN, leukocyte IFN. Also depending on the type of stimulus applied to induce IFN synthesis, e.g. viral or antigenic, and the acid-lability of the IFNs so induced, IFNs were classified as type I and type II. Thus, type I IFNs included virally induced fibroblast and leukocyte IFN whose activity was resistant to acid (pH 2), whereas type II IFN, also referred to as immune IFN, was acid-labile IFN produced by lymphocytes following antigenic or mitogenic stimulation. In 1978, an international nomenclature committee introduced an alternative system of IFN designation based on the letters of the Greek alphabet. Leukocyte IFN became IFNα, fibroblast IFN became IFNβ, and type II (immune) IFN became IFNγ. (Figure 5.1) This system is now universally accepted. IFNα and IFNβ are known to have immunoregulatory or immunomodulatory activities, but their molecular characterization and most aspects of their biology will be covered in the next chapter. The present chapter is be mainly concerned with IFNγ but, where relevant, a comparison of the immunoregulatory activities of IFNγ and IFNα/β will be given.

Interferon gamma

In the late 1960s, it was discovered that lymphocytes can produce an IFN species, IFNγ, in response to stimulation with plant lectins such as PHA or conA, which act as mitogens. The antiviral activity of this IFN was substantially reduced following treatment with acid at pH 2, and this distinguished it from the acid-resistant, virally induced IFNs. Further research showed that

IFNγ was mainly the product of T-lymphocytes, and that it could also be produced by T-lymphocytes in response to their cognate antigens. In the latter case, the activation of T-lymphocytes requires binding of antigen, presented by accessory cells, e.g. macrophages, in combination with MHC molecules, to the T-cell receptor, in a manner identical to that previously described in Chapter 4 (see pp. 119–25).

There is now some evidence for monocyte/macrophage involvement generally in the induction of IFNγ synthesis. For instance, monocyte/macrophage IL-1 probably stimulates T-cell IL-2 synthesis, and possibly IL-2 in turn is required for IFNγ induction. Other cells of lymphoid origin such as NK cells have also been shown to produce IFNγ, but its production by non-lymphoid cells has never been conclusively demonstrated. Nevertheless, certain T-cell-derived tumour cell lines and T-cell hybridomas may produce IFNγ constitutively at low levels, or at higher levels following appropriate stimulation.

Until the early 1980s the major source of human IFNγ was lectin (mitogen)-induced peripheral blood mononuclear cells (PBMC) or splenocytes (or murine splenocytes for murine IFNγ). IFNγ was difficult to purify from medium conditioned by activated T-lymphocytes, and while physicochemical and antigenic properties had been established which distinguished it from IFNα/β, little was known at the time about its molecular characteristics. However, by 1982 Yip and Vilcek had, by re-extracting active IFNγ from polyacrylamide gels used to separate proteins of differing molecular weight, strong evidence that IFNγ was a dimer (MW 45–50000) of glycosylated subunits (MW 25000 or 20000), the heterogeneity probably reflecting varying levels of glycosylation. No knowledge of the amino acid sequence was available then, but, despite this, gene cloners succeeded in isolating human IFN cDNA in 1982 or thereabouts. The molecular cloning of IFNγ cDNA was achieved by isolating poly(A)$^+$ RNA from activated lymphocytes or splenocytes, preparing cDNAs from this and linking them into bacterial plasmids for amplification in *E.coli*, and subsequently using re-extracted plasmid DNA as a hybridization probe to bind IFNγ mRNA, release of this and translation in *Xenopus* oocytes led to identification of bacteria containing IFNγ cDNA. Nucleotide sequencing of the latter showed that it contained an open reading frame of 166 codons. At first it was thought that the mature IFNγ polypeptide was 146 amino acids long (MW 17140) with the first N-terminal 20 amino acids forming the signal sequence in the 166 amino acid precursor, but later research has shown that the first N-terminal amino acid is a blocked pyroglutamic acid residue, thus giving a signal sequence of 23 amino acids and a 143 amino acid mature IFNγ (see Figure 6.1, Chapter 6). The latter contains two potential N-linked glycosylation sites (Asn 25 and 97) of which both are used for the 25 kDa subunit and one only for the lower molecular weight 20 kDa molecules of native, dimeric IFNγ. It is probable that most IFNγ secreted by activated T-cells is in the form of a homodimer between two 25 kDa subunits, but heterogeneity is possible not only from variations in glycosylation, but also from differential cleavage of up to 13 amino acids from the C-terminal ends of subunits. The role of the oligosaccharide side chains is not known;

non-glycosylated IFNγ derived from *E.coli* containing IFNγ cDNA appears to be fully biologically active.

Mouse IFNγ, which was cloned about one year after human IFNγ, has been shown to contain 133 amino acids (MW 15 500) and is approximately 40 per cent homologous to the human molecule. In fact, the difference in structure is large enough for there to be essentially no cross-species reactivity between human and mouse IFNγ. However, rat IFNγ, whose primary sequence is also known, is much more homologous to mouse IFNγ, and mouse and rat IFNγ are interchangeable with regard to activity in mouse and rat cells. The smaller mouse/rat IFNγ molecules are also extensively glycosylated and form dimers of approximately 38 kDa.

Human IFNγ contains a high proportion of basic amino acids but no cysteine residues, and therefore no intrachain disulphide bridges are possible. On the basis of a method for predicting secondary structure, the IFNγ molecule would appear to contain both α-helices and β-strands. However, there is as yet no information from X-ray crystallographic studies as to the three-dimensional structure of IFNγ.

The gene for human IFNγ contains four exons and three introns and is located on chromosome 12. The equivalent mouse gene is located on chromosome 10. The exon–intron organization of the IFNγ gene is similar to that of other cytokines such as IL-2, IL-4, and GM-CSF, although at the protein level IFNγ shares little or no homology with other cytokines. In addition, there is an inducible transcriptional enhancer in the 5′ flanking region, proximal to the coding nucleotide sequence, which is similar to that contained in the 5′ flanking regions of the IL-2 gene and the IL-2R (Tac) gene. It is likely that IFNγ gene-expression is controlled by the binding of nuclear transcription factors to this enhancer region.

Both IFNγ and IFNα/β induce antiviral activity, but it is clear that not only are these molecules very different structurally, but also that they have separate cell-surface receptors. Once purified hrIFNγ became available, characterization of the IFNγ receptor (IFNg-R) was made possible. Binding studies with ^{125}I-hrIFNγ demonstrated the presence of high-affinity receptors with a K_d of $3–10 \times 10^{-9}$M in many different cell types, including fibroblasts, monocytes, macrophages, lymphocytes, epithelial cells, keratinocytes, and a wide variety of tumour cell lines, e.g. melanoma. Numbers of receptors per cell ranged from around 100 to 10 000: T-lymphocytes have about 500 receptors, macrophages about 5000. Similar receptors have also been demonstrated in many murine cell types. Since human IFNγ does not normally bind to mouse cells, in other words to the murine IFNg-R, it has been possible by the use of human × murine cell hybrids, which retain only a proportion of the full set of human chromosomes, to locate the gene coding for human IFNg-R to a particular human chromosome. Thus, ^{32}P-hrIFNγ was shown to bind only to those human × murine cell hybrids that retained human chromosome 6, suggesting that a gene on this chromosome codes for human IFNg-R. More specific analysis has located the human IFNg-R to the long arm(q) of chromosome 6. However, while cell hybrids containing human chromosome 6 specifically bound human IFNγ, they did not respond in any measurable way that IFNγ responsive cells would normally do following IFNγ stimulation, e.g. by the development of an antiviral state. This has suggested that there are other human-specific components of IFNg-R besides that encoded by the chromosome-6 gene. Evidence to support this belief has been obtained with human × murine hybrids which retain human chromosomes 6 and 21 together. These hybrids were shown to respond to human IFNγ by the expression of MHC antigens. It is, however, not yet clear what human chromosome 21, which is also known to contain the gene(s) for the human IFNα/β receptor (IFNa/b-R) contributes to IFNg-R. Possibly, the IFNa/b-R molecule itself plays some role in the transduction of signals from the IFNg-R, but there is presently no evidence for this.

Chemical cross-linking experiments with ^{125}I-hrIFNγ and responsive human cells have revealed the presence of a putative receptor glycoprotein of 90–100 kDa. More recently, this IFNg-R glycoprotein has been purified from human fibroblasts, from the B-lymphoblastoid cell line, Raji, and from placental tissues, and shown to be a 90–95 kDa moiety. Partially purified 95 kDa IFNg-R was used to raise monoclonal antibodies (moabs) and these moabs have been used in IFNg-R characterization studies. Such moabs have identified a further 55 kDa IFNγ-binding protein, but this was probably a degradation product of the 95 kDa glycoprotein.

Using a rabbit polyclonal antihuman IFNg-R (derived from Raji cells), Aguet and colleagues have recently molecularly cloned IFNg-R cDNA by a novel cloning strategy. In this case, poly(A)$^+$ RNA was isolated from Raji cells and the cDNA prepared from it cloned into λ-phage gt10, following which fusion proteins were expressed and those containing IFNg-R identified by immunoreactivity with the rabbit antiserum. This then led to isolation of IFNg-R cDNAs and oligonucleotide sequencing to determine the primary amino acid sequence of the encoded polypeptide chain. It was found that IFNg-R cDNA contained an open reading frame of 1515 bases which included coding for the 489 amino acids of the IFNg-R precursor. From hydropathy plots, which pinpoint regions of hydrophobic amino acids, the first 17 N-terminal amino acids probably form a signal sequence and a 21 amino acid hydrophobic domain in the middle of the polypeptide probably corresponds to the transmembrane segment. The extracellular domain of 229 amino acids has five potential N-linked glycosylation sites and a preponderance of serine residues which could be potential sites of O-glycosylation. Extensive glycosylation of the extracellular domain probably accounts for the discrepancy between the apparent MW of 90 000 of the purified native IFNg-R from Raji cells and the MW of approximately 54 000 calculated for the predicted full-length polypeptide chain. The primary amino acid sequence of IFNg-R does not appear to be significantly homologous to that of any known protein, and the function of the large intracellular domain (222 amino acids) is not yet known. Thus, IFNg-R may represent a unique receptor-type (see Figure 7.2, Chapter 7).

The chromosomal localization of the human IFNg-R gene to the long arm of chromosome 6 by somatic cell hybrid analysis has been confirmed by using the IFNg-R cDNA as a hybridization probe in cell hybrids containing chromosome 6 or segments thereof. In addition, IFNg-R cDNA was used to isolate its nuclear gene and the latter transfected into mouse L1210 cells which are normally unresponsive to human IFNγ. A number of transfectants were isolated that expressed IFNg-R, but responses usually associated with IFN stimulation, e.g. increased MHC antigen expression, could not be conclusively demonstrated. Therefore, as in cell hybrids containing human chromosome 6, there appears to be a requirement for an additional species-specific element for signal transduction to ensue. Whether this has anything to do with the co-expression of IFNa/b-R, as previously mentioned (p. 148), remains to be determined.

Following IFNγ binding to its receptor, the receptor complex is rapidly internalized by endocytosis, and there is some evidence that IFNγ is transported into the nucleus. Whilst it is widely believed that IFNγ triggers cellular responses from the plasma membrane via its surface receptor, it may also act intracellularly. One research group has recently shown that IFNg-R may be by passed by transfecting normally unresponsive mouse L-cells with DNA coding for human IFNγ without its signal sequence. Human IFNγ thus accumulates in the cytoplasm — it cannot be secreted without a signal sequence — and has been shown to induce various IFNγ-specific responses, e.g. induction of the antiviral state and of enzymes such as $(2'-5')$ oligo-adenylate synthetase and protein kinase associated with the antiviral mechanism, and increased expression of MHC class I and class II antigens. This strongly suggests that IFNg-R at the cell surface confers species specificity since, when the heterologous human IFNγ was present in mouse L-cell cytoplasm, the normal species specificity of the cellular response was lost. It also suggests that events involving

1 the endocytosis of the IFNγ–IFNg-R complex, or
2 alternative modes of signal transfer inside the cytoplasm, or
3 binding of internalized IFNγ to nuclear receptors, and not merely those occasioned by cell surface IFNg-R occupancy,

are largely responsible for IFNγ-mediated effects. This does not explain why when the human IFNg-R gene is transfected into mouse cells there are no IFNγ-mediated responses, unless the receptor complex, and thus human IFNγ, cannot be internalized in this case for some unknown reason. Obviously, there is much to clarify here, but it would seem that IFNγ is unusual in the manner it stimulates cellular responses. For example, by contrast, IFNα when introduced into the cytoplasm does not evoke typical IFN-mediated responses and thus appears to be strictly surface-receptor-dependent for activity.

The early events following IFNg-R occupancy are not well documented. There is preliminary evidence that signal transduction triggers Ca^{2+} mobilization and translocation of PKC in murine macrophages. Phosphorylation of IFNg-R has also been demonstrated following IFNγ binding, but the role of this phosphorylation remains to be elucidated. Proto-oncogenes, e.g. c-*myc* and c-*fos*, may also be induced or inhibited by IFNγ, but their expression appears to be a late response, taking place days after the initial stimulus, associated with the appearance of cell-surface differentiation markers. A number of genes are, however, induced in macrophages relatively early, within 30 minutes of stimulation, principal among them being those coding for MHC class II (human HLA-DR) antigens. The expression of MHC class II antigens in macrophages is triggered by relatively low doses of IFNγ, at the level of a few pg/ml, whereas the development of macrophage cytotoxic functions and the antiviral state appear to require much higher doses and probably prolonged exposure to IFNγ. This apparent differential stimulation possibly reflects differences at the level of signal transmission pathways. Alternatively, whereas one response requires signal transduction via the plasma membrane IFNg-R, others may require internalized, intracellular IFNγ–IFNg-R complexes and/or binding of IFNγ to nuclear receptors. On the evidence of neutralization of specific IFNγ activities with monoclonal antibodies, the IFNγ molecule may contain separate domains, each responsible for a particular function or subset of functions. For example, some moabs appear to neutralize the antiproliferative effect of IFN γ, but not its antiviral effect. This may represent a dosage effect, however, and such observations need verification.

Immunoregulatory activity of IFNγ

Macrophages
One of the main functions of IFNγ appears to be a macrophage activating factor (MAF). However, a note of caution should be sounded here for the following reason: Macrophages are extremely heterogeneous, with diverse morphology, location, and function. Following production in the bone marrow, monocytes enter the circulation and emigrate to various tissues throughout the body. In these tissues, they differentiate into mature macrophages, often becoming dendritic in appearance, and occupy interstitial sites associated with epithelia. Depending on their tissue location, they are differently named. Thus macrophages of bone are called osteoclasts; macrophages in the skin, Langerhans cells; in the liver, Kupffer cells; and in the central nervous system, microglial cells. Such tissue-adherent 'fixed' macrophages differ from populations of loosely adherent macrophages found in the peritoneal cavity and in the alveolar space. The latter are usually more rounded in morphology with few plasma-membrane-extended processes, and probably perform different functions from those of tissue-adherent macrophages.

Virtually all of the studies using IFNγ as a MAF have been carried out *in vitro* with purified alveolar or peritoneal macrophages, or with peripheral blood monocytes differentiated into macrophages in culture, or with monocytoid cell lines. The characteristics of these macrophages or 'macrophage-like' cells probably do not fully represent those of tissue-adherent macrophages, and the functions and differentiation markers induced by IFNγ *in vitro* may not correspond to those induced *in vivo*. However, it is clear from extensive investigations *in vitro* that IFNγ is likely to be a differentiation stimulus for macrophages and other cell types. For example, as previously mentioned, IFNγ and probably IFNs in general are potent regulators of MHC antigens, the latter being of central importance in the immune response to foreign (non-self) antigens. Both IFNγ and IFNα/β can up-regulate the expression of MHC class I (HLA-A, -B, -C) antigens, but IFNγ is by far the most effective inducer of *de novo* synthesis of MHC class II (HLA-DR, -DP, -DQ) antigens. Thus, the effect of IFNγ stimulation in macrophages is to increase the expression of both MHC class I and class II antigens, class I being required for recognition of foreign antigen by CTLs and class II being required for recognition of foreign antigen by T_H-cells. IFNγ has also been demonstrated to increase MHC antigen expression in other antigen-presenting 'accessory' cell types, e.g. endothelial cells, and in various cultured normal and tumour cell lines.

In addition to MHC antigens, IFNγ may modulate the synthesis or expression of a number of other cell-surface antigens, complement components, pro-coagulant and chemotactic proteins, intracellular enzymes, and inflammatory mediators in macrophages. For example, IFNγ up-regulates the expression of the cell-surface receptor (FcR) for IgG and thus increases antibody-mediated cellular cytotoxicity (ADCC) by macrophages. Simultaneously, various CD antigens may be up- or down- regulated. Adherence proteins and receptors for plasminogen and urokinase, involved in fibrinolysis, may also increase. In contrast, IFNγ has been shown to up-regulate melanocyte-stimulating hormone (MSH) receptors in melanoma tumour cells.

The secretion of a number of biologically active proteins is also modulated by IFNγ. For example, secretion of components of the complement pathways such as C2 and factor B is enhanced in macrophages by IFNγ. Transient synthesis of IP-10, a cytokine structurally homologous to a family of proteins with chemotactic activities (see IL-8, pp. 163–8) and more prolonged synthesis of IP-30, a secreted protein of unknown function, are also observed following IFNγ-stimulation of macrophages.

The induction of MHC class II synthesis has been correlated to the prior Ca^{2+} mobilization effected by IFNγ stimulation. This activation step may be mimicked by calcium ionophore A23187 and platelet activating factor (PAF). However, this step in itself is insufficient to trigger macrophage cytotoxic functions. It does nevertheless 'prime' macrophages to respond to second stimulants such as bacterial LPS. 'Secondary' activation by LPS appears to be mediated via PKC activation, since diacylglycerol and phorbolesters, e.g. PMA, which are known to act on PKC, may replace LPS. PKC activation is itself Ca^{2+} dependent, and calcium and calmodulin antagonists inhibit macrophage cytotoxicity. Thus, there are similarities between macrophage activation, LPS plus IFNγ, and the dual stimulant model of lymphocyte activation, e.g. antigen plus IL-1 in T-lymphocytes, antigen plus IL-4 in B-lymphocytes.

One of the main functions of IFNγ appears to be to prime macrophages to mount a respiratory burst, i.e. rapid production of oxygen radicals and hydrogen peroxide, in response to various stimuli acting at the cell surface. For example, synergy of IFNγ and LPS considerably enhances the respiratory burst. The release of superoxide (O_2^-) and hydrogen peroxide (H_2O_2) by macrophages contributes to their toxic activities towards bacteria and intracellular pathogens (see Chapter 6). In addition, IFNγ markedly augments the LPS-stimulated production by macrophages of cytokines such as IL-1, TNFα, and IL-6 which themselves have immunoregulatory and cytotoxic properties. IL-1 and TNFα may also act in an autocrine manner to stimulate production of more IL-1 and TNFα. Increased production of cytokines by IFNγ LPS–stimulated macrophages is inhibited by glucocorticoids which are known also to inhibit differentiation.

In monocytic cell lines, e.g. HL60 and U937, IFNγ may induce terminal differentiation, i.e. the tumour cells adopt the macrophage phenotype. During the differentiation process, a number of cell-surface markers, e.g. MHC antigens, gene products, e.g. TNFα, and functions characteristic of activated macrophages, may be expressed or induced. For these reasons, monocytic cell lines are often proposed as models of macrophage activation and differentiation, although it should be noted that their continuous growth in culture may have in many cases radically altered their sensitivity and nature of responses to cell surface stimuli such as LPS.

T-lymphocytes
T-lymphocytes are the major producers of IFNγ, but it is clear that since they bear IFNg-R that they can respond to IFNγ-autocrine or paracrine stimulation. The responses of T-cells to IFNγ appear to differ from those triggered in macrophages and other cell types. For instance, IFNγ does not induce MHC class II antigen expression in T-cells, although it may increase MHC class I. Further, IFNγ is unable to induce an antiviral state in T-cells and, in contrast to its antiproliferative effect in some tumour cells, probably acts as a proliferation stimulus for T-cells. For the latter, it probably provides the T-cell with the ability to respond to further exogenous mitogenic stimuli rather than being directly mitogenic itself. For functionally differentiated T-cells such as CTL, IFNγ appears to be required as a maturation factor for the expression of full cytotoxic potential.

B-lymphocytes
In resting B-lymphocytes, IFNγ may act as a co-stimulant for proliferation (see Chapter 4). In this regard, IFNγ has been shown to enhance the PMA-induced proliferation of a B-cell prolymphocytic leukaemia. In addition to its putative role in B-cell proliferation, IFNγ has also been shown to increase IgM secretion by both resting and activated B-lymphocytes *in vitro*. In many instances, the action of IFNγ has been found to oppose that of IL-4. For example, IL-4 stimulates mature B-cells to produce IgG1 and IgE, but suppresses IgG2a, whereas IFNγ enhances IgG2a secretion and inhibits IgG1 and IgE production. Thus, the relative amounts of IL-4 and IFNγ produced during an immune response may control the selection of Ig isotypes secreted.

Granulocytes and other cells
IFNγ and IFNs in general have been demonstrated to have marked inhibitory effects on the growth of normal haemopoietic progenitor cells, at least *in vitro*. IFNs suppress the proliferation and/or differentiation of haemopoietic cells at the level of colony- or burst-forming units, e.g. CFU-GEMM, BFU-E, etc. (see Chapter 3). Since T-lymphocytes produce IL-3 and GM-CSF which stimulate progenitor cell proliferation/differentiation as well as the inhibitory IFNγ, based on *in vitro* observations, the relative amounts of these cytokines produced during an *in vivo* immune response may regulate the rate of haemopoietic cell production.

For mature polymorphonuclear phagocytes, e.g. neutrophils, IFNγ probably acts in a similar way to its activation of macrophages. For instance, IFNγ has been reported to up-regulate FcR expression and thus enhance ADCC by neutrophils and eosinophils. Furthermore, IFNγ has been shown to potentiate the respiratory burst of neutrophils to different stimuli.

The potential contributory role of IFNγ in inflammatory reactions, e.g. cell-mediated hypersensitivity, will be discussed later in this chapter (pp. 168–70). Antiviral, antimicrobial and antitumour activities of IFNγ will be considered in Chapter 6.

Tumour necrosis factors

Introduction
An association between endotoxin, the LPS component of the cell walls of Gram-negative bacteria, and antitumour activity has long been recognized. As long ago as the late 1880s, regression of tumours had been observed in patients recovering from bacterial infections or where patients were intentionally injected with bacterial toxins. Subsequently, it was found that endotoxins induced haemorrhagic necrosis of certain transplanted tumours in mice. However, in the early 1950s it was demonstrated that endotoxin *per se* did not kill tumour cells *in vitro*, and this led to the suggestion that the observed haemorrhagic necrosis of tumours *in vivo* was due to endotoxin-induced hypotension and consequent vascular collapse and ischaemia in the tumour itself. More recently, Carswell and colleagues, working in the USA in 1975, identified a cytotoxin (CTX) in the sera of mice infected with Bacille Calmette-Guérin (BCG) and subsequently treated with endotoxin. They called this CTX tumour necrosis factor (TNF) because of its ability to induce selective tumour necrosis. It has been subsequently demonstrated that activated macrophages (mononuclear phagocytes) are the major cellular sources of TNF. A second type of CTX has also been isolated from the culture supernatants of antigen- or mitogen-stimulated peripheral blood leukocytes (PBL) and this was first called lymphotoxin (LT). This CTX, produced mainly by activated T-lymphocytes, has been found to have virtually identical biological activity to TNF; both have tumoricidal activity against a range of tumour cells *in vitro*.

Molecular characterization
The molecular relationship between the macrophage-derived CTX, TNF, and the T-lymphocyte-derived CTX, LT, remained unknown until about the mid-1980s. Partially purified CTX proteins derived from stimulated human leukocytes suggested extensive heterogeneity of molecular species, particularly of LT. However, isolation and purification of CTX from certain cell lines, e.g. HL60, RPMI 1788, strongly indicated that TNF and LT activities could be attributed to two distinct homogeneous proteins. Cell-line-derived TNF (apparent MW 45 000), was shown to be composed of three identical monomeric subunits (MW 17 000), each containing one internal disulphide bridge. In contrast, the subunit of LT was found to have a somewhat higher MW (20 000–25 000), owing to the attachment of N-linked oligosaccharides, and contained no disulphide bonds. The observed heterogeneity of LT derived from PBL possibly resulted from high levels of aggregation of its subunits.

At about the same time as these biochemical characterizations, the application of rDNA techniques led to the successful cloning and expression in *E.coli* of TNF and LT from genetic material obtained from cell lines. The nucleotide sequences of the cloned cDNA coding for TNF and LT confirmed the amino acid sequences deduced from chemical analysis of their respective monomeric protein molecules. In addition, it was learnt that TNF was synthesized in human cells as a precursor product of 233 amino acids, and that the monomeric protein of 157 amino acids (MW 17 356) resulted following cleavage of an unusually long 'leader' polypeptide from the N-terminus. By contrast, LT, in common with many other secreted proteins, is synthesized with an N-terminal signal polypeptide of 24 amino acids which is cleaved to produce the 171 amino acid monomeric protein (MW 18 664). Excluding the leader (signal) sequences, TNF and LT have 36 per cent of their amino acids in common; this homology increases to 51 per cent when conservative replacements of amino acids are taken into account (Figure 5.2). Thus, from an evolutionary point of view TNF and LT may be regarded as distantly related proteins which probably arose from a common ancestral gene (cf. IFNα/β). This molecular relationship between TNF and LT and their common biological activities has led to them being renamed TNFα and TNFβ respectively. Quite unexpectedly, TNFα has been recently found to be identical to 'cachectin', a hormone which suppresses lipoprotein lipase activity, and is frequently referred to as such.

The primary structures of mouse TNFα and TNFβ have also been recently determined and found to show much the same degree of homology as their human counterparts. Mouse TNFα monomeric protein contains 156 amino acids (there is an additional leader sequence of 79 amino acids in the precursor molecule), an intramolecular disulphide bond and, in contrast to human TNFα, one potential N-linked glycosylation site. Nevertheless, mouse and human TNFα are approximately 80 per cent homologous overall in amino acids and share several structural features. For example, both molecules contain two cysteine residues in the same positions, indicating that the

```
                                                   10
LT                            L  P  G  V  L  T  P  S  A  A  Q  T  A  R  Q  H  P  K


      20                    30                    40
LT    M  H  -  L  A  H  S  T  L  -  K  P  A  A  H  L  I  G  D  P  S  K  Q  N  S  L  L  W  -  -
TNF   V  R  S  S  R  T  P  S  D  K  P  V  A  H  V  V  A  N  P  Q  A  E  G  Q  L  Q  W  L  N


            50                    60                    70
LT    -  R  A  N  T  D  R  A  F  L  Q  D  G  F  S  L  S  N  N  S  L  L  V  P  T  S  G  I  Y  F
TNF   R  R  A  N  -  -  -  A  L  L  A  N  G  V  W  L  R  D  N  Q  L  V  V  P  S  E  G  L  Y  L


            80                    90                    100
LT    V  Y  S  Q  V  V  F  S  G  K  A  Y  S  P  K  A  T  S  S  P  L  Y  L  A  H  E  V  Q  L  F
TNF   I  Y  S  Q  V  L  F  K  G  Q  G  C  -  P  -  -  S  T  -  H  V  L  L  T  H  T  I  S  R  I


            110                   120
LT    S  S  Q  Y  P  F  H  V  P  L  L  S  S  Q  K  M  V  Y  -  -  -  -  P  -  G  L  Q  E  -  D
TNF   A  V  S  Y  Q  T  K  V  N  L  L  S  A  I  K  S  P  C  Q  R  E  T  P  E  G  A  E  A  K  P


      130                   140                   150
LT    W  L  H  S  M  Y  H  G  A  A  F  Q  L  T  Q  G  D  Q  L  S  T  H  T  D  G  I  P  H  L  V
TNF   W  Y  E  P  I  Y  L  G  G  V  F  Q  L  E  K  G  D  R  L  S  A  E  I  N  R  P  D  Y  L  D


      160                   170
LT    L  S  P  S  T  -  V  F  F  G  A  F  A  L
TNF   F  A  E  S  G  Q  V  Y  F  G  I  I  A  L
```

Figure 5.2 Comparison of amino acid sequences of human TNFα and β showing maximum alignment.

disulphide bond which they form is highly conserved among the TNFα of different animal species. Additionally, the two regions at each side of these cysteines are highly conserved between mouse and human TNFα, suggesting that these domains are of functional importance. Mouse TNFβ is 169 amino acids long and shows approximately 74 per cent overall homology with human TNFβ.

The three-dimensional structure of hrTNFα has recently been elucidated,

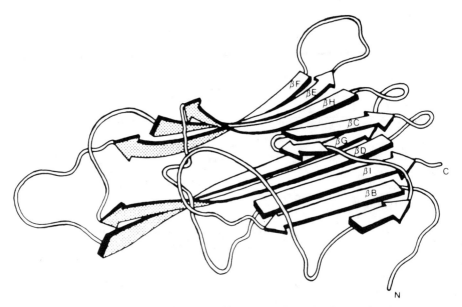

Figure 5.3 Schematic stereo diagram of human TNFα. The β-strands are shown as thick arrows. The TNF trimer threefold axis would be horizontal in this orientation. (Reprinted with permission from Jones *et al.*, *Nature* **338**, p.227; copyright 1989 Macmillan Magazines Ltd.)

and shows marked differences to the three-dimensional structures of two other cytokines, IL-1 and IL-2. This indicates that similarities in biological activities among these cytokines are not governed by protein structures. Further, in contrast to the monomeric structure of IL-1 and IL-2, TNFα is trimeric. Each TNFα monomer of 157 amino acids contains several β-strands and is folded up into a wedge-shape (Figure 5.3). This β-barrel or jelly-roll configuration is shared by many viral coat proteins, e.g. foot and mouth disease virus VP3 and satellite tobacco necrosis virus. The three TNFα monomers pack together around a threefold axis to form a cone-like molecule, the top of which is probably involved in receptor binding. It is likely that TNFβ also adopts a similar structure, despite seemingly large differences in primary amino acid sequence between TNFα and TNFβ.

In humans and mice, TNFα and TNFβ have single copy genes of similar size (approximately 3 kbp) which are closely linked on human chromosome 6 (short arm) and mouse chromosome 17 respectively. Each gene has four exons and three introns, a gene organization that is common among cytokines. Only in the fourth exon, which codes for about 80 per cent of the mature, monomeric proteins, is there greater than 50 per cent homology in nucleotide sequences between TNFα and TNFβ genes. Comparison of the 5′ untranslated flanking regions of these genes has revealed conserved structural features, e.g. Goldberg–Hogness TATA sequences involved in promoting transcription initiation, which appear to be similar to a number of other genes specifically expressed in activated leukocytes and which may thus play a role in control of genes. Of particular interest has been the discovery that the TNFα and TNFβ genes map within the MHC gene-locus. This has allowed the tying together, at least at the genetic level, of secreted cytokines that display effector and regulatory functions and membrane proteins that function as cell surface recognition structures. Evidence is now accumulating to suggest that this association has functional significance and does not merely reflect the coincidental clustering of genes.

Production of tumour necrosis factors
Mononuclear phagocytes (monocytes/macrophages) are the major cellular producers of TNFα. Bacterial endotoxin, LPS, appears to be one of the most potent inducers of TNFα production *in vitro* and *in vivo*. It is clear, however, that other substances, e.g. cell wall components of mycobacteria, certain viruses (e.g. Sendai virus), other cytokines (e.g. IL-1, IL-2) and some chemicals (e.g. phorbolesters) also act as inducers and that production of TNFα may also be effected by other cell types, e.g. NK cells, T-lymphocytes, mast cells, fibroblasts, etc. In addition, certain monocytic cell lines (e.g. HL-60, U-937), T-cell hybridomas, and retrovirus (HTLV-1) transformed cell lines produce TNFα spontaneously and/or in response to phorbolester stimulation. Further, cytokines such as IFNγ and M-CSF may 'prime' cells for the synthesis of TNFα and thus lead to enhanced production following, for example, LPS stimulation. Following induction, TNFα is rapidly synthesized and released into the extracellular milieu. However, there is growing evidence that TNFα may also exist in a plasma-membrane bound form, similar to that described for IL-1 (see p. 112).

Whereas most cell types appear capable of producing TNFα, the production of TNFβ is probably restricted to T- and B-lymphocytes and perhaps some LGL. Production of TNFβ occurs following mitogenic or antigenic activation of T-lymphocytes. Both T_H lymphocytes and CTL have been shown to produce TNFβ in response to mitogens. In addition, cloned T-lymphocytes, certain T-cell hybridomas, retroviral (HTLV-1) transformed T-cell lines, and certain B-lymphoblastoid cell lines (RPMI 1788) may produce TNFβ spontaneously and/or following antigenic, mitogenic or phorbolester stimulation. In contrast to TNFα, synthesis of TNFβ appears generally to be at a relatively slow rate following induction, with production continuing over a lengthier period of time.

There are several reports of other CTXs whose relationship to the cloned human TNFα and β proteins remains uncertain. For instance, CTXs produced by the LukII B-lymphoblastoid cell line, by the monocytic leukaemia cell line THP-1, and by particular HTLV-1-transformed cell lines, all appear to be biochemically distinct from either TNFα or TNFβ. Other novel CTXs, produced by cloned NK and CTL, have also been described. Some, but not all, of these novel CTXs are apparently immunochemically related to either TNFα or TNFβ. The relationship of TNFα, TNFβ or other novel CTXs to other factors reported to have cytotoxic action, e.g. natural killer cytotoxic factor (NKCF) or leukoregulin (LR), remains enigmatic.

Receptors and mechanism of action
Despite marked differences in primary amino acid sequences, TNFα and TNFβ probably are similar in three-dimensional structure. This is also reflected by the finding that they share a common cell surface receptor. The TNF receptor (TNF-R) is present on many normal and tumour cell types, and is probably ubiquitous. Its numbers vary from a few hundred up to about 20 000 per cell. One exception is the resting T-lymphocyte which does not bind TNF until activated, when several hundred TNF-R are subsequently expressed. Although the dissociation constant, K_d, for TNF binding to TNF-R appears to vary among different cell types, there is probably only one class of receptors. Cross-linking studies in murine cells have revealed two cell surface proteins, 95 kDa and 75 kDa, which appear to be involved in TNF-R. Cross-linking of radiolabelled human TNFα to human cells has revealed a 100 kDa TNF–TNF-R complex, suggesting a major receptor component of 60–80 kDa. The TNF-R has yet to be molecularly cloned. Differences in structure of TNF-R among animal species appear to be minor, since human TNF binds to mouse and rabbit cells as well as human ones, and other animal TNFs also exhibit a similar low degree of species specificity. There is, however, recent evidence suggesting an *in vitro* species preference of human and murine TNFα; human TNFα was found to bind more strongly to human cells than did mouse TNFα, and vice versa. In one instance where murine TNFα has been found to provide a proliferative stimulus for a cultured T-cell line, both binding and activity appeared to be strictly species specific, i.e. human TNFα did not bind to these cells and thus had no effect on proliferation. IFNγ, and to a lesser extent IFNα/β, may act on TNF-R bearing cells to significantly increase, by two–threefold, the amount of TNF-R. It has been proposed that such an increase may explain, at least in part, the frequently observed synergistic activities of TNF and IFNγ although to date there has been little supportive evidence for this contention. On the other hand, activators of PKC such as phorbolesters in combination with Ca^{2+} ionophore A23187 decrease expression of TNF-R. Furthermore, LPS, which activates macrophages via a PKC-dependent pathway, has been shown to trigger internalization of TNF-R. This suggests that PKC may have a physiological role in mediating cell sensitivity to TNF.

Besides expression of TNF-R, cell responsiveness to TNF will be controlled by post-receptor signal transmission pathways. Little, however, is presently known about the underlying molecular mechanisms involved in TNF-specific signalling pathways. Early events following TNF-R occupancy include increased plasma membrane fluidity and permeability with subsequent Ca^{2+} influx (but without apparent mobilization of intracellular Ca^{2+} stores), activation of phospholipase A_2 with resultant production of arachidonic acid and prostaglandin E_2, and activation of respiratory burst oxidase, the plasma membrane enzyme responsible for O_2^- production. Activation of respiratory burst oxidase probably requires protein phosphorylation of certain plasma membrane substrates. TNFα has recently been shown to induce the serine phosphorylation of at least one 26 kDa cytosolic protein in U937 monocytic cells, suggesting that TNF can activate protein kinases. The biochemical links between protein phosphorylation induced by TNF and signal transfer to the cell nucleus with the subsequent induction of particular genes have get to be elucidated. In common with IL-1, TNFα has been shown to induce the transient expression of c-*fos* and c-*myc*, at least in cultured fibroblasts. Again like IL-1, TNFα has been shown to induce PDGF-A chain mRNA in fibroblasts, although PDGF-B (c-*sis*) was not co-expressed. Presently, it is unclear whether the mitogenic effect of TNFα in normal fibroblasts is due to directly mediated TNFα effects *per se* or to the induced expression of other mitogenic cytokines. Nonetheless, it is apparent that following stimulation with TNFα that several proteins associated with the proliferative response are induced. For instance, it has recently been shown that TNFα induces the synthesis of ornithine decarboxylase, an enzyme involved in spermidine formation which is almost certainly involved in cell growth. In addition, TNFα has been demonstrated to increase the number of EGF-R in human fibroblasts and this may be functionally related to its mitogenic action. Furthermore, in murine NIH 3T3 fibroblasts, TNFα induces amplified expression of the c-*neu* proto-oncogene product, which is related to the c-*erb*B product, i.e. EGF-R, and probably acts as a growth factor receptor. Thus, in many ways the effects of TNFα in normal, proliferation-responsive cells are typical of the growth-promoting cytokines previously described in this book. Other examples of TNFα and TNFβ acting as proliferation stimuli are discussed below in the wider context of their actions on leukocytes.

Immunoregulatory effects of tumour necrosis factor

T- and B-lymphocytes
The biological activities of TNFα/β and IL-1, as is becoming apparent, are quite similar in many instances (Table 5.1). Thus, for lymphocytes TNFα and TNFβ can, like IL-1, act as co-stimulants for cell proliferation. TNFα may interact with activated T-cells, which express TNF-R, and regulate both growth and functional activities of these cells, which in turn regulate B-cell growth and differentiation. In addition, TNFα as well as IL-1 may enhance the proliferation of lectin-stimulated thymocytes and mature T-lymphocytes. TNFα has been shown to induce IL-2Rα (Tac) in certain T-cell lines, e.g. YT, and this mechanism may also be involved in thymocyte and T-lymphocyte proliferation. In high doses, TNFα has also been shown to enhance the proliferation of IL-2-dependent T-cells and increase their IFNγ production. Both TNFα and TNFβ have been demonstrated to augment B-cell proliferation and to enhance Ig secretion induced by IL-2. TNFα and TNFβ, which are known to up-regulate MHC antigen expression, particularly class I molecules, in several different cell types including fibroblasts, endothelial cells, and various tumour cells, may also modulate cell-surface MHC expression in

Table 5.1   Actions of TNFα and TNFβ: comparison with IL-1

Target cell	Action(s) of TNFα/β	Actions of IL-1 (+ or −)
T-lymphocytes, B-lymphocytes	Regulation of proliferative and functional responses	+
Monocytes/ macrophages	Synthesis of IL-1, IL-6, PAF, chemotactic peptides ROI production	±
	Differentiation of myeloid/ promyelomonocyte cell lines	+
	Inhibition of intracellular microbes	±
Neutrophils	Inhibition of progenitor proliferation	−
	Secretion of ROI intermediates	−
	Enhancement of phagocytosis and ADCC	+?
	Adhesion to vascular endothelium	+
	Degranulation	+
Eosinophils	Toxicity to schistosomes	+?
Endothelium	Induction of procoagulant activity (decreased activation of protein C, decreased synthesis of plasminogen activator, increased synthesis of plasminogen activator inhibitor)	+
	Induction of IL-1, IL-6, prostacyclin, and GM-CSF synthesis	+
	Increased expression of class I MHC antigens	−
	Increased expression of adhesion antigens for monocytes and neutrophils	+
	Morphological changes (in conjuction with IFN$_\gamma$)	+
Fibroblasts, synoviocytes	Increased proliferation	+
	Synthesis of PGE-2, PDGF-A, collagenase, IL-1, IL-6	+
	Expression of class I MHC antigens	+
	Antiviral activity	−
	Transient induction of c-*fos*, c-*myc*	+
Chondrocytes	Decreased synthesis of proteoglycans, increased proteoglycanase, collagenase	+
Adipocytes	Decreased synthesis of lipoprotein lipase	+
	Inhibition of adipsin (serine protease)	?
Skeletal myocytes	Membrane depolarization	?

Hepatocytes	Modulation acute-phase protein expression	+
	Depression of cytochrome P450	?
Tumour cells	Cytotoxicity	±
	Antiviral activity	−
	Enhanced class I and class II MHC gene expression	±
	Increased ornithine decarboxylase activity	?
	Modulation of oncogene expression	?
Pancreatic islets	Enhanced class II MHC antigen expression (in conjunction with IFN$_\gamma$)	+
In vivo, loci of action not certain	Haemorrhagic necrosis of certain tumour types	±
	Accumulation of neutrophils	+
	Stimulation of G/M-CSF activity	+
	Suppression of erythropoiesis	?
	Fever induction	+
	Hypotension	+

lymphocytes. In this respect, they possibly synergize with the enhancing actions of IFNγ, as has been found for murine Ly-6 surface antigen (a complex involved in cell activation) expression in thymocytes and T-lymphocytes. Like IFNγ, TNFα and TNFβ also probably act as maturation factors for the development of the cytolytic function of CTL and natural cytotoxic cells, i.e. non-MHC restricted lymphocytes such as LAK cells, in general. These immuno-enhancing effects of TNFs are again probably potentiated by IFNγ, but in contrast are almost certainly antagonized by the action of TGFβ.

Macrophages and granulocytes
The effects mediated by TNFα and TNFβ on haemopoiesis are complex (Table 5.1). In most cases reported, TNFs have suppressive effects on the *in vitro* development of early haemopoietic progenitors, e.g. CFU-GM, and these inhibitory actions on proliferation are enhanced by IFNγ. Erythroid progenitors (e.g. BFU-E) are also growth-inhibited by TNFα. This antiproliferative action of TNF is in marked contrast to its growth-promoting activity for mitogen-activated lymphocytes, but is in keeping with its antitumour activity which will be discussed in the next chapter. The mechanism of action of the TNF-mediated suppression of haemopoietic progenitor cell growth is

not known. However, *in vivo*, TNFα has unexpectedly been shown to induce granulopoiesis. This could possibly arise as the result of TNF-mediated induction of CSF secretion.

In more mature normal myeloid cells, acute and chronic myeloid leukaemia cells and leukaemia-derived cell lines, there is evidence that TNFα or TNFβ alone, or synergistically with IFNγ, may induce differentiation. TNF-mediated inhibition of cell proliferation is often accompanied by terminal differentiation, e.g. the differentiation of HL-60 myelomonocytic leukaemia cells into morphologically and functionally mature macrophage-like cells, and preceded by inhibition of c-*myc* proto-oncogene expression. In the case of chronic myeloid leukaemia (CML), the tumour cells may constitutively produce TNFα and this could be involved in autocrine growth inhibition and differentiation, and may account for the more controlled tumour cell growth in this chronic malignancy.

TNFα, which is the major cytokine product of activated macrophages, may act on monocytes/macrophages in an autocrine manner to enhance various functions, e.g. cytotoxicity to tumour cells, and to induce the expression of a number of other immunoregulatory and inflammatory mediators (Table 5.1). For instance, TNFα may act back on monocytes/macrophages to increase its own synthesis together with that of IL-1, IL-6, M-CSF, and GM-CSF. TNFα also stimulates peritoneal macrophages to synthesize and release PAF, a family of cell-derived lipid inflammatory mediators, having as their basic structure acetyl-glycerol-ether-phosphorylcholine, with a wide range of biological activities. Production of PAF is probably dependent on TNF-mediated phospholipase A_2 activation, the enzyme being necessary to hydrolyse 2-lyso-PAF to active PAF. TNFα has also been demonstrated to increase macrophage arginase activity resulting in the production and release of ornithine and its decarboxylated byproduct, putrescine, which are thought to have immunopotentiating effects.

Granulocytes are shortlived (2–3 days) phagocytic cells which are rapidly produced by the bone marrow. They are able to adhere to and penetrate the endothelial cells lining blood vessels, and are well known to be involved in defence and inflammatory mechanisms. TNFα and TNFβ have been shown to stimulate neutrophil (90 per cent of granulocytes) functions including phagocytosis, degranulation, and respiratory burst activity (Table 5.1). Phagocytosis probably depends on the TNF-induced enhanced expression of cell surface molecules, a complex termed CDw18 in neutrophils, which are required for optimal adherence to target cells or particles. In this respect, it is also probable that cell surface molecules on vascular endothelial cells which are involved in adherence or attraction of neutrophils are up-regulated by TNF (see pp. 168–70). Neutrophil-mediated ADCC has also been shown to be increased by TNFs, possibly by activation of oxidative metabolism. This may be responsible for neutrophil-mediated inhibition of the growth of micro-organisms such as *Candida albicans*. TNF may also activate eosinophils to kill or inhibit, in the presence of antibody, parasites such as blood-stage malaria and schistosomules (schistosomiasis).

Soluble chemoattractant proteins: interleukin-8

Macrophages present at the site of tissue injury or infection are largely responsible for the initiation of host defence mechanisms. To amplify the local immune response, they secrete and respond to a variety of mediators including cytokines. Circulating granulocytes form a reservoir of phagocytic and cytolytic cells which can be recruited to sites of tissue injury by soluble chemoattractant proteins produced by macrophages and endothelial cells. Several of the cytokines previously discussed, e.g. IL-1, TNFα, and GM-CSF, have been described as having chemotactic activity for neutrophilic granulocytes. However, these cytokines are only weakly chemotactic, if at all, *in vitro*, but it is likely they act *in vivo* by increasing expression of neutrophil and endothelial cell adherence proteins and/or stimulating the production of

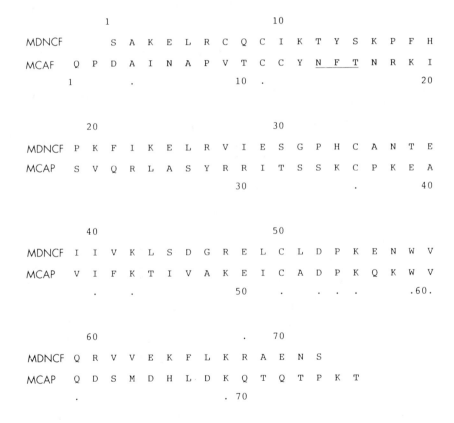

Figure 5.4 Comparison of primary sequences of MDNCF and MCAF/MCP-1 showing maximum alignment. The underlining indicates a potential N-glycosylation site in MCAF only.

soluble chemoattractant proteins. In fact, it is becoming apparent that IL-1 and TNF stimulate macrophages to produce several related proteins having chemotactic properties for neutrophils and other leukocytes.

One of the principal chemotactic proteins having specificity for neutrophils and known as macrophage-derived neutrophil chemotactic factor (MDNCF) has recently been molecularly cloned. This factor is also known by a variety of other names, which will not be mentioned here to avoid confusion. Macrophage-derived MDNCF cDNA codes for a polypeptide of 99 amino acids of which the first 27 N-terminal residues form a signal sequence. The 72 amino acid mature MDNCF has four cysteines, which are probably involved in intrachain disulphide bond formation, but there are no potential N-linked glycosylation sites (Figure 5.4). Comparison of the deduced amino acid sequence of MDNCF with those of known proteins has revealed that it shows significant homology with a number of inflammatory or mitogenic proteins. These include platelet factor 4, β-thromboglobulin, connective tissue-activating peptide III, 9E3 (a protein induced by RSV transformation and associated with proliferating fibroblasts), and the IFNγ-induced macrophage IP-10 (see p. 151). In MDNCF and all of these related proteins, the positions of the four cysteines are perfectly conserved.

A second monocyte/macrophage-derived chemotactic protein has also been molecularly cloned recently (1988). This has been called either mono-cyte chemotactic and activating factor (MCAF) or monocyte chemoattrac-tant protein-1 (MCP-1) and was cloned from the human promyelocytic cell line, THP-1, or from a human glioma cell line, U-105MG. MCAF/MCP-1 cDNA codes for a polypeptide of 99 amino acids, which includes an N-terminal 23 amino acid sequence. The 76 amino acid mature MCAF/MCP-1 (MW 8681) has four cysteines, which are probably involved in disulphide bridge formation, and one potential site for N-glycosylation (Figure 5.4). MCAF/MCP-1 shows greatest homology (42 of 76 amino acid residues, 55 per cent) with a murine competence protein factor, JE, cloned from a PDGF-stimulated mouse fibroblast line, and therefore it has been suggested that MCAF-MCP-1 is the human equivalent (homologue) of JE. There are however at least four more proteins that are strongly related to MCAF/MCP-1, e.g. murine macrophage inflammatory protein (MIP, 25 per cent homolo-gous) in which the positions of the four cysteines are precisely conserved. MCAF/MCP-1 is also related to MDNCF with which it shares 21 per cent homology, but the positions of the four cysteines differ somewhat between these two chemoattractant proteins. In all it may be considered that MCAF/ MCP-1 and MDNCF each belong to separate sub-families of a broad group of chemotactic and mitogenic proteins.

The full range of biological activities of MDNCF, MCAF/MCP-1 and other proteins in this category has yet to be determined. The production of these proteins has been found to be widespread among different cell types, includ-ing monocytes/macrophages, lymphocytes, fibroblasts and endothelial cells, in response to a variety of stimuli, e.g. LPS, IL-1, TNFα, PHA, etc. The specificity of individual proteins for particular cell types, however, remains

Table 5.2 Molecular characteristics of immunoregulatory and inflammatory human cytokines and their receptors. For details of IL-1α/β and IL-6, see Table 4.2

Cytokine	Precursor (aa)	Mature protein (aa)	Glycosylation	Disulphide bonds	Chromosome assignment	Receptors
IFNγ	166	143 (45 kDa dimer)	N-linked	0	12	90 kDa glycoprotein (gene on chromosome 6)
TNFα	233	157 (45–50 kDa trimer)	—	1	6	60–80 kDa glycoprotein (details unknown)
TNFβ	195	171 (60 kDa trimer)	N-linked	0	6	Same as TNFα
MDNCF	99	72 (8.5 kDa)	—	2	unknown	unknown
MCAF/MCP-1	99	76 (8.7 kDa)	N-linked	2	unknown	unknown

uncertain. MDNCF has been shown to be chemotactic for neutrophils, but not monocytes. Nevertheless, more recent investigations have demonstrated that MDNCF is a chemotactic and activating factor for T-lymphocytes and for this reason it has been called interleukin-8 (IL-8). In contrast, MCAF/MCP-1 does not attract neutrophils, but probably acts as a chemotactic and activating factor for blood monocytes. Much obviously remains to be clarified, but it appears certain that stimuli which activate macrophages such as LPS generate cytokines, among which some act as chemoattractants for the accumulation of more effector cells, neutrophils and monocytes, at sites of tissue injury. Such cytokines, including MDNCF (IL-8) and MCAP/MCP-1, further act as inflammatory mediators by binding to receptors on their respective target cells to induce respiratory burst responses and degranulation, resulting in the generation of superoxide (O_2^-) anion and hydrogen peroxide, and the release of lysosomal enzymes.

A summary of the molecular characteristics of the human cytokines and their receptors covered in this chapter is given in Table 5.2.

5.3   Inflammatory reactions

Introduction

Tissue injury and encounters with pathogenic stimuli triggger off a number of endogenous host defence mechanisms that virtually always lead to inflammation. This occurs locally due to the release of several different pre-formed substances by endothelial cells, connective-tissue cells, tissue macrophages, and mast cells. These 'early' mediators of inflammatory reactions include vasodilatory molecules such as bradykinin and histamine which increase blood supply to affected areas, and which increase capillary permeability in the local vasculature. Complement components, e.g. C5a, and the products of blood coagulation are also produced. Together, these inflammatory mediators account for the resultant swelling (oedema), reddening (erythema) and pain (algesia) in the inflamed area, e.g. in skin lesions (Figure 5.5). Such acute inflammation may occur without the overt involvement of the immune system. However, some substances released by pathogenic stimuli themselves (e.g. bacteria) or by cells at the focus of inflammation are chemotactic for neutrophils and macrophages. These lead to the egress of neutrophils and blood monocytes from the blood supply and their accumulation at the site(s) of inflammation. Once there, these cells become activated, e.g. blood monocytes differentiate into functional macrophages with enhanced microbicidal and cytotoxic capabilities, in response to cytokines produced by local tissue cells such as endothelial cells or resident tissue macrophages. Thus, host defence mechanisms become amplified, and when cellular processes are overstimulated by the continuous production of mediators at high level, tissue damage and destruction may result. Further, should the pathogenic stimuli be of such intensity that massive production of inflammatory mediators occurs, their spillage into the circulation can cause acute-phase responses and fever as

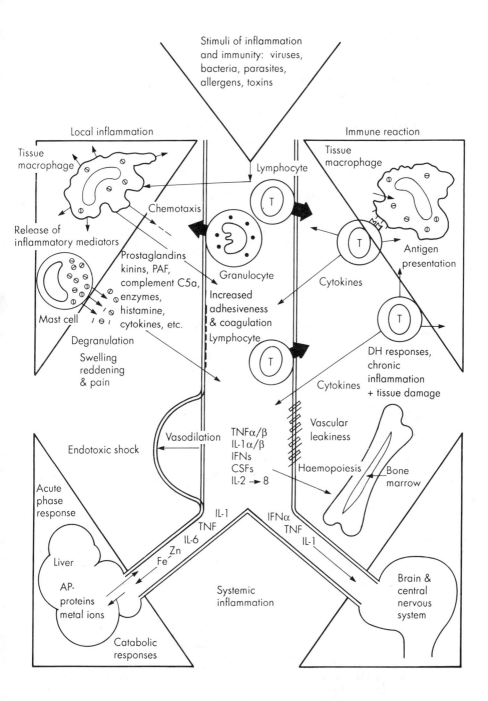

Figure 5.5   Acute and immune-based inflammatory reactions.

well as detrimental systemic changes, e.g. endotoxic shock, which threaten the well-being of the host.

Activated macrophages and neutrophils 'burn, puncture, and poison' pathogenic microorganisms at sites of inflammation and remove these pathogenic stimuli by phagocytosis and digesting them. In doing so, such cells, macrophages in particular, may then present processed foreign antigens in combination with MHC molecules to T-lymphocytes to initiate immune responses (Figure 5.5). Thus, T_H cells become activated and release cytokines, such as IFNγ, IL-3, and IL-6, which in turn stimulate

1   B-cells to proliferate and secrete antibodies,
2   the growth and differentiation of haemopoietic precursors, and
3   the activation of CTL, macrophages, and granulocytes.

By a combination of humoral (antibody) and cell-mediated processes, pathogenic stimuli may then be eliminated. Coincidentally, cytokines produced by T-lymphocytes and macrophages may stimulate tissue repair and wound healing.

If, however, the immunogenic stimulus, i.e. antigen presentation, persists, then again this may lead to overproduction of cytokines and other inflammatory mediators resulting in cell-mediated delayed hypersensitivity responses and chronic inflammatory disease in some cases (Figure 5.5). In the latter case, T-lymphocytes may become activated by self-antigens and give rise to autodestruction of host tissues and autoimmune disease.

Effects of cytokines on the vascular endothelium

The infiltration of damaged or infected tissues by neutrophils and macrophages is an important feature of acute inflammation. As has already been discussed (see pp. 163–6), there are at least two cytokines, MDNCF and MCAF/MCP-1, which act as chemoattractants for neutrophils and macrophages respectively. These and other chemotactic substances released at inflammatory sites probably account for the accumulation from the blood supply of neutrophils and macrophages. However, it is also necessary to 'hold' these phagocytic and cytotoxic cells at sites of inflammation so that they may adhere to the endothelial linings of blood vessels and subsequently move through the vessel wall into the inflamed tissue(s). It is now clear that soluble mediators, including certain cytokines, are involved in the processes which increase adherence between neutrophils and vascular endothelial cells (Figure 5.5).

It has already been mentioned that TNFα and TNFβ induce and/or enhance expression of neutrophil–CDw18 antigen complex, which is important in adherence to endothelial cells and microorganisms. Endothelial cells themselves also respond to TNFs and IL-1 by becoming markedly more adhesive for neutrophils, monocytes, and lymphocytes, thus providing a localized substratum for infiltrating inflammatory leukocytes. Both endothelial leukocyte adhesion molecule-1 (ELAM-1), which serves to bind neutrophils, and intercellular adhesion molecule-1 (ICAM-1) which serves to bind lymphocytes and monocytes, are induced by TNF, IL-1 and possibly IFNγ (ICAM-1 only) in endothelial cells *in vitro*. ELAM-1 is not expressed normally, but is found in high amounts in the endothelial cells of capillary vessels during ongoing acute inflammation, suggesting that the *in vitro* findings with cytokines are directly relevant to the *in vivo* situation.

The vascular endothelium is also involved in procoagulant activity and the deposition of fibrin to form clots, a response to pathogenic and neoplastic stimuli. TNF appears to be a principal mediator of such inflammatory stimuli in that it causes the induction of procoagulant activity and at the same time inhibits an endothelial cell co-factor activity for the anticoagulant protein C pathway. This alteration of endothelial cell haemostatic properties leading to clot formation may potentially limit pathological processes such as infection and tumour growth. The procoagulant effects produced by TNF-stimulation may be mimicked by IL-1, and it would appear that for all intents and purposes the actions of TNF and IL-1, although they act through different cell surface receptors, are nearly identical in endothelial cells (see Table 5.1 for a comparison of TNF and IL-1 activation).

TNF and IL-1 have been demonstrated to stimulate the production *in vitro* of a number of endothelial cell mediators that could be involved in acute inflammation. For example, they induce production of prostacyclin (PGI_2) which is known to be a potent inhibitor of platelet aggregation and a powerful vasodilator. It has been hypothesized that TNF-induced PGI_2 production may have a role in producing depressed blood pressure or shock. It is difficult to reconcile this effect with the procoagulant/clotting responses mentioned above. Possibly, undue vasodilation only occurs at high TNF levels such as would be present during bacterial sepsis. TNF and IL-1 also induce the synthesis of PAF, a mediator with diverse biological activities associated with platelet aggregation, neutrophil degranulation, increased vascular permeability and hypotension (Figure 5.5). PAF may be responsible for endotoxin-induced hypotension and shock, as well as vascular 'leakiness' which is often found accompanying acute inflammation. In addition, TNF and IL-1 may induce their own synthesis together with that of PDGF-A chains and GM-CSF; PDGF has been implicated in wound healing and GM-CSF up-regulates haemopoietic cell production.

Besides enhancing adhesion molecules such as ELAM-1 and ICAM-1, cytokines, and principally IFNs, increase the expression of endothelial cell MHC antigens. It is possible that endothelial cells, as well as macrophages and dendritic cells, are capable of presenting foreign antigens to T-lymphocytes and this results in the initiation of so-called 'immune inflammation'. TNFα/β, and IFNα/β, but not IL-1, stimulate the increased expression of MHC class I molecules in endothelial cells. IFNγ alone or in synergy with TNFα or TNFβ induces the *de novo* synthesis of MHC class II molecules, the latter being required for binding T_H cells via the T-cell (antigen) receptor. In the presence of IL-1, also produced by endothelial cells, bound T_H cells are activated, proliferate, and secrete several immunoregulatory cytokines which can act on other leukocytes. MHC class II expression, which occurs 12–24 hours after IFNγ stimulation, appears to persist as long as IFNγ remains present. This may mean there is a delay in the recruitment of additional T_H cells, but when these are activated the cytokines they produce and/or the secondary perivascular infiltrate of activated neutrophils, macrophages plus CTL which recognize antigen in combination with MHC class I molecules, may initiate hypersensitivity reactions (Figure 5.5). The latter are known as delayed hypersensitivity (DH) responses. *In vitro*, cytokines such as TNF or IL-1 in synergy with IFNγ cause profound changes in the morphology of endothelial cells. They lose their normal polygonal morphology and contact inhibition, and become elongated and overlapping resulting in holes or gaps appearing in the monolayer. It has been hypothesized that these cytokine-induced morphological changes in endothelial cells represent the *in vitro* equivalent of *in vivo* DH reactions, including changes in cell shape and increased vascular permeability.

Immediate hypersensitivity and allergic reactions will be covered in Chapter 7.

Acute phase responses

In the cases of more profound systemic injury or infection, the host responds by a well-recognized series of humoral and cellular reactions known collectively as the acute (inflammatory) phase (AP) response. The AP response is characterized by leukocytosis, alterations in plasma metal ion and steroid concentrations, increased vascular permeability, and fever. In addition, the liver responds by a dramatic change in the synthesis of several plasma proteins as well as by increasing uptake of amino acids and metal ions such as iron and zinc. The plasma proteins include α_1-acid glycoprotein, α_1-antitrypsin, α_1-antichymotrypsin, haptoglobulin, haemopexin, fibrinogen, C-reactive protein, complement components (C3 and factor B), and serum amyloid A protein (in humans). mRNA levels for these proteins increase markedly within a few hours of traumatization. Subsequently, 'acute-phase' proteins are secreted in abundance and plasma levels rise accordingly (Figure 5.5).

It is almost certain that monocytes/macrophages which play a pivotal role in local acute inflammation are the major cellular sources of factors mediating AP responses. Monocytes/macrophages respond to a number of 'noxious' stimuli by secreting certain immunoregulatory and potentially inflammatory cytokines. Principal among these cytokines are IL-1, TNFα, and IL-6. IL-1 was previously known as endogenous pyrogen (EP) and it is clear that its systemic release, together with that of TNFα, leads to fever induction. Both IL-1 and TNF are known to stimulate prostaglandin synthesis, and it is believed that increased prostaglandin PGE_2 secretion in or near the anterior hypothalamus of the brain is responsible for fever induction (Figure 5.5).

The effects of TNF and IL-1 on the vascular endothelium with respect to its increased adhesiveness and permeability have been dealt with in a preceding section (p. 168). However, the identity of a putative 'hormone-like' mediator produced at the site of injury and travelling via the circulation to the liver to effect AP protein synthesis remained unknown until fairly recently. Both TNF and IL-1 appeared to increase AP protein secretion *in vivo*, but their effects on AP protein synthesis in cultured hepatocytes (liver cells) were found to be minimal. This suggested that liver synthesis of AP proteins was controlled by a separate cytokine, probably one that was induced by TNF or IL-1. Researchers working in the field of hepatocyte stimulation also knew that monocytes/macrophages were a major cellular source of what they termed hepatocyte-stimulating factor (HSF). The similarity in the induction characteristics of HSF and IL-6 eventually led, with the molecular cloning and expression of the latter in large amounts, to the discovery that IL-6 was identical to HSF, or was a major component of it. IL-6 is now known to be produced by monocytes/macrophages and a variety of other cell types, including endothelial cells, in response to LPS, TNF, or IL-1 and has been found in raised levels in the plasma in a variety of patients with severe injuries or infections or following major surgery. *In vitro*, IL-6 (HSF) stimulates hepatocytes and hepatoma cell lines to produce many or all of the major AP proteins. Therefore, it would appear that IL-6 is the strongest candidate for the 'hormone-like' factor which mediates liver AP protein production. It remains possible that other cytokines such as IL-1 act independently to modulate liver protein synthesis, positively or negatively, or to act as co-stimulants with IL-6 to synergistically increase the synthesis of particular AP plasma proteins.

Chronic inflammation

Chronic inflammation results from the prolonged persistence of immunogenic stimuli, e.g. when a micro-organism is not completely eradicated, or from the continuous release of inflammatory cytokines by certain tumour cells, e.g. IL-6 from myelomas. Alternatively, T-lymphocytes may have become sensitized to self-antigens leading to endogenous cytokine release, chronic inflammation and tissue damage as found in auto-immune diseases. Besides many of the manifestations of acute inflammation, chronic inflammation is also characterized by tissue wasting and erosion. Certain actions of cytokines again link them strongly to the underlying causes of chronic inflammation. For instance, TNFα is now known to be identical to a hormone associated with tissue wasting (cachexia) called cachectin. The latter, a macrophage product, and recombinant TNFα have been shown to inhibit lipoprotein lipase, an enzyme responsible for fat storage, in cultured adipocytes (fat cells). Thus, it is possible that TNFα (cachectin) could contribute to the cachexia and weight loss frequently associated with chronic invasive diseases, e.g. chronic parasitic disease and cancer. Indeed, administration of TNFα (cachectin) to mice has been demonstrated to induce anorexia (loss of appetite) and an ensuing weight loss. Nevertheless, it is not certain that TNFα decreases fat storage *in vivo*, and thus other cytokines, e.g. IL-1 and mediators may be involved in cachexia.

Tissue erosion probably results mainly from the cytolytic actions of activated leukocytes, but cytokines may directly induce certain degradative
enzymes that compound cell-mediated damage. For example, TNF and IL-1
stimulate synovial cells and other connective tissue cells to secrete collagenase, an enzyme that functions to disrupt extracellular collagen matrices. In
addition, TNF and IL-1 stimulate cartilage resorption and inhibit synthesis of
proteoglycan, the essential matrix component of cartilage. Also, IL-1β has
been shown to be identical to osteoclast-activating factor (OAF), a mediator
responsible for inducing osteoclastic bone-resorbing activity. TNFα and
TNFβ act similarly, but are less potent than IL-1β. Taken together, these *in
vitro* findings suggest that TNFs and IL-1s may be instrumental in causing the
osteolysis and cartilage degradation that accompany some malignant and
rheumatoid diseases.

Further reading

Interferon gamma

Alfa, M.J. and Jay, F.T. (1988) Distinct domains of recombinant human IFN-γ
responsible for anti-viral effector-function. *Journal of Immunology* **141**, 2474.

Aguet, M., Dembic, Z., and Merlin, G. (1988) Molecular cloning and expression of
the human interferon-γ receptor. *Cell* **55**, 273.

Boyd, A.W., Tedder, T. F., Griffin, J.D., *et al.* (1987) Pre-exposure of resting B cells
to interferon-γ enhances their proliferative response to subsequent activation
signals. *Cellular Immunology* **106**, 355.

Cassatella, M.A., Cappelli, R., Bianci, V.D., *et al.* (1988) Interferon-gamma activates
human neutrophil oxygen metabolism and exocytosis. *Immunology* **63**, 499.

Celada, A. (1988) The interferon gamma receptor. *Lymphokine Research* **7**, 61.

Celada, A. and Schreiber, R.D. (1987) Internalization and degradation of receptor-
bound interferon-γ by murine macrophages: demonstration of receptor recycling.
Journal of Immunology **139**, 147.

De Maeyer, E. and De Maeyer-Guignard, J. (1988) *Interferons and Other Regulatory
Cytokines*. John Wiley, New York.

Devos, R., Cheroutre, H., Taya, Y., *et al.* (1982) Molecular cloning of human
immune interferon cDNA and its expression in eukaryotic cells. *Nucleic Acid
Research* **10**, 2487.

Finkelman, F.D., Katona, I.M., Mossman, T.R., and Coffman, R.L. (1988) IFN-γ
regulates the isotypes of Ig secreted during *in vivo* humoral immune responses.
Journal of Immunology **140**, 1022.

Ganser, A., Carlo-Stella, C., Greher, J., *et al.* (1988) Effect of recombinant interferons alpha and gamma on human bone-marrow-derived megakaryocytic progenitor cells. *Blood* **70**, 1173.

Gordon, S., Keshav, S., and Chung, L.P. (1988) Mononuclear phagocytes: tissue
distribution and functional heterogeneity. *Current Opinion in Immunology* **1**, 26.

Gray, P.W. and Goeddel, D.V. (1982) Cloning and expression of the human immune
interferon gene. *Nature* **298**, 859.

Gray, P.W. and Goeddel, D.V. (1983) Cloning and expression of murine immune
interferon cDNA. *Proceedings of the National Academy of Sciences USA* **80**,
5842.

Hemmi, H. and Breitman, T.R. (1987) Combinations of recombinant human interferons and retinoic acid synergistically induce differentiation of the human pro-myelocytic leukaemia cell line HL-60. *Blood* **69**, 501.

Hogan, M.M. and Vogel, S.N. (1988) Inhibition of macrophage tumoricidal activity by glucocorticoids. *Journal of Immunology* **140**, 513.

Kameyama, K., Tanaka, S., Ishida, Y., and Hearing, V.J. (1989) Interferons modulate the expression of hormone receptors on the surface of murine melanoma cells. *Journal of Clinical Investigation* **83**, 213.

Koide, Y., Ina, Y., Nezu, N., and Yoshida, T.O. (1988) Calcium influx and the Ca^{2+}-calmodulin complex are involved in interferon-γ-induced expression of HLA class II molecules on HL-60 cells. *Proceedings of the National Academy of Sciences USA* **85**, 3120.

Landolfo, S., Gariglio, M., Gribaudo, G., *et al.* (1988) Interferon-γ is not an antiviral, but a growth-promoting factor for T lymphocytes. *European Journal of Immunology* **18**, 503.

Langer, J.A. and Pestka, S. (1988) Interferon receptors. *Immunology Today* **9**, 393.

Lotz, M. and Zuraw, B.L. (1987) Interferon-γ is a major regulator of C1-inhibitor synthesis by human blood monocytes. *Journal of Immunology* **139**, 3382.

Luster, A.D. and Ravetch, J.V. (1987) Biochemical characterization of a γ-interferon-inducible cytokine (IP-10). *Journal of Experimental Medicine* **166**, 1084.

Luster, A.D., Weinshank, R.L., Feinman, R., and Ravetch, J.V. (1988) Molecular and biochemical characterization of a novel γ-interferon inducible protein. *Journal of Biological Chemistry* **263**, 12036.

MacDonald, H.S., Kushnaryov, V.M., Sedmak, J.J., and Grossberg, S.E. (1986) Transport of γ-interferon into the cell nucleus may be mediated by nuclear membrane receptors. *Biochemical and Biophysical Research Communications* **138**, 254.

Maudsley, D.J. and Morris, A.G. (1987) Rapid intracellular calcium changes in U937 monocyte cell line: transient increases in response to platelet-activating factor and chemotactic peptide but not interferon-γ or lipopolysaccharide. *Immunology* **61**, 189.

Messadi, D.V., Pober, J.S., and Murphy, G.F. (1988) Effects of recombinant γ-interferon on HLA-DR and DQ expression by skin cells in short term organ culture. *Laboratory Investigation* **58**, 61.

Nathan, C.F. (1987) Secretory products of macrophages. *Journal of Clinical Investigation* **79**, 319.

Naylor, S.L., Sakaguchi, A.Y., Shows, T.B., *et al.* (1983) Human immune interferon gene is located on chromosome 12. *Journal of Experimental Medicine* **57**, 1020.

Petroni, K.C., Shen, L., and Guyre, P.M. (1988) Modulation of human polymorphonuclear leukocyte IgG Fc receptors and Fc receptor-mediated functions of IFN-γ and glucocorticoids. *Journal of Immunology* **140**, 3467.

Rinderknecht, E., O'Connor, B.H., and Rodriguez, H. (1984) Natural human interferon: complete amino acid sequence and determination of sites of glycosylation. *Journal of Biological Chemistry* **259**, 6790.

Sancéau, J., Sondermeyer, P., Béranger, F., *et al.* (1987) Intracellular human γ-interferon triggers an antiviral state in transformed murine L cells. *Proceedings of the National Academy of Sciences USA* **84**, 2906.

Sariban, E., Mitchell, T., Griffin, J., and Kufe, D.W. (1987) Effects of interferon-γ on proto-oncogene expression during induction of human monocytic differentiation. *Journal of Immunology* **138**, 1954.

Sauerwein, R.W., van der Meer, W.G.J., and Aarden, L.A. (1987) Induction of proliferation of B prolymphocytic leukaemia cells by phorbol ester and native or recombinant interferon-γ. *Blood* **70**, 670.

Siegel, J.P. (1988) Effects of interferon-γ on the activation of human T lymphocytes. *Cellular Immunology* **111**, 461.

Stewart, W.E., II. (1978) *The Interferon System.* Springer-Verlag, New York.

Svedersky, L.P., Benton, C.V., Berger, W.H., *et al.* (1984) Biological and antigenic similarities of murine interferon-γ and macrophage-activating factor. *Journal of Experimental Medicine* **159**, 812.

Yip, Y.K., Barrowclough, B.S., Urban, C., and Vilcek, J. (1982) Molecular weight of human gamma interferon is similar to that of other human interferons. *Science* **215**, 411.

Tumour necrosis factors

Aggarwal, B.B., Henzel, W.J., Moffat, B., *et al.* (1985) Primary structure of human derived lymphotoxin from 1788 lymphoblastoid cell line. *Journal of Biological Chemistry* **260**, 2334.

Aggarwal, B.B., Kohr, W.J., Hass, P.E., *et al.* (1985) Human tumour necrosis factor: production, purification and characterization. *Journal of Biological Chemistry* **260**, 2345.

Bakouche, O., Ichinose, Y., Heicappell, R., *et al.* (1988) Plasma membrane-associated tumour necrosis factor: a non-integral membrane protein possibly bound to its own receptor. *Journal of Immunology* **140**, 1142.

Barber, K.E., Crosier, P.S., and Watson, J.D. (1987) The differential inhibition of hemopoietic growth factor activity by cytotoxins and interferon-gamma. *Journal of Immunology* **139**, 1108.

Beutler, B., Greenwald, D., Hulmes, J.D., *et al.* (1985) Identity of tumour necrosis factor and the macrophage secreted factor cachectin. *Nature* **316**, 552.

Camussi, G., Bussolino, F., Salvidio, G., and Baglioni, C. (1987) Tumour necrosis factor/cachectin stimulates peritoneal macrophages, polymorphonuclear neutrophils and vascular endothelial cells to synthesize and release platelet activating factor. *Journal of Experimental Medicine* **166**, 1390.

Dröge, W., Benninghoff, B., and Lehmann, V. (1987) Tumour necrosis factor augments the immunogenicity and the production of L-ornithine by peritoneal macrophages. *Lymphokine Research* **6**, 111.

Ferrante, A., Nandonskar, M., Bates, E.J., *et al.* (1988) Tumour necrosis factor beta (lymphotoxin) inhibits locomotion and stimulates the respiratory burst and degranulation of neutrophils. *Immunology* **63**, 507.

Bock, G. and Marsh, J. (eds.) (1987) *Tumour Necrosis Factor and Related Cytotoxins.* Ciba Foundation Symposium **131**, Wiley, Chichester.

Gray, P.W., Aggarwal, B.B., Benton, C.V., *et al.* (1984) Cloning and expression of cDNA for human lymphotoxin, a lymphokine with tumour necrosis activity. *Nature* **312**, 721.

Hackett, R.J., Davis, L.S., and Lipsky, P.E. (1988) Comparative effects of tumour necrosis factor-α and IL-1β on mitogen-induced T cell activation. *Journal of Immunology* **140**, 2639.

Hori, K., Ehrke, M.J., Mace, K., *et al.* (1987) Effect of recombinant human tumour necrosis factor on the induction of murine macrophage tumoricidal activity. *Cancer Research* **47**, 2793.

Hudziak, R.M., Lewis, G.D., Shalaby, M.R., *et al.* (1988) Amplified expression of the HER2/ERBB$_2$ oncogene induces resistance to tumour necrosis factor α in NIH3T3 cells. *Proceedings of the National Academy of Sciences USA* **85**, 5102.

Jelinek, D.F. and Lipsky, P.E. (1987) Enhancement of human B cell proliferation and differentiation by tumour necrosis factor-α and interleukin-1. *Journal of Immunology* **139**, 2870.

Johnson, S.E. and Baglioni, C. (1988) Tumour necrosis factor receptors and cytocidal activity are down-regulated by activators of protein kinase C. *Journal of Biological Chemistry* **263**, 5686.

Jones, E.Y., Stuart, D.I., and Walker, N.P.C. (1989) Structure of tumour necrosis factor. *Nature* **338**, 225.

Kehrl, J.H., Alvarez-Mon, M., Delsing, G.A., and Franci, A.S. (1987) Lymphotoxin is an important T-cell-derived growth factor for human B cells. *Science* **238**, 1144.

Kournatzki, E., Kapp, A., and Uhrich, S. (1988) Modulation of human neutrophil granulocyte functions by recombinant tumour tumour necrosis factor and recombinant human lymphotoxin. Promotion of adherence, inhibition of chemotactic migration and superoxide anion release from adherent cells. *Clinical and Experimental Immunology* **74**, 143.

Larrick, J.W., Graham, D., Toy, K., *et al.* (1987) Recombinant tumour necrosis factor causes activation of human granulocytes. *Blood* **69**, 640.

Le, J. and Vilcek, J. (1987) Tumour necrosis factor and interleukin-1: cytokines with multiple overlapping biological activities. *Laboratory Investigation* **56**, 234.

Lee, J.C., Truneh, A. Smith, M.I., and Tsang, K.Y. (1987) Induction of interleukin 2 receptor (Tac) by tumour necrosis factor in YT cells. *Journal of Immunology* **139**, 1935.

Lin, J.-X. and Vilcek, J. (1987) Tumour necrosis factor and interleukin-1 cause a rapid and transient stimulation of c-*fos* and c-*myc* mRNA levels in human fibroblasts. *Journal of Biological Chemistry* **262**, 11908.

Malek, T.R., Danis, K.M., and Codias, E.K. (1989) Tumour necrosis factor synergistically acts with IFN gamma to regulate Ly-6A/E expression in T lymphocytes, thymocytes and bone marrow cells. *Journal of Immunology* **142**, 1929.

Owen-Schaub, L.B., Gutterman, J.U., and Grimm, E.A. (1988) Synergy of tumour necrosis factor and interleukin 2 in the activation of human cytotoxic lymphocytes. *Cancer Research* **48**, 788.

Palombella, V.J., Yamashiro, D.J., Maxfield, F.R., *et al.* (1987) Tumour necrosis factor increases the number of epidermal growth factor receptors on human fibroblasts. *Journal of Biological Chemistry* **262**, 1950.

Paulson, Y., Austgulen, R., Hofsli, E., *et al.* (1989) Tumour necrosis factor-induced expression of platelet-derived growth factor A-chain messenger RNA in fibroblasts. *Experimental Cell Research* **180**, 490.

Pennica, D., Nedwin, G.E., Hayflick, J.S., *et al.* (1984) Human tumour necrosis factor: precursor structure, expression and homology to lymphotoxin. *Nature* **312**, 724.

Ransom, J.H., Evans, C.H., McCabe, R.P., *et al.* (1985) Leukoregulin, a direct-acting anticancer immunological hormone that is distinct from lymphotoxin and interferon. *Cancer Research* **45**, 851.

Schütze, S., Scheurich, P., Pfizenmaier, K., and Krönke, M. (1989) Tumour necrosis factor signal transduction: tissue-specific serine phosphorylation of a 26-kDa cytosolic protein. *Journal of Biological Chemistry* **264**, 3562.

Shalaby, M.R., Aggarwal, B.B., Rindernecht, E., *et al.* (1985) Activation of human polymorphonuclear neutrophil functions by gamma interferon and tumour necrosis factor. *Journal of Immunology* **135**, 2069.

Stauber, B.G. and Aggarwal, B.B. (1989) Characterization and affinity cross-linking of receptors for human recombinant lymphotoxin (tumour necrosis factor-β) on a human histocytic lymphoma cell line, U-937. *Journal of Biological Chemistry* **264**, 3573.

Stauber, G.B., Aiyer, R.A., and Aggarwal, B.B. (1988) Human tumour necrosis factor-α receptor: purification by immunoaffinity chromatography and initial characterization. *Journal of Biological Chemistry* **263**, 19098.

Stone-Wolff, D.S., Yip, Y.K., Chroboczek-Kelker, H., *et al.* (1984) Inter-relationships of human interferon gamma with lymphotoxin and monocyte cytotoxin. *Journal of Experimental Medicine* **159**, 828.

Trinchieri, G., Rosen, M., and Perussia, B. (1987) Induction of differentiation of human myeloid cell lines by tumour necrosis factor in co-operation with 1α, 25-dihydroxyvitamin D3. *Cancer Research* **47**, 2236.

Zucali, J.R., Elfenbein, G.J., Barth, K.C., and Dinarello, C.A. (1987) Effects of human interleukin-1 and tumour necrosis factor on human T lymphocyte colony formation. *Journal of Clinical Investigation* **80**, 772.

Soluble chemoattractant proteins: interleukin-8

Furutani, Y., Nomura, H., Notake, M., *et al.* (1989) Cloning and sequencing of the cDNA for human monocyte chemotactic and activating factor. *Biochemical and Biophysical Research Communications* **159**, 249.

Larsen, C.G., Anderson, A.O., Appella, E., *et al.* (1988) The neutrophil-activating protein (NAP-1) is also chemotactic for T lymphocytes. *Science* **243**, 1464.

Matsushima, K., Morishita, K., Yoshimura, T., *et al.* (1988) Molecular cloning of a human monocyte-derived neutrophil chemotactic factor (MDNCF) and the induction of MDNCF mRNA by interleukin-1 and tumour necrosis factor. *Journal of Experimental Medicine* **167**, 1883.

Samanta, A.K., Oppenheim, J.J., and Matsushima, K. (1989) Identification and characterization of specific receptors for monocyte-derived neutrophil chemotactic factor (MDNCF) on human neutrophils. *Journal of Experimental Medicine* **169**, 1185.

Strieter, R.M., Kunkel, S.L., Showell, H.J., *et al.* (1988) Endothelial cell gene expression of a neutrophil chemotactic factor by TNF-α, LPS and IL-1β. *Science* **243**, 1467.

Van Damme, J., Beeumen, J.V., Opdenakker, G., and Billiau, A. (1988) A novel, NH$_2$-terminal sequence-characterized human monokine possessing neutrophil chemotactic, skin-reactive, and granulocytosis-promoting activity. *Journal of Experimental Medicine* **167**, 1364.

Yoshimura, T., Yuhki, N., Moore, S.K., *et al.* (1989) Human monocyte chemoattractant protein-1 (MCP-1). *FEBS Letters* **244**, 487.

Effects of cytokines on vascular endothelium

Cavender, D.E., Edelbaum, D., and Ziff, M. (1989) Endothelial cell activation induced by tumour necrosis factor and lymphotoxin. *American Journal of Pathology* **134**, 551.

Cotran, R.S. (1987) New roles for the endothelium in inflammation and immunity. *American Journal of Pathology* **129**, 407.

Dinarello, C.A. (1987) The biology of interleukin 1 and comparison to tumour necrosis factor. *Immunology Letters* **16**, 227.

Lapierre, L.A., Fiers, W., and Pober, J.S. (1988) Three distinct classes of regulatory cytokines control endothelial cell MHC antigen expression. *Journal of Experimental Medicine* **167**, 794.

Male, D. and Pryce, G. (1988) Synergy between interferons and monokines in MHC induction on brain endothelium. *Immunology Letters* **17**, 267.

Morrison, D.C. (1987) Endotoxins and disease mechanisms. *Annual Reviews of Medicine* **38**, 417.
Pober, J.S. (1988) Cytokine-mediated activation of vascular endothelium: physiology and pathology. *American Journal of Pathology* **133**, 426.
Steinman, R.M. (1988) Cytokines amplify the function of accessory cells. *Immunology Letters* **17**, 197.
Van Hinsbergh, V.W.M., Kooistra, T., van den Berg, E.A., *et al.* (1988) Tumour necrosis factor increases the production of plasminogen activator inhibitor in human endothelial cells *in vitro* and in rats *in vivo. Blood* **72**, 1467.

Acute-phase responses

Baumann, H., Richards, C., and Gauldie, J. (1987) Interaction among hepatocyte-stimulating factors, interleukin-1 and glucocorticoids for regulation of acute phase plasma proteins in human hepatoma (HepG2) cells. *Journal of Immunology* **139**, 4122.
Baumann, H., Onorato, V., Gauldie, J., and Jahreis, G.P. (1987) Distinct sets of acute phase plasma proteins are stimulated by separate human hepatocyte-stimulating factors and monokines in rat hepatoma cells. *Journal of Biological Chemistry* **262**, 9756.
Gauldie, J., Richards, C., Harnish, D., *et al.* (1987) Interferon beta-2/B-cell stimulatory factor type 2 shares identity with monocyte-derived hepatocyte-stimulating factor and regulates the major acute phase protein response in liver cells. *Proceedings of the National Academy of Sciences USA* **84**, 7251.
Houssiau, F.A., Bukasa, K., Sindic, C.J.M., *et al.* (1988) Elevated levels of the 26k human hybridoma growth factor (interleukin 6) in cerebrospinal fluid of patients with acute infection of the central nervous system. *Clinical and Experimental Immunology* **71**, 320.
Jirik, F.R., Podor, T.J., Hirano, T., *et al.* (1989) Bacterial lipopolysaccharide and inflammatory mediators augment IL-6 secretion by human endothelial cells. *Journal of Immunology* **142**, 144.
Marinkov, S., Jahreis, G.P., Wong, G.G., and Baumann, H. (1989) IL-6 modulates the synthesis of a specific set of acute phase plasma proteins *in vivo. Journal of Immunology* **142**, 808.
May, L.T., Ghrayeb, J., Santhanam, U., *et al.* (1988) Synthesis and secretion of multiple forms of beta-2-interferon/B cell differentiation factor 2/hepatocyte-stimulating factor by human fibroblasts and monocytes. *Journal of Biological Chemistry* **263**, 7760.
Morrone, G., Ciliberto, G., Olivero, S., *et al.* (1988) Recombinant interleukin 6 regulates the transcriptional activation of a set of human acute phase genes. *Journal of Biological Chemistry* **263**, 12554.
Ramadori, G., Van Damme, J., Rieder, H., *et al.* (1988) Interleukin 6, the third mediator of acute-phase reaction, modulates hepatic protein synthesis in human and mouse; comparison with interleukin-1 beta and tumour necrosis factor-alpha. *European Journal of Immunology* **18**, 1259.
Rappolee, D.A. and Webb, Z. (1988) Secretory products of phagocytes. *Current Opinion in Immunology* **1**, 47.

Chronic inflammation

Beutler, B. and Cerami, A. (1988) The common mediator of shock, cachexia, and tumour necrosis, in *Advances in Immunology* **42** (Dixon, F.J. ed.) Academic

Press, San Diego, p.213.

Canalis, E. (1987) Effects of tumor necrosis factor on bone formation *in vitro*. *Endocrinology* **140**, 827.

Dinarello, C.A. (1989) Interleukin-1 and its biologically related cytokines, in *Advances in Immunology* **44** (Dixon, F.J., ed.) Academic Press, San Diego, p.153.

Ikebe, T., Hirata, M., and Koga, T. (1988) Effects of human recombinant tumour necrosis factor alpha and interleukin-1 on the synthesis of glycosaminoglycan and DNA in cultured rat costal chondrocytes. *Journal of Immunology* **140**, 827.

Le, J. and Vilcek, J. (1987) Tumor necrosis factor and interleukin-1: cytokines with multiple overlapping biological activities. *Laboratory Investigation* **56**, 234.

Mahony, S.M. and Tisdale, M.J. (1988) Induction of weight loss and metabolic alterations by human recombinant tumour necrosis factor. *British Journal of Cancer* **58**, 345.

Price, S.R., Olivecrona, T., and Pekala, P.H. (1986) Regulation of lipoprotein lipase synthesis in 3T3-L1 adipocytes by cachectin. *Biochemical Journal* **240**, 601.

Solis-Herruzo, J.A., Brenner, D.A., and Chojkier, M. (1988) Tumor necrosis factor alpha inhibits collagen gene transcription and collagen synthesis in cultured human fibroblasts. *Journal of Biological Chemistry* **263**, 5841.

6

Antiviral, antimicrobial, and antitumour cytokines

6.1 Introduction

The last three chapters have covered a number of cytokines which are able to activate cells to respond positively to tissue injury, microbial infection, and invasive neoplasia. Principally, macrophages, granulocytes, and lymphocytes of the immune system are activated by particular cytokines to orchestrate and amplify immune and inflammatory responses that lead to the destruction, inactivation, and elimination of noxious and potentially pathogenic stimuli. These activated cells 'fight off' infectious microbes by various humoral and cell-mediated mechanisms. For example, activated mature B-lymphocytes or plasma cells secrete antibodies which bind to viral particles or bacteria to form immune complexes which can be cleared from the body. Activated macrophages and granulocytes phagocytose micro-organisms and may kill infected or tumour cells by their several cytotoxic/cytolytic actions, e.g. release of reactive oxygen intermediates, degranulation, and secretion of cytotoxic mediators such as TNF. Functional CTL may kill infected cells by first recognizing microbial antigens presented in combination with MHC class I molecules on the cell surface through binding to the T-cell antigen receptor, and then puncturing them by inserting 'perforins' into the plasma membrane. While the defensive activities of cytokine-stimulated cells against extracellular pathogens and infected host cells undoubtedly play a major part in the eradication of pathogenic micro-organisms, cytokines also have effects that directly inhibit the replication of intracellular pathogens. Some cytokines already discussed, e.g. IFNγ, TNF, GM-CSF, IL-4, have this inhibitory action, but there is a major group of cytokines, IFNγ and IFNβ, which are of prime importance for the inhibition of viral replication, and which probably have other protective roles. IFN was discovered in 1957 as an inhibitor of infectious virus production, but has subsequently been shown to have many activities that also affect cell growth, differentiation and function. Thus IFN, which is now known to consist of a relatively large number of molecularly related species (to be described below) has biological characteristics typical of cytokines.

Cancer or tumour cells have aberrant phenotypic and genotypic characteristics that distinguish them from normal diploid cells. The abnormal, unregulated proliferation of tumour cells predisposes them to certain chemical cytotoxic drugs and, as is becoming increasingly apparent, to growth inhibition and cytolysis by a number of cytokines. The latter include IFNα, IFNβ, and IFNγ, TNFα and TNFβ, IL-1 and the recently characterized oncostatin M. The antitumour properties of these cytokines will be covered in the latter part of this chapter.

6.2   Interferons alpha and beta

Nomenclature

The designation of IFNs was described in Chapter 5, but will be reiterated here for the sake of clarity. Based on the producer-cell type and antigenic properties of IFN, three different types of IFN were originally defined. These were known as leukocyte-, fibroblast-, and immune-IFNs and these names were used throughout the 1960s and 1970s. Additionally, based on physicochemical properties, IFNs, as defined above, were subdivided into two types: type I IFN was resistant to pH_2 (acid) inactivation and included both leukocyte- and fibroblast-IFN, whereas type II IFN was acid-labile and synonymous with immune-IFN. However, in 1978, an International Nomenclature committee re-designated leukocyte-IFN as IFNα, fibroblast-IFN as IFNβ, and immune-IFN as IFNγ. This nomenclature system was unfortunately devised before the full extent of the heterogeneous nature of IFNs and their intermolecular relationships were revealed by rDNA methods. When this happened, shortcomings of the α, β, γ system were emphasized, and led to the confusing use by different research groups of alternative nomenclature systems, particularly for IFNα. In this chapter, the different molecular species of IFNα are referred to as subtypes and designated by Arabic numerals: IFNα1, IFNα2, etc. In addition, two-letter prefixes are used to denote the species' origin. Thus for human, HuIFNα, for mouse, MuIFNα, for bovines, BoIFNα, etc. IFNβ is not heterogeneous in man, but is often referred to as IFNβ1. Rather unfortunately, in 1980, the name IFNβ2 was used to describe what was then thought to be a second subtype of human IFNβ. The eventual molecular cloning of the cDNA of this cytokine has revealed that it shows only very weak sequence homology to human IFNβ (Figure 6.1), but has sequence identity with BSF-2, subsequently renamed IL-6 (see Chapter 4). Human recombinant IL-6 (formerly IFNβ2, BSF-2) in comparison with human recombinant IFNβ, and indeed with other IFNs in general, has very low antiviral activity and its claim to be an IFN is therefore slight. There are however in other species, e.g. bovines, multiple subtypes of IFNβ which share a high degree of sequence homology and for which the β1, β2, β3 terminology would be appropriate. In contrast, the designation of IFNγ has remained simple, there being only one gene and one (glyco)protein in all species thus far examined.

There are one or two other complications regarding IFN nomenclature, but these will be dealt with as they arise in the text to follow.

Molecular characterization of interferon alpha and interferon beta

All IFNs are inducible, secreted proteins or glycoproteins (monomeric MW ~20 000). However, the main stumbling block to their molecular characterization was that they could only be obtained in very small quantities from mammalian cells. Thus, only following the advent of gene-cloning methods in the late 1970s, approximately 20 years after the first isolation of IFN, was the complexity of IFNs at the molecular level revealed. IFN mRNA-containing poly(A)$^+$ RNA preparations from appropriately stimulated human cells were used to synthesize cDNAs which were then inserted into bacterial plasmids. The latter were used to transform *E.coli* and subsequently IFN cDNA-containing bacteria were identified, cloned, and grown up to mass culture. IFN cDNAs were then re-isolated, sequenced, and attached to bacterial promoters to ensure high levels of expression.

Partial amino acid sequences for both IFNα and IFNβ had been determined with small amounts of these proteins, purified from medium conditioned by IFN-producing cells, prior to molecular cloning. Sequencing of IFN cDNAs permitted the full amino acid sequences of a number of IFNs to be inferred, and these were found to be in broad agreement with N-terminal amino acid sequences deduced from IFN proteins. However, the major outcome from the sequencing of IFN cDNAs was the discovery of substantial molecular heterogeneity within the IFNα type. It now appears that there are probably as many as 23 different human IFNα genes and pseudogenes, giving rise to a family of at least 16 closely related proteins known as subtypes. Most of these IFNα subtypes are predicted to contain 166 amino acids (165 in the case of the IFNα2 subtype), but a more recently cloned member is predicted to have 172 amino acids (Figure 6.1). Rather confusingly, the latter has been designated IFNαII, and even IFNω by one group! All the IFNα subtypes, including the larger-sized one, are synthesized in human cells with an N-terminal signal sequence of 23 amino acids which is cleaved off before secretion. Most IFNα subtypes do not contain sites for N-linked oligosaccharides, but there is some evidence for carbohydrates being associated with IFNα, possibly via O-linked glycosylation. The molecular weight of IFNα subtypes is approximately 18 500, although apparent molecular weights in sodium dodecyl sulphate (SDS)-polyacrylamide gels vary from 17 000 to 26 000.

All human IFNα subtypes are highly related in primary structure. Among the subtypes with 166 amino acids, one of the largest divergences of primary

Figure 6.1   Amino acid sequence comparison of human IFNs. Asterisks indicate positions of amino acid identity among IFNα1, α2, αII(ω), β1 and β2 (IL-6).

<pre>
                  *   *   *

α1   L A V K K Y F R R I T L Y L T E K K Y S P C A W E V V R A

α2   L A V R K Y F Q R I T L Y L K E K K Y S P C A W E V V R A

αII(w)   L T L R R Y F Q G I A V Y L K E K K Y S D C A W E V V R M

β1   L H L K R Y Y G R I L H Y L K A K E Y S H C A W T I V R V

β2 (IL-6) L L T - - - - - - - - - - - - - - K L Q A Q N Q W L Q D M T

γ   I Q V M A E L - - - - - - - - - - - - S P A A K T G K R K

                       *   * *

α1   - - E I M R S L S L S T N L Q E R L R R K E¹⁶⁶

α2   - - E I M R S F S L S T N L Q E S L R S K E¹⁶⁵

αII(w)   - - E I M K S L F L S T N M Q E R L R S K D A D L G SS¹⁷²

β1   - - E I L R N F Y F I N R L T G Y L R N¹⁶⁶

β2 (IL-6) T H L I L R S F K E F - - L Q S S L R A L R Q M¹⁸⁴

γ   - - R -.- - - - - - S Q M L - F R G R R A S Q¹⁴³
</pre>

<pre>
β2 (IL-6)   -28 M N S F S T S A F G P V A

β2 (IL-6) F S L G L L L V L P A A F P A P¹V P P G E D S K D V A A P

                                                  *

α1   -23M A S P F A L L M V L V V L S C K S S C S L G¹C D L P

α2   M A L T F A L L V A L L V L S C K S S C S V G¹C D L P

αII(w)   M V L L L P L L V A L P L C H C G P C G S L S¹C D L P

β1   -21M T N K C L L Q I A L L L C F S T T A L S¹M S Y N L L

β2 (IL-6)   H R Q P L T S S E R I D K Q I R Y I L D G I S A L R K E T

γ   -23M K Y T S Y I L A F Q L C I V L - G S L G C Y C Q¹D P
</pre>

```
                            *                                    *
α1      E T H S L D N R R T L M L L A Q M S R I S P S S C L M D R
α2      Q T H S L G S R R T L M L L A Q M R K I S L F S C L K D R
αII(w)  Q N H G L L S R N T L V L L H Q M R R I S P F L C L K D R
β1      G F L Q R S S N F Q C Q K L L W Q L N G R L E Y C L K D R
β2 (IL-6) C N K S N M C E S S K E A L A E N N L N L P K M A E K D -
γ       Y V K E A E N L K K Y F N A G H S D V A D N G T L F L G I


                  *                 *                                    *
α1      H D F G F P Q - E E F D G N Q F Q K A P A I S V L H - E L
α2      H D F G F P Q - E E F - G N Q F Q K A E T I P V L H - E M
αII(w)  R D F R F P Q - E M V K G S Q L Q K A H V M S V L H - E M
β1      M N F D I P E - E I K Q L Q Q F Q K E D A A L T I Y - E M
β2 (IL-6) G C F Q S G F N E E T C L V K I I T G L L E F E V Y L E Y
γ       L K N W K E E - S D R K I M Q S Q I V S F Y F K L - - - -


                  *     *             * *
α1      I Q Q I F N L F T T K D S S A A W D E D L L D K F C T E L
α2      I Q Q I F N L F S T K D S S A A W D E T L L D K F Y T E L
αII(w)  L Q Q I F S L F H T E R S S A A W N M T L L D Q L H T E L
β1      L Q N I F A I F R Q D S S S T G W N E T I V E N L L A N V
β2 (IL-6) L Q N R F - - - - - - E S S E E Q A R A V Q M S T K V L I
γ       F K N F K D D Q S I Q K S V E T I K E D M N V K F F N S N


                  *
α1      Y Q - Q L N D L E A C V M Q E E R V G E T P L M N A D S I
α2      Y Q - Q L N D L E A C V I Q G V G V T E T P L M K E D S I
αII(w)  H Q - Q L Q H L E T C L L Q V V G E G E S A G A I S S P A
β1      Y H - Q I N H L K T V L E E K L E K E D F T R G K L M S S
β2 (IL-6) Q F L Q K K A K N L D A I - - - - - - T T P D P T T N A S
γ       K K - K R D D F E K L T N Y S V T D L N V Q R K A I H E L
```

structures is the 28 (17 per cent) amino acid difference found between IFNα1 and IFNα2 (Figure 6.1). The subtype with 172 amino acids (IFNαII or IFNω) is somewhat less related at about 56 per cent homology to IFNα1 (Figure 6.1). However, the positions of the four cysteines involved in intrachain disulphide bridge formation are precisely conserved in all IFN subtypes. The three-dimensional structure of IFN-α has yet to be determined, but computer predictions based on hydropathy profiles suggest that it has a high α-helix content (*c.* 60 per cent) (Figure 6.2). IFNα subtypes of other animal species show a similar degree of heterogeneity to human ones, but individual subtypes have diverged somewhat from their human counterparts during evolution. The numbers of subtypes and their sizes are also variable among different species, although the positions of four cysteine residues are universally conserved. For example, MuIFNα subtypes, for which ten different cDNAs have been cloned and expressed, contain 166 or 167 amino acids, or exceptionally 162 (MuIFNα4). MuIFNα subtypes are only about 40 per cent homologous to their human counterparts. This means there is considerable species preference in biological activity, i.e. MuIFNα is only weakly active in human cells, and HuIFNα subtypes, with one or two exceptions, are poorly active in mouse cells. (This species preference is not always so profound; HuIFNα subtypes are highly active in bovine cells, for example.) Unlike the HuIFNα subtypes, most MuIFNα subtypes contain one N-linked glycosylation site and are probably glycoproteins in their native state.

Genes for HuIFNα subtypes have been shown to be clustered together and located on the short arm of chromosome 9. The equivalent site for MuIFNα genes is mouse chromosome 4. All of the IFNα genes are intron-less, which is unusual among cytokine genes.

Human IFNβ, sometimes called HuIFNβ1, contains 166 amino acids, is preceded by a 21 amino acid N-terminal signal sequence, and shows only 29 per cent homology with HuIFNα2, i.e. 118 (71 per cent) differences out of 166 amino acids (Figure 6.1). In common with the HuIFNα subtype genes, the gene for HuIFNβ is intron-less and is also closely linked to HuIFNα genes on chromosome 9. It is clear that genes for IFNα subtypes and IFNβ evolved from a common ancestor. Unlike HuIFNα proteins, HuIFNβ contains an N-linked oligosaccharide side chain (Asn, p80), and thus is a glycoprotein, its apparent molecular weight in SDS-polyacrylamide gels being approximately 21 000. HuIFNβ contains only three cysteine residues and only one of the two disulphide bridges found in HuIFNα subtypes is conserved (p31–p141). In contrast, MuIFNβ has 161 amino acids, contains three potential N-linked glycosylation sites (the molecular weight of native glycoprotein is 34 000), but only a single cysteine and thus no possibility of on intramolecular disulphide bond. It is about 60 per cent homologous to HuIFNβ but there is no cross-species reactivity. For bovine (Bo) IFNβ, there are at least three distinct genes coding for three highly related 165 amino acid BoIFNβ glycoproteins; these might be legitimately called BoIFNβ1, β2, and β3.

While HuIL-6 (IFNβ2) does not appear to fit into the classical type I IFN (IFNα + IFNβ) family, aligning the amino acid sequence with those of

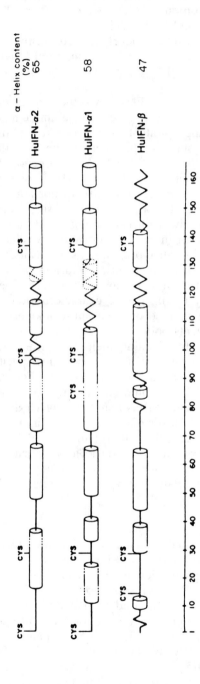

Figure 6.2 Secondary structure predictions for HuIFNα and HuIFNβ. Residues were scored for their relative tendencies to exist in four possible states (α-helix, extended chain, reverse turn, and coil) based on values for each amino acid obtained by examination of 26 protein crystal structures. Only α-helix (barrels) and extended chain (β-strands, zigzags) are shown since they are predicted most accurately. Stretches equally likely to be in α-helix or extended chain are shown with these structures dotted and superimposed. Regions with moderate helical potential which might be strengthened by adjoining helical regions are shown as dotted connections between helices. (From Zoon and Wetzel, 1984, *Handbook of Experimental Pharmacology* **71**, 79; reprinted with permission from Springer-Verlag, Berlin.)

IFNα1, IFNα2, IFNαII, and IFNβ to give maximum correspondence of amino acids, as in Figure 6.1, gives 17 positions of identity among them all and 28 positions of identity between IL-6 and IFNβ. This suggests a distant evolutionary relationship. IFNγ appears also to be poorly related to either the type I IFN family or IL-6, but unlike IL-6 does have distinct antiviral activity. The molecular characterization of IL-6 and IFNγ has been described in Chapters 4 and 5 respectively.

From an antigenic point of view, human IFNs vary sufficiently in structure from their animal counterparts that they can be used as immunogens for raising IFN-specific antisera in appropriate animals. Further, HuIFNβ is sufficiently dissimilar to HuIFNα subtypes for there to be essentially no cross-reaction between anti-HuIFNβ and anti-HuIFNα, a distinction that was recognized early between the fibroblast and leukocyte-IFNs of the older nomenclature system. As expected, neither anti-HuIFNβ nor anti-HuIFNα recognizes the molecularly unrelated HuIFNγ. Rather surprisingly the HuIFN-αII (ω) subtype is antigenically distinct from most or all of the other HuIFNα subtypes, which are however themselves antigenically related.

As the availability of more highly purified preparations of IFN increased in the 1980s, the possibility of preparing moabs against the various IFNs became evident. Large numbers of anti-IFN moabs have subsequently been developed and have been extremely useful for the characterization and immunoassay of IFNs. (It should be pointed out that anti-cytokine moabs in general have been important reagents both for the antigenic identification/characterization of cytokines and for defining their biological activities.) Moabs raised against a particular type of IFN are very highly specific, and cross-reactivity with other IFN types has rarely been observed. For example, a moab raised against HuIFNα2 does not bind either HuIFNβ or HuIFNγ. Such a moab may however bind other HuIFNα subtypes which display the equivalent antigenic determinant of HuIFNα2. Nevertheless, a moab raised against HuIFNαII (ω) does not recognize other HuIFNα subtypes, thus confirming its antigenic dissimilarity with these latter. The specificity of some moabs is often so great that even minor differences in structure, e.g. a single amino acid change between closely related subtypes, can be detected.

Induction of IFNα and IFNβ

There are many ways in which normal cells may be stimulated to produce IFN. The major cell sources and stimuli are shown in Table 6.1. This, however, encompasses only a simplistic view of IFN induction and production, since it is known that several cell types respond to stimuli by producing a mixture of IFNs. For instance, virally induced human diploid fibroblasts produce mainly HuIFNβ, but also produce a minor amount of HuIFNα. Cells of the immune system produce IFNα, IFNβ, or IFNγ depending on the induction stimulus. For example, T-lymphocytes produce mainly IFNγ following mitogenic or antigenic stimulation, but if these cells are virally infected, they may produce IFNα and/or IFNβ. It should be pointed out that

Table 6.1   Production of IFN by normal human cells

Interferon type	Alternative name	Major producer cells	Stimuli for production
IFNα (sub-classes I and II)	Leukocyte IFN	Null lymphocytes, monocytes/ macrophages	Viruses, bacteria, xenogenic or allogeneic tumour cells, virally infected cells, B-cell mitogens
IFNβ1	Fibroblast IFN	Fibroblasts, epithelial cells	Viruses, polynuc-leotides
IFNβ2	26 kDa protein B-cell stimula-tory factor 2 (BSF-2) IL-6	Fibroblasts, monocytes	Polynucleotides, cyto-kines (e.g. TNF, IL-1)
IFNγ	Immune IFN	T-lymphocytes, NK cells	Allogeneic cells or virally infected syngeneic cells, foreign antigens, T-cell mitogens

other cytokines, e.g. IL-2 or TNF, may be co-produced with IFNs in response to common stimuli.

Besides normal cells, a range of tumour-derived cell lines are known to be IFN producers. For example, paramyxoviral infection (e.g. Sendai virus) of the human B-lymphoblastoid cell line Namalwa induces the production of a mixture of IFNα subtypes and a minor amount of IFNβ, this mixture often being referred to as 'lymphoblastoid IFN'. The osteosarcoma-derived fibrob-last cell line MG63 has been found to be a good producer of HuIFNβ following induction by polyI:C or virus. It is likely that the nature of the IFNs produced by normal and tumour cells is subject to genetic control which influences transcription of IFN genes, translation of IFN mRNAs, and post-translational modifications to IFN proteins.

Normally, IFNα and IFNβ genes are not expressed. However, inducibility appears to reside in the IFN genes themselves, since when a HuIFNα gene is transferred into a mouse cell, where it integrates with the mouse genome, it remains inducible by viruses. By examining various IFN gene constructs, DNA sequences in the 5′ non-coding region have been delineated which appear to control inducibility. These have been called IFN gene regulatory elements (IRE). It is probable that the IRE is a transcriptional enhancer, similar to those found in other cytokine genes, which operates in response to direct binding of nuclear transcription factors. It is thought that upon induc-tion two repressor proteins are removed from 'positive response domains' in the 5′ non-coding region, followed by association or binding of nuclear transcription factors, the second of which may be identical to NF-κB, for which potential binding sites are present in a number of genes involved in the immune response, and which allows IFN mRNA transcription to proceed.

Although there are many IFN inducers, e.g. viruses, double-stranded RNAs, growth factors (cytokines), etc, the signalling pathways and the molecular mechanisms leading to IFN gene transcription are not known. However, the fact that double-stranded RNA itself, which is often an intermediate in viral genome replication of RNA-containing viruses, is able to induce IFN gene expression, suggests that double-stranded RNA is the 'proximal inducer'. The question that remains is whether double-stranded RNA interacts with the repressor proteins bound to the IFN gene IRE or with nuclear transcription factor elements in the cytoplasm, but there is as yet no unambiguous evidence to answer this. It is also not clear whether double-stranded RNA is unique as a 'proximal inducer' or whether there are other molecules which could perform the same function.

Following induction, transcription of IFN mRNAs continues only for a brief period of a few hours before the IFN genes are fully 'shut-down' again. The reasons for this renewed repression of IFN genes remain unanswered. Transcription of IFN mRNAs, particularly that of IFNβ, may however, be enhanced by blockers of protein synthesis such as cycloheximide. The simplest explanation of this enhanced transcription is that the inhibition of protein synthesis curtails the production of IFN gene repressor proteins, although cycloheximide may also stabilize IFNβ mRNA in as yet unknown ways.

IFNα and IFNβ receptors: structure–activity relationships of IFNs

Receptors for IFNα and IFNβ appear to be ubiquitous, and it is almost certain that all the IFNα subtypes and IFNβ share a common receptor. This receptor is distinct from the IFNγ receptor (IFNg-R) and human × mouse hybrids, in which human chromosomes are segregated, have indicated that the IFNα/β receptor (IFNa/b-R) gene is located on chromosome 21. Binding studies with ^{125}I-labelled IFNα or IFNβ have demonstrated the presence of a few thousand high-affinity receptors per cell for many cell types. Chemical cross-linking studies with radiolabelled IFNα or IFNβ to receptor-bearing cells have led to the identification of a 150 kDa complex; the size of the putative receptor is therefore around 130 kDa. It is likely that this receptor is a cell-surface glycoprotein, since binding of IFNα is lost following protease-treatment of cells. Molecular cloning of the IFNa/b-R has yet to be accomplished, despite several years of intensive research effort (but see p. 226).

Since the three-dimensional structures of IFNα and IFNβ and the molecular structure of their cell surface receptor have yet to be elucidated, it is currently unknown how signalling mechanisms operate. However, it is known that substitution of particular single amino acids in IFN molecules, using genetic manipulation techniques, may either deleteriously affect activity or alter the degree of species specificity, i.e. the activity in heterologous species cells. Thus, the magnitude of the cellular response may depend in part on how well particular IFNs bind to or 'fit' the receptor. In general, it appears that structurally intact IFN molecules are required to stimulate cellular responses; denatured or fragmented IFNs are inactive. While a few amino acids may be removed from the N- and C- terminals of IFNα subtypes without dramatic loss of activity, the intactness of intramolecular disulphide bonds is probably essential for structural integrity and fully biologically active molecules. However, glycosylation as in IFNβ and MuIFNα subtypes is unnecessary for biological activity, at least *in vitro*.

It is currently unclear which amino acids of IFNα or IFNβ are involved in the interaction with receptor molecules. Most evidence to date, where hybrid and substituted IFNα molecules have been investigated, suggests that amino acids in positions 10–44, 80–86, and 121, 125, and 132 are important for binding to receptors. Thus, it is probable that amino acid residues in both the N- and C-terminal halves of IFNα are required for biological activity. The question that remains unanswered is why there are so many structurally distinct IFNα subtypes when there is apparently only a single population of receptors. IFNα subtypes and IFNβ are qualitatively similar in the cellular responses they evoke, although there are quantitative differences in activity amongst these IFNs. For example, recombinant HuIFNα1 appears to be much less potent than recombinant HuIFNα2 in the induction of antiviral activity in human cells *in vitro*. This observation may again reflect how well these HuIFNα subtypes 'fit' the IFNa/b-R, and there is some evidence that HuIFNα1 has reduced avidity for this. Nevertheless, the problem of biochemical redundancy of IFNα subtypes remains. It has been speculated that the functions of individual IFNα subtypes are subtly different and mediated by a common receptor which, however, has a mosaic of 'pressure pads' in its binding site. The slightly varying overall shapes of IFNα subtypes would then determine which 'pressure pad' was triggered and ultimately the nature and strength of the cellular response. Such a model assumes a multichannel receptor giving rise to differential activation of independent, intracellular signalling pathways and offers an attractive explanation of the pleiotypic effects of IFNs. Regrettably, there is as yet no evidence to substantiate this hypothetical model.

Modes of action of IFNα and IFNβ; comparison with IFNγ

Antiviral activity
Antiviral effects in cells are expressed several hours after interaction of IFNs with their specific receptors at the cell surface. However, it is not yet known what the transmembrane or intracellular signals are that cause the reprogramming of nuclear genes necessary for the establishment of the antiviral state, or indeed for the other manifestations/phenomena associated with IFN–cell interactions. It is clear that the development of the antiviral state, which probably reflects an integral part of the overall cellular response to IFNs, is dependent upon protein synthesis; a dozen or so proteins are induced by IFNα or IFNβ in human fibroblasts. This set of proteins is also induced by

IFNγ indicating some similarity in the activation pathways of IFNα and IFNγ. However, IFNγ induces several additional proteins, besides the common set, suggesting that it activates cells differently in some respects to IFNα. The development of the antiviral state is rapid, a matter of a few hours, in cells treated with IFNα or IFNβ, but the induction of antiviral activity by IFNγ is by contrast much slower (more than six hours). It has been suggested that IFNγ actually induces IFNα/β, and that it is the latter which is responsible for antiviral action by autocrine stimulation. The recent finding by one group that IFNγ-stimulated mouse L-929 cells produce MuIFNα and that the development of the antiviral state in these cells is blocked by poly- or monoclonal antibodies which specifically neutralize the effects of MuIFNα lends strong support for this suggestion. Such results, however, have been rarely, if ever, observed by others in the past and verification is required to prove that the antiviral action of IFNγ is indirect. A similar suggestion has been made to explain the antiviral activity of TNFα and TNFβ, but to date, while the expression of IL-6 mRNA is readily detected in TNF-stimulated fibroblasts, expression of IFNβ mRNA has not been unequivocally found. Nevertheless, antibodies to IFNβ have been found to block TNF-mediated antiviral activity.

Several genes and proteins activated by IFNs have been identified, but only those which have been implicated as playing a role in the inhibition of viral replication will be covered in this section. The best characterized are those which affect protein synthesis. One enzyme known as 2,5A-synthetase is induced in some cells and is activated in the presence of double-stranded RNA, often a by-product of viral transcription, to catalyse a reaction leading to the formation of an unusual oligonucleotide known as 2-5A (Table 6.2). This substance acts as a potent inhibitor of protein synthesis by indirectly activating an endonuclease which in turn degrades mRNA (Figure 6.3). Although both IFNα/β and IFNγ induce 2,5A-synthetase, its appearance is relatively late when induced by IFNγ, and this would fit with its slower induction of the antiviral state. In some IFN-treated cells, activation of a protein kinase leads to the phosphorylation of a peptide initiation factor, eIF2, involved in polyribosomal translation of mRNA (Table 6.2). The phosphorylated eIF2 is inactive and hence protein synthesis is inhibited (Figure 6.3). While these two pathways clearly affect protein synthesis in general, it is not understood how they specifically inhibit viral protein synthesis. Part of the explanation might be that any inhibitory effects on protein synthesis will more profoundly affect the rapid replication of relatively simple, intracellular pathogens such as viruses than the slower, more complex, processes involved in cell growth.

While inhibition of viral protein synthesis is likely to diminish the replication of all infectious viruses, certain other IFN-induced effects may affect the replication of particular viruses. For example, the MuIFNα induced synthesis of a nuclear protein called Mx appears to specifically inhibit influenza virus replication in mouse cells (Table 6.2). IFNs also induce changes in the structure and fluidity of cell membranes and these may limit the assembly and budding processes associated with the late replicative stages of enveloped

Table 6.2   Proteins induced by interferons

Protein	Function	Induction by IFNα/β	IFNγ
2,5A-synthetase	dsRNA-dependent synthesis of ppp (A2p) n-A (2–5A); activator of RNase F	+	+
Protein kinase	Phosphorylation of peptide initiation factor eIF-2α	+	+
MHC class I (HLA-A, B, C)	Antigen presentation to CTL	+	+
MHC class II (HLA-DR)	Antigen presentation to T_H-lymphocytes	±	+
Indoleamine 2, 3 dioxygenase	Tryptophan catabolism	−	+
Guanylate-binding proteins	GTP, GDP binding	+	+
Mx	Specific inhibition of influenza virus	+	−
IP-10	Related to chemotactic IL-8-like proteins	±	+
Metallothionine	Metal detoxification	+	+
TNF receptor	Cell surface receptor for TNF	±	+
IL-2 receptor	T-lymphocyte receptor for IL-2	−	+
Intercellular adherence molecule (ICAM-1)	Endothelial cell adhesion protein	−	+
Immunoglobulin Fc-receptor (Ig-FcR)	Ig binding by macrophages/neutrophils	±	+
Thymosin β 4	Induction of terminal transferase in B lymphocytes	+	?
Nuclear transcription factors	Induction of IFN-responsive genes	+	+

viruses, e.g. retroviruses. In fact, IFNs may induce multiphase antiviral effects where viral functions are inhibited at particular stages of the viral replicative cycle. The outcome of such antiviral activity will depend both on the type of virus and the type of cell, and probably also on the type of IFN.

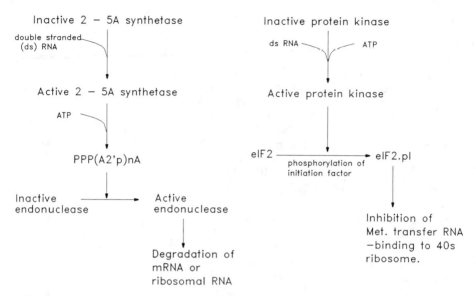

Figure 6.3   Translation inhibitory pathways activated by IFN treatment of cells.

Antiproliferative effects

All IFNs, at doses usually greater than those required for antiviral activity, have demonstrable antiproliferative effects in many cell lines grown *in vitro*, including both normal and tumour cells. Generally, cell-cycling (the time interval required for completion of the cell cycle) may be shown to be increased in the presence of IFN, but it is as yet unclear which of several potential mechanisms are involved. The effect of IFN on overall RNA and protein synthesis appears to be limited. Nevertheless, selective action of IFN has been shown on certain proteins — some are induced, e.g. 2,5A-synthetase, while others are inhibited, e.g. c-MYC. Obviously, enzymes such as 2,5A-synthetase and endonucleases (see above) which inhibit protein synthesis generally may play a role in IFN-induced cytostasis and, interestingly, higher levels of these have often been found in resting or growth-arrested cells than in proliferating cells. Another enzyme that is affected by IFNs is ornithine decarboxylase. This catalyses the first rate-limiting step in polyamine synthesis. Polyamines are crucial for the regulation of numerous cellular processes, e.g. protein synthesis, and thus the observed decrease in ornithine decarboxylase activity in IFN-treated cells may inhibit proliferation. (Note that other cytokines such as TNF increase ornithine decarboxylase activity in proliferation-responsive cells.) Similarly, synthesis of calmodulin, the major intracellular calcium-binding protein, is also inhibited in IFN-treated cells. Calmodulin binds to and activates several Ca^{2+}-dependent enzymes and has been shown to play an important part in controlling cell proliferation both *in vitro* and *in vivo*. IFNs may also limit growth by acting as antagonists of the proliferation-stimulatory effects of growth factors, e.g. insulin, PDGF, EGF; a decrease in numbers of plasma-membrane receptors for these mediators often follows IFN treatment. Finally, IFNs are potent inhibitors of oncogene expression in transformed and tumour cell lines, e.g. c-*myc* in the human B-lymphoblastoid cell line Daudi by HuIFNα.

The situation regarding inhibition of cell proliferation by IFNs is thus likely to be complex. There are also quantitative and qualitative differences in the capacity of individual IFN types and subtypes to decrease cell proliferation. For example, HuIFNα2 appears to be more potent generally than HuIFNα1 and the proliferation of Daudi cells, which is highly susceptible to the inhibitory effects of HuIFNα/β, is, despite the presence of IFNg-R in Daudi cells, unaffected by HuIFNγ. In other tumour cell lines, the antiproliferative effects (also antiviral effects) of IFNα/β may be enhanced synergistically by the simultaneous addition of IFNγ. Other cytokines, e.g. TNFs, may also potentiate, and therefore augment, the antiproliferative action of IFNs; the combination of IFNγ and TNFα is particularly effective in certain tumour cell lines. The availability of other factors, e.g. insulin and essential metabolites normally required for cell growth and mitogenesis, will also affect the antiproliferative action of IFNs.

Differentiation and immunomodulation
The antiproliferative activity of IFNs is often linked to their effects on differentiation or development of cell phenotype. For example, the inhibition of c-*myc* oncogene expression in the promyelomonocytic cell line HL-60 precedes terminal differentiation into macrophage-like cells and cessation of cell division. However, long-term *in vitro* cultivation of some tumour cells in the presence of IFNα/β frequently leads to an apparent 'reversion' of cell phenotype towards non-tumorigenicity without dramatic changes in pro-liferation rate. Such 'reverted' cell have increased cell volume, morphologi-cally resemble normal cells and exhibit contact-inhibited growth, although oncogene, e.g. H-*ras*, expression may or may not be affected. Some of these changes reflect underlying IFN-induced alterations to the cytoskeleton and cell membrane. IFNs are known to increase significantly microtubules and actin-containing fibres and to alter the distribution of cell surface fibronectin, changes which may be expected to affect cell shape and plasma membrane rigidity. Furthermore, IFNs have been shown to cause rapid alterations in the phospholipid composition of cell membranes, which possibly also increase membrane rigidity.

An IFN-induced effect on the plasma membrane of major biological importance is the increased expression of MHC antigens in many cell types, including immunocytes (leukocytes). The MHC antigens are cell-surface glycoproteins which are essential for reactions of immune recognition of foreign, non-self, antigens. All IFN types stimulate expression of MHC class I (e.g. HLA-A, B, C) molecules and release of β2-microglobulin in lympho-cytes (Table 6.2). IFNγ appears to be the most potent IFN in this respect and, in contrast to most IFNα subtypes and IFNβ, is able to induce *de novo* synthesis of MHC class II (e.g. HLA-DR) molecules in antigen-presenting cells such as macrophages and endothelial cells. Under certain conditions IFNα/β may antagonize the MHC class II-inducing capacity of IFNγ. IFNs may also variably induce/enhance MHC class I and/or class II expression in tumour cells and virally infected cells, both *in vitro* and *in vivo*, and thus increase their recognition by CTL. IFN-inducible genes, such as MHC antigen genes, contain IFN response sequences in their 5' flanking regions and are regulated by inducible transcription factors.

IFNs also appear to be involved in the differentiation of CTL. For example, IFNγ has been shown to be a necessary factor for the maturation to cytotoxicity of CTL. In addition, IFNα has been shown to induce rearrangement of T-cell antigen receptor α-chain genes and again maturation to cytotoxicity of CTL *in vitro*.

Another differentiation antigen, the IgG-Fc receptor (FcR) on macrophages is also increased following stimulation with IFNα/β or IFNγ (Table 6.2). The capacity of macrophages to affect ADCC and FcR-mediated phagocytosis is thus enhanced. The effects of IFNγ on MHC class II antigens and FcR have been shown to be enhanced by vitamin D_3, a differentiation inducer, and to be antagonized by glucocorticoids, which are known to inhibit macrophage differentiation.

Besides the IFN-induced differentiation involving modulation of cell surface antigen expression, many other IFN-induced effects on the functional behaviour of cells have been described. For example, IFNs may regulate antibody production by B-lymphocytes. In low concentrations, IFNα/β appear to enhance IgG synthesis, but in high concentrations they are inhibitory. IFNγ in contrast may act as a co-stimulant for proliferation in resting B-cells and as an Ig isotype switch in antibody-producing plasma cells (see Chapter 5). IFNs also have profound effects in NK cells. These are a heterogeneous population of lymphoid cells, morphologically identified as LGL, with respect to

1   a number of cell surface antigens such as FcR, a variety of T-lymphocyte markers (e.g. CD1, CD8, CD10, CD11) and the monocyte/macrophage marker OKM1, and
2   target cell specificity.

NK cells are capable of carrying out a variety of cytotoxic and immunoregulatory functions *in vitro*. As well as being able to kill virally infected cells and certain tumour cell targets in the absence of antibody and without restriction by MHC antigens, they are also active in regulating proliferative and/or functional responses of a range of normal cell types, including B-lymphocytes, thymocytes, and certain haematopoietic progenitor cells. NK cells are believed to have antitumour effects *in vivo*, although compelling evidence to support this belief remains elusive. IFNs and other cytokines, e.g. IL-2, can markedly increase the *in vitro* cytotoxic activity of NK cells against virally infected cells, allogeneic tumour cells, and certain tumour cell lines, e.g. the erythroleukaemic line K562. IFNα/β and IL-2 appear to be much more effective in augmenting NK cell cytotoxic function than is IFNγ. Activated NK cells produce a range of cytokines, including IFNγ, TNFα, and an uncharacterized cytotoxin known as NKCF, which have various immuno-regulatory and protective roles.

6.3 Antiviral cytokines

Viruses in general, by their replicative processes, trigger cellular responses that are 'designed' to restrict viral replication and the spread of infectious progeny viruses to other cells. IFNs, and perhaps one or two other cyto-kines, are important antiviral mediators whose synthesis and secretion is induced by viral replication. IFNs act locally at the focus of infection to protect cells from infectious progeny virus particles by inducing a cellular 'antiviral state'. The latter is probably a part of the overall cellular response to IFNs, as IFNs are known to profoundly affect cellular metabolic processes and thus likely to inhibit both viral and cellular proliferation. Of the other cytokines, only TNFα and TNFβ have antiviral activity, and this only in certain circumstances. TNFα has been shown to induce a set of nine proteins in human fibroblasts, two of which appear to be in common with those proteins induced by IFNα. Possibly one of these common proteins is 2,5A-synthetase, which is known to be induced by both IFNα and TNFα, and for which there is evidence for a role in reducing viral mRNA translation. In contrast, IL-1α which induces seven of the nine proteins induced by TNFα, does not induce any proteins in common with those induced by IFNα, and has not been found to induce antiviral activity. However, it should be noted that while IFNα and IFNγ have antiproliferative effects in human fibroblasts, TNFα and IL-α have growth stimulatory effects, in the same cells.

The induction of nuclear transcription factors necessary for the prolifera-tive response may in some circumstances render cells permissive for viral replication. For example, TNFα induces the nuclear transcription factor NF-κB in T-cells and monocytes, and this factor appears to activate the HIV genome for transcription. Thus, the antiviral effects, if any, of cytokines depends critically on the type of virus and its mode of replication.

The antiviral activities of different IFN types, mixtures, and single cloned recombinant species can differ for individual viruses, and also depend on the 'virus–cell system' investigated, indicating that multiple molecular mechan-isms of IFN action exist, as has already been exemplified (see pp. 189–92). While viruses are incredibly diverse regarding their structure and strategy of replication, most viruses are inhibited in one way or another by IFNs. Thus, the macromolecular synthesis of many virus families, including picornavir-idae, rhabdoviridae, orthomyxoviridae, reoviridae, poxviridae, adenoviridae, herpesviridae, and retroviridae, is inhibited by one or more mechanisms induced by IFNs. It is regrettably not possible to give a comprehensive account of the antiviral actions of particular IFNs on different viruses in this chapter. However, it is pertinent to give a few examples to illustrate relevant antiviral mechanisms induced by IFNs.

Small RNA viruses, picornaviridae, are among those most susceptible to the inhibitory antiviral actions of IFNs. For two viruses in this family, namely Mengovirus and encephalomyocarditis virus (EMCV), the effect of IFNα/β treatment is to inhibit the synthesis of viral polypeptides. This inhibitory effect has been shown to correlate well with the induction of 2,5A-synthetase activity. When the antisense RNA of 2,5A-synthetase is introduced into cells, enzyme activity cannot be induced (presumably the antisense RNA and the normal 2,5A-synthetase-coding mRNA combine to form a non-translatable double-stranded hybrid) by IFN, and EMCV protein synthesis is not inhibited following infection. Conversely, in cells constitutively expressing high levels of 2,5A-synthetase, Mengovirus protein synthesis is inhibited. Thus, the 2,5A-synthetase system is probably the major effector of inhibition of picornavirus replication through indirect degradative cleavage of viral mRNA by 2,5A-activated endonuclease, although this has not been unequivocally demonstrated. For rhabdoviridae, e.g. vesicular stomatitis virus (VSV), identification of the precise inhibitory mechanism(s) which prevents viral macromolecular synthesis has proved more elusive. IFNα/β have been variously reported to inhibit VSV replication by inhibiting

1   VSV transcription, or
2   cap methylation of VSV mRNA transcripts or
3   translation of VSV mRNAs, or
4   glycosylation of the VSV coat protein.

This apparent diversity of IFN-induced antiviral effects may in part be a reflection of the use of different cell types in which such studies were performed. For example, in human fibroblasts IFNα-induced inhibition of VSV replication is probably mediated via reduction of viral mRNA transcription, whereas in the human U-cell line the inhibition appears to occur solely at the level of viral mRNA translation. The latter has been associated with the IFN-induced protein kinase which is responsible for phosphorylating, and thus inactivating, the eIF-2 peptide initiation factor. Co-infection of VSV-infected, IFN-treated cells with vaccinia virus, a member of the poxviridae, blocks induction of this protein kinase and leads to 'rescue' of VSV replication. In contrast, IFNγ appears to inhibit VSV replication by a mechanism which does not overtly affect either viral RNA or protein synthesis. The 'unique' antiviral mechanisms induced by IFNα and IFNγ respectively have been found to be synergistic for the inhibition of VSV replication in human U-cells.

In the case of influenza virus, a member of the orthomyxoviridae, IFNα/β appears to inhibit viral replication in mouse cells by induction of a 75 kDa protein called Mx. Influenza virus has a nucleus-located phase in its replicative cycle, and Mx probably inhibits early primary transcription to form viral mRNAs. Only cells isolated from mice carrying Mx[+] gene can be protected by IFNα from influenza virus infection, but by contrast Mx cannot be induced by IFNγ. The replication of other viruses, e.g. VSV, is not affected by the presence in cells of the Mx protein. An 'Mx-like' protein has been described for humans, but it is not yet clear whether this plays the same role in preventing influenza virus replication in human cells as does Mx in mouse cells.

The antiviral effects of IFNs and other cytokines on HIV replication are being intensively studied. To date, *in vitro* studies have indicated that IFNα/β inhibit HIV replication in PBL and in T-cell and monocyte cell lines, whilst IFNγ is less effective, especially in PBL and T-cell lines. However, synergistic inhibitory effects have been observed between IFNγ and GM-CSF in monocytic cell lines, e.g. U-937. In addition, TNFα has been reported to reduce the susceptibility of the human T-cell line HUT-78 to HIV infection, again a synergistic inhibitory effect being observed in combination with IFNγ. Nevertheless, in apparent contradiction to these results, more recent investigations strongly suggest that TNFα may enhance replication of HIV *in vitro*. This difference in the TNFα susceptibility of HIV replication is probably explainable by the varying responses to TNFα in the different cell types used in the current studies, and once more emphasizes the complexity of cytokine–virus–cell interactions. The molecular mechanisms underlying the IFNα/β inhibition of HIV replication are not known. By comparison, in cells infected with Molony murine leukaemia virus, another retrovirus, antiviral action of IFNs appears to be mediated by inhibition of viral assembly. In other cases, early events before proviral integration, or expression of retroviral oncogene, or post-translational processing of viral precursor polypeptides, are inhibited in IFN-treated cells. The involvement of various antiviral mechanisms in the inhibition of replication of different viruses is summarized in Table 6.3.

There is a diversity of IFN-inducible antiviral mechanisms, which potentially can inhibit the growth of a wide range of viruses, but whose efficiencies are however dependent upon the type of IFN, the type of virus, the type of cell, and the experimental conditions under which such investigations are performed. *In vivo*, further layers of complexity may be added. Besides the direct antiviral actions of IFNs, viral replication will be subject to humoral and various cell-mediated antiviral processes, as well as compartmental and micro-environmental (e.g. thermoregulatory) restrictions. Antiviral antibodies, if present, provide prophylactic protection; prior vaccination with certain inactivated or attenuated viruses will induce neutralizing antibodies that block reinfection with the same or related virus as contained in the vaccine. Ideally, vaccines should also induce virus-specific CTL which persist in the circulation (memory CTL) and which clear any secondary viral infections that break through antibody neutralization.

Acute virus infections may be envisaged to follow a pattern of events, although there is some variation, leading to a temporal sequence of host-mediated responses. Typically, in the absence of antibody, a virus replicates in its target tissue(s) to give a burst of infectious virus progeny particles known as viraemia. During this time, infected cells respond by secreting IFNα/β and other cytokines, and these may limit the local spread of infectious virus. Two or three days after onset of infection, virus shedding reaches its

Table 6.3   Antiviral mechanisms applying to different virus families

Virus family	Genome	Mechanisms induced by IFN
Papovaviridae (includes SV40, polyoma)	DNA	Inhibition of uncoating of virions, before early transcription
Picornaviridae (includes rhinoviruses, poliovirus, encephalomyocarditis virus, Coxsackie virus)	RNA (+ sense)	2,5-A-synthetase system, inhibition of viral polypeptide synthesis
Rhabdoviridae (includes VSV, rabies virus)	RNA (− sense)	2,5-A-synthetase system and/or eIF-2α initiation factor-protein kinase, inhibition of viral polypeptide synthesis. Also inhibition of cap methylation of viral transcripts, and inhibition of glycosylation of viral envelope protein
Orthomyxoviridae (influenza viruses)	RNA (− sense)	Mx protein, inhibition of early nuclear-phase transcription of viral mRNAs (IFNα/β only)
Reoviridae (various serotypes, bovine diarrhoea virus)	RNA	2,5-A-synthetase system, inhibition of early viral protein synthesis leading to inhibition of second-stage uncoating of viral RNA in cores. Maybe more complex
Adenoviridae (various serotypes)	DNA	Resistant to IFNα/β through production of two small virus-associated (VA)-RNAs which inhibit activation of eIF-2α protein kinase
Herpesviridae (herpes simplex, chickenpox)	DNA	Inhibition of translation of HSV early mRNA into HSV early proteins — 2,5A-synthetase system? (macrophages). In fibroblasts, late stage of viral replication inhibited, e.g. inhibition of viral glycoproteins and assembly
Retroviridae RSV, HTLV-1	RNA	*Acute infections*: IFNs act at early stage, e.g. preventing synthesis or integration of proviral DNA *Chronic infections*: IFNs act at late stage, e.g. inhibition of viral assembly

maximum rate and this is often accompanied by IFNs and other cytokines being found in the circulation. At this stage, fever may be induced, probably as a direct result of the pyrogenic properties of circulating cytokines, e.g. IFNα. Some viruses have been found to replicate poorly at elevated temperatures, and thus fever should be regarded as a protective response. Further, systemic IFNα/β activates NK cells which may directly lyse virus-infected cells in the absence of antibody and the involvement of the MHC complex. Activated NK cells themselves secrete cytokines, including IFNγ and TNFα, which activate macrophages and T-lymphocytes besides inducing/enhancing MHC antigen expression to increase presentation and recognition of viral antigens. About one week after infection commenced, sites of viral replication are infiltrated by CTL and virally infected cells specifically lysed. At about two weeks, antibodies to the virus start to appear in the circulation, and these combine with any remaining released viral particles and subvirion debris to form immune complexes which are removed from the circulation by phagocytic cells. ADCC by macrophages and neutrophils of any virally infected cells that still remain also then becomes possible. Individuals previously exposed to a particular virus or recently vaccinated against the virus could be expected to resist reinfection more strongly because of increased production of IFNs from primed or sensitized leukocytes, the presence of antibodies and greater numbers of virus-specific CTL, and the possibility of ADCC.

As has been discussed, cytokines, particularly IFNs, may be intimately associated with each stage of host defence mechanisms against viral infections. That they are essential mediators of host defence mechanisms is inferred mainly from their actions *in vitro*, but there is also strong circumstantial evidence from *in vivo* studies to confirm their crucial involvement. For example, mice injected with neutralizing antibodies against IFNα/β are markedly more susceptible to certain viral infections and show more severe symptoms. Further, cells isolated from animals or humans with active viral infections are found to manifest the antiviral state *in vitro* without the addition of exogenous IFN. Animals with deficient immune systems or patients undergoing immunosuppressive therapy have low numbers of circulating leukocytes and have a greatly increased risk of viral infections and reactivation of latent viruses, e.g. cytomegalovirus and herpes zoster (chickenpox) virus. Certain strains of inbred mice show genetically linked deficiency of IFNα/β production and are more susceptible to certain viruses than mouse strains able to produce normal high levels of IFN. Interestingly in this regard, some children are peculiarly susceptible to rhinovirus (common cold) infections and this too has been linked with deficient IFNα/β production.

Other evidence for the protective role of IFNs against viral infections comes from clinical studies in which high doses of IFN were evaluated for their prophylactic or therapeutic use in certain virus diseases. This will be discussed in Chapter 9, which deals with the clinical applications of IFNs and other cytokines.

6.4   Antimicrobial cytokines

A vast range of micro-organisms, including bacteria, mycoplasma, rickettsiae, chlamydia, protozoa, and fungi, have been reported to induce IFN synthesis. This, as in the case of viruses, suggests that IFNs and probably other cytokines are critically involved in activating host defensive responses against microbial infections. However, IFNs have little or no apparent effects in isolated cultured microorganisms, probably because such prokaryotic cells lack IFN receptors. Thus, IFNs and other cytokines are much more likely to affect the growth of micro-organisms which replicate intracellularly in host cells. Nevertheless, such parasitic micro-organisms have their own membrane-bound macromolecular synthetic apparatus and therefore are not likely to be affected by IFN-induced effects that inhibit the replication of 'naked' viruses, which is totally host-cell dependent. Alternative IFN-induced mechanisms are thus suggested for controlling/inhibiting the growth of intracellular pathogenic micro-organisms, and these are mainly of the indirect cell-mediated, phagocytic and cytolytic variety. There are however a few direct effects of IFNs which may limit intracellular replication of certain micro-organisms, without the participation of cell-mediated immune mechanisms, and these will be described first.

One enzyme, not so far discussed, called indoleamine 2,3-dioxygenase (IDO) is induced by IFNs, and in particular by IFNγ (Table 6.2), and probably has a crucial role in inhibiting the growth of certain intracellular micro-organisms. IDO catalyses the conversion of tryptophan, one of eight essential amino acids, to N-formylkynurenine. The rapid catabolism of tryptophan in IFN-treated cells inhibits microbial growth by tryptophan deprivation. For example, the replication of the obligate intracellular protozoon *Toxoplasma gondii*, which can invade almost all body cells, is inhibited by IFNγ and appears to be regulated by the availability of tryptophan. Similarly, *in vitro*, IFNγ-mediated inhibition of chlamydial growth in human epithelial cells and fibroblasts appears also to depend on activation of IDO and the resultant tryptophan 'starvation'. This inhibitory mechanism probably does not apply to all cells, e.g. inhibition of *Chlamydia* in murine systems, or appear to affect the replication of other groups of micro-organisms, e.g. rickettsial growth in IFNγ-treated fibroblasts. IFNγ does however induce other inhibitory mechanisms which decrease rickettsial growth. These probably require host–cell protein synthesis, but are as yet poorly characterized.

Besides playing a pivotal role in immunoregulatory and inflammatory responses, the macrophage is a host cell for many micro-organisms, including *Toxoplasma gondii*, *Leishmania* (another family of protozoan parasites which grow only in monocytes/macrophages), *Trypanosoma cruzi*, *Mycobacteria*, e.g. *M. tuberculosis*, and *Legionella pneumophila*, the causative agent of Legionnaires' disease. Some of these micro-organisms are sensitive to macrophage-derived respiratory burst oxidative metabolites, e.g. hydrogen peroxide. IFNs, and especially IFNγ, activate macrophages leading to increased respiratory burst and the synthesis of reactive oxygen intermediates (ROI). The latter involves the consumption of exogenous oxygen and its conversion by respiratory burst oxidase, in combination with a cytochrome b pathway in the plasma membrane, firstly to O_2^- (superoxide anion), and subsequently to highly reactive hydroxyl radicals, singlet oxygen, and hydrogen peroxide, which are potentially toxic to micro-organisms. It should be noted that O_2^- is a necessary co-factor for the IDO-mediated catabolism of tryptophan to N-formylkynurenine, and that these antimicrobial pathways are therefore interlinked and may act cooperatively in some instances. For example, oxidative killing of *Leishmania donovani* may occur during parasite entry into macrophages, or the parasite may be killed intracellularly by oxidative and non-oxidative mechanisms. That IFNγ is the cytokine that activates cells to kill *L.donovani* in this way is supported by the finding that neutralizing anti-IFNγ antibodies administered to mice increased the parasite numbers. However, the interactions between IFNγ-induced non-specific immune responses and replicative stages of protozoan parasites are likely to be much more complex than indicated above. In the case of malarial infections, malaria sporozoites, introduced into the host by the bite of *Anopheles* mosquitoes, invade the liver hepatocytes and there multiply rapidly, enclosed in a structure known as the exoerythrocytic form (EEF). When the EEF ruptures, thousands of merozoites enter the circulation to infect red blood cells (erythrocytes) and continue the malarial life cycle. IFNγ has been shown to be effective in inhibiting malarial parasite replication *in vitro*, but only at the intrahepatocytic-EEF stage. IFNα/β was much less effective, and IL-1 treatment was effective only when applied before sporozoite infection *in vitro*. However, *in vivo*, IFNγ and TNFα probably activate macrophages and neutrophils to release ROI which kill the intraerythrocytic malaria parasites. Substances which 'scavenge' ROI have been found to increase malarial replication suggesting that T-cell-dependent, macrophage-derived mediators, e.g. TNFα, are central to host antimalarial actions. The more complex interaction between T-cell- and macrophage-derived cytokines and cerebral malaria will be outlined in Chapter 8.

For bacterial and mycobacterial infections, evidence for a crucial role of IFNγ is less conclusive. In the case of *Legionella pneumophila*, replication in macrophages is inhibited by IFNγ treatment, but intracellular bacteria are not killed. Similarly, IFNγ may induce antimycobacterial activity in murine macrophages, but is singularly ineffective in doing so in human macrophages. It would appear in many instances that IFNγ is not the only cytokine with antimicrobial activity. Possibly other macrophage-activating cytokines such as IL-2, IL-4, TNFα, and GM-CSF either individually, or in combination with IFNγ, induce stronger intracellular antimicrobial mechanisms.

In vivo, the involvement of specific immune mechanisms adds an additional tier of antimicrobial effector systems. For instance, the release of chemoattractants and microbial antigen presentation by macrophages and endothelial cells recruits and activates T_H lymphocytes, which release a number of cytokines necessary for inducing/enhancing/maintaining T-cell functions and the recruitment and activation of phagocytic cells, i.e. monocytes and neutrophils, and CTL. (T-cell cytotoxicity does not appear to be a predominant host defence mechanism against micro-organisms, as it is in viral infections.) The continuous release of cytokines at the focus of infections leads to a large accumulation of such leukocytes which initiate the formation of granulomas — nodular-like tissue masses characteristic of infections caused by obligate or facultative intracellular microorganisms, especially mycobacteria, e.g. *M.*

tuberculosis, *M. leprae* (leprosy), *Leishmania*, and *Listeria monocytogenes*. Granulomas represent a cell-mediated chronic inflammatory response to persistent infection(s) present in various anatomical sites, which probably prevent dissemination of the infectious microbe while permitting macrophage- and neutrophil-mediated destruction of the microbes. The generation of ROI by macrophages/neutrophils in response to IFNγ, TNFα/β, and other activating cytokines is probably responsible, at least in part, for their microbicidal action. For example, patients with chronic granulomatous disease, who are inherently deficient in the respiratory burst oxidase system, suffer from repeated severe bacterial infections of the deep tissues. If the infectious microbes are not cleared, and persist over long periods, the continued production of ROI can result in tissue damage and destruction.

For extracellular pathogenic micro-organisms, it is probably true that cell-mediated responses are more likely to occur in the presence of antibodies. These bind to the micro-organism and serve as an opsonin. (Opsonization is the process whereby particles are coated with substances, e.g. antibodies, which render them more readily phagocytosed.) IFNγ is known to increase the expression of Ig-FcR in monocytes/macrophages and neutrophils, and thus facilitates the immobilization and phagocytosis of opsonized micro-organisms. Once engulfed, the micro-organisms are killed by the actions of a variety of hydrolytic lysosomal enzymes, toxic ROI, and growth inhibitors, e.g. lactoferrin, which sequesters iron necessary for microbial replication. A number of secreted enzymes produced by macrophages, e.g. lysozyme and neutral proteases, may be important for inhibiting the growth of micro-organisms in the extracellular milieu.

Neutrophil-mediated ADCC has also been shown to be increased by TNFα/β. This may be responsible for neutrophil-mediated inhibition of the growth of micro-organisms such as *Candida albicans*. TNFs may also activate eosinophils to kill or inhibit, in the presence of antibody, parasites such as blood-stage malaria and schistosomules (schistosomiasis), although the release of ROI may be equally important for their parasiticidal activity.

6.5   Antitumour cytokines

Some cytokines, as been instanced at the beginning of this chapter, have direct antiproliferative effects in both normal and tumour cell types. IFNα/β can induce cytostasis in a number of normal and tumour cells, although relatively high concentrations may be necessary to bring this about. IFNα/β has only very rarely been reported as acting as a growth factor. On the other hand, cytokines such as IFNγ, TNFα/β, IL-1, and TGFβ, which often induce mitogenic activity in some normal cells, are also known to be potent antiproliferative agents in other normal cells, e.g. haemopoietic progenitors, and in certain tumour cell lines. TNF was so named because of its tumoricidal action against a range of tumour cells *in vitro* and *in vivo*. Novel cytokines, e.g. oncostatin M (Table 6.4) and amphiregulin (see Chapter 7), are still being

Table 6.4   Properties of human oncostatin M

Molecular properties	M_r 28 000,
	228 amino acids (5 cysteines)
	Glycoprotein
	N-terminal sequence Ala-Ala-Ile-Gly-Ser-Cys-Ser-Lys-Glu-Tyr^{10}-Arg-Val-Leu-Leu-Gly^{15}
	No homology to other known cytokines
Producer cells	Activated T-lymphocytes
	Monocytic cell lines, e.g. U-937
Receptors	Widespread among normal and tumour cell types
	M_r = 150 000 − 160 000
Biological properties	Growth stimulatory for normal human fibroblasts
	Growth inhibitory for many, but not all, tumour cells having receptors
	Synergistic growth inhibition with TNFα or TGFβ

discovered. These appear to have a duality of function, i.e. they stimulate proliferative responses in normal cells, but inhibit the proliferation of some, but by no means all, tumour cell lines grown *in vitro*. In most instances, the antiproliferative activity of cytokines is fairly restricted, and there may or may not be overlap of effects. For example, TNF is cytostatic/cytotoxic for murine L-929 cells but has little, if any, effect in human A375 melanoma cells, whereas for IL-1 the reverse is true. In contrast, the cytostatic/cytotoxic effects of TNF and IFNγ have been often demonstrated to be synergistic in certain tumour cell lines.

The 'antitumour' cytokines stimulate a variety of cellular responses, as is evident from the preceding chapters, and just as in the case of antiviral effects, it has been extremely difficult to pinpoint the molecular mechanisms which underlie antiproliferative effects in individual tumour cell lines. IFNs have been shown to inhibit expression of oncogenes such as c-*fos* and c-*myc*, and to induce the synthesis of several enzymes, some of which probably are involved in the antiproliferative response. The 2,5A-synthetase system and the IFN-induced protein kinase, which have been associated with antiviral mechanisms, presumably could play a role in controlling cell proliferation through their inhibitory effects on protein synthesis. The IFNγ induction of IDO, which catalyses the breakdown of tryptophan, one of the essential amino acids, could indirectly inhibit protein synthesis and thus lead to curtailment of cell growth and proliferation. A correlation between cell proliferation and IDO activity has indeed been demonstrated in the oral carcinoma cell line KB and the WiDr colon adenocarcinoma, the IFNγ-induced cytostatic effect being reversed by raising the concentration of exogenous tryptophan. Thus, IDO might mediate the antitumour effect of IFNγ, besides its antimicrobial action (see Section 6.4). In contrast, DNA polymerases and ornithine decarboxylase are other enzymes whose activities are strongly inhibited by IFNs, and which possibly contribute to their antiproliferative action. In addition, the IFN-induced effects on the cytoskeleton, e.g. increased microtubular and actin fibres, and on the plasma membrane, e.g. increased rigidity and altered phospholipid content, together with the IFN-mediated down-regulation of plasma membrane receptors for growth-stimulating cytokines such as EGF, all may potentially influence the antiproliferative reponse (Figure 6.4).

TNFα/β have direct cytotoxic action in a limited number of tumour cell lines. Certain murine cell lines, e.g. the long-established mouse L-929 line and the more recently isolated murine fibrosarcoma line WEHI164 clone 13, are extremely sensitive to TNF-mediated cytotoxicity. In comparison, long-established human tumour cells in culture show widely differing responses to the cytotoxic action of TNF. Most, in common with normal diploid fibroblasts, are relatively resistant to TNF, but some at least, including a few lines derived from breast and lung carcinomas, are highly susceptible. Additionally, it has been reported that tumour cells derived from a single human renal cell carcinoma exhibit a heterogeneous response to the cytotoxic effects of hr TNFα. For a number of human tumour lines, e.g. myelogenous leukaemia cell lines, the effects of TNF are cytostatic rather than cytotoxic. TNF-mediated inhibition of cell proliferation is often accompanied by terminal differentiation, e.g. the differentiation of HL-60 myelomonocytic leukaemia cells into morphologically and functionally mature monocyte-and/or macrophage-like cells, and preceded by inhibition of oncogene, e.g. c-*myc*, expression.

The mechanism of TNF-mediated cytotoxicity is as yet incompletely understood. It would appear that TNF-induced activation of arachidonic acid metabolism is involved since inhibitors of this, such as aspirin or indomethacin, inhibit cytotoxic activity. It has been suggested that the early activation of phospholipase A2, which cleaves phospholipids into lysophospholipid and arachidonic acid, is responsible for initiating the events leading to cell death. Nevertheless, it is not clear which step(s) of the metabolic pathway leading to the formation of arachidonic acid and its derivatives, e.g. prostaglandins, thromboxanes, leukotrienes, etc., are necessary for cytotoxicity. Certainly, the pathway of conversion of arachidonic acid to prostaglandin results in the generation of free radicals, which are highly chemically reactive intermediates and by-products. The finding that nuclear DNA becomes fragmented in TNF-treated cells is reminiscent of the end result of free-radical attack on DNA (Figure 6.4). Possibly cells which are susceptible to TNF-mediated cytotoxicity are inefficient in removing potentially harmful free radicals. Certain inhibitors of macromolecular synthesis, e.g. cycloheximide (protein synthesis) and actinomycin D (DNA-dependent RNA synthesis, inhibition of mRNA synthesis) are known to significantly enhance the cytotoxic action of TNF. This suggests that certain proteins play a protective role, which may include free-radical removal; for example, superoxide dismutase and glutathione peroxidase scavenge superoxide anions and hydrogen peroxide, respectively. Alternatively, TNF may induce DNA fragmentation by an alteration in nuclear membrane permeability leading to exposure of DNA to digestion by cytoplasmic endonucleases, a mechanism that has also been suggested to explain CTL killing of tumour cell targets. It is clear that there must be subtle differences in the activation pathways of TNF and IL-1, although they share many biological properties, since IL-1 is rarely cytotoxic to TNF-susceptible cells, and indeed may inhibit the cytotoxicity of TNF.

The mechanism(s) by which IL-1 and other antitumour cytokines cause cytostasis or cytotoxicity is not known. Possibly they work by inducing the synthesis of other cytokines which are the effectors of cytostatic/cytotoxic actions. For instance IL-1 can induce TNF, TNF can induce IFNβ, and IFNγ may induce IFNα. It has even been reported that TGFβ may mediate the antiproliferative effect of IFNα in a human breast carcinoma cell line. It appears virtually certain that autocrine inhibitory circuits mediated by cytokines have antiproliferative effects in some tumour cells. Up-regulation of antitumour cytokines and/or their receptors by other cytokines could therefore markedly increase cytostatic/cytotoxic effects (Figure 6.4). For example, IFNγ and TNF exhibit synergistic cytotoxic activity in some tumour cell lines and part of this increased cytotoxicity may be reflected in the observed IFNγ-mediated increase in TNF-R. Further, a genetically engineered hybrid IFNγ × TNFβ protein molecule has enhanced cytotoxicity compared to either cytokine alone; this suggests a novel, receptor-mediated, synergistic mechanism. On the other hand, IFNα down-regulates the numbers of EGF-R (also insulin receptors) in some cell lines, and thus may raise the threshold necessary for EGF/TGFα-stimulated mitogenesis. There are obviously many kinds of cytokine-mediated growth-regulatory loops which could account for some of their antitumour actions, but the outcome of treatment with any particular cytokine will depend on a host of variables, including the cell type and its ability to produce and respond to different cytokines and other mediators, the presence of growth regulatory substances in the culture medium, and environmental conditions such as temperature.

In vivo, there are several indirect mechanisms whereby cytokines may exert antitumour effects. Some of these, such as cell-mediated toxicity, can be demonstrated *in vitro*. For example, isolated macrophages may be activated by LPS and IFNγ to recognize and kill certain tumour cells in culture by a mechanism that requires direct cell-to-cell contact. It is not clear how macrophages recognize neoplastic cells, but this seems to occur by a process independent of MHC antigen expression, species-specific antigens, tumour-specific antigens, phases of the cell cycle and many phenotypic aspects, e.g. metastatic potential, associated with tumour cells. It has been hypothesized that macrophages may be able to discriminate between normal and tumour cells by recognizing changes at the cell surface occasioned by the different membrane phospholipid composition in tumour cells as compared to normal cells. As to the actual mediators of macrophage cytotoxicity, TNFα appears to be a strong candidate. Evidence to support TNFα as a macrophage tumoricidal agent stems from several observations. Firstly, sensitivity to

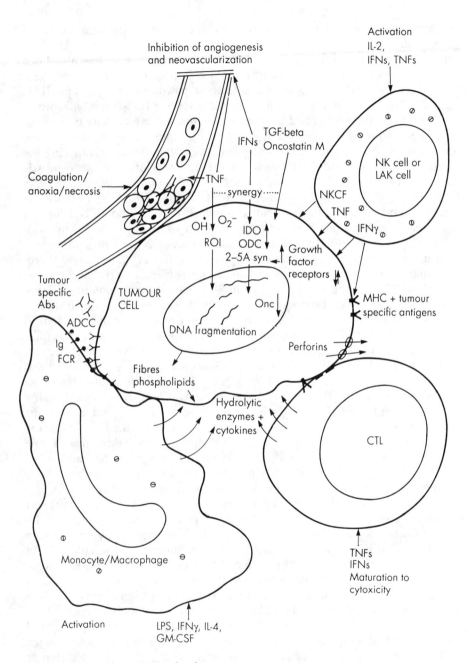

Figure 6.4   Antitumour mechanisms.

macrophage tumoricidal activity corresponds with sensitivity to purified recombinant TNFα. Secondly, macrophage cytotoxicity may be neutralized by anti-TNFα-specific antibodies, and thirdly, tumour cell killing is increased if target cells are pre-incubated with IFNγ (i.e. IFNγ potentiates TNF-mediated cytotoxicity — see the previous paragraph). It is, however, presently unclear whether TNF is secreted by macrophages on tumour cell contact, or is associated with the macrophage plasma membrane. Most reports to date suggest that TNF may function as a membrane-associated cytotoxin in macrophage-mediated cytotoxicity. Release of TNF may be incidental to the latter. It should be pointed out that macrophages may also kill tumour cells by TNF-independent mechanisms (Figure 6.4).

NK cells may also kill some allogeneic tumour targets (Figure 6.4) by a similar mechanism involving TNFα, but the most widely used NK target cells, the K562 erythroblastoid cell line, is resistant to TNF-mediated cytotoxicity. Thus, TNF may only correspond to an NKCF in a situation where the target cells are susceptible to TNF. (It should be noted that other less well-characterized cytotoxins, distinct from TNF, have also been called NKCF.) It has been suggested that lysis of several NK-susceptible target cells by TNF, which takes approximately 20 hours, requires the presence of additional agents that are sublethally toxic and/or inhibitory to macromolecular synthesis, e.g. Cr^{51} used to label target cells may damage them.

Besides acting as an effector molecule of NK-cell-mediated cytotoxicity, TNFα may also activate NK cells to further increase their innate cytotoxic functions. This is also a property of other cytokines, including IFNs and IL-2. When PBL are incubated in the presence of IL-2, a population of them becomes markedly more cytotoxic to tumour cells, including autologous targets. These natural cytotoxic (NC) cells, often referred to as LAK cells, are mostly contained in the heterogeneous LGL population, but possibly might also include some CTL. The action of IL-2 in boosting NK and LAK cell cytotoxicity is probably partly indirect, through the induction and auto-crine/paracrine stimulation of other cytokines such as IFNγ and TNFα. In fact, IL-2 and TNFα have been shown to act synergistically in the generation of LAK cells. In contrast, the action of TGFβ is to antagonize the activation of LAK cells by TNFα.

The role of NK cells and LAK cells in non-specific killing of tumour cells *in vivo* is controversial. It has been suggested that NK cells take part in immune surveillance to recognize and destroy any potential tumorigenic cells, but there is little direct evidence to support this suggestion. In cancer patients treated with IFNα, NK cell activity is boosted transiently, but on the whole does not correlate well with tumour regression. On the other hand, 'tumour infiltrating lymphocytes' (TIL), which probably include some LAK cells, have been shown to be highly cytotoxic to the autologous tumour cells themselves. Furthermore, cancer patients receiving back their own IL-2-activated LAK cells frequently do show an initial regression in their tumour(s). However, activated LAK cells produce many cytokines and other mediators which may activate other host antitumour mechanisms, and it is difficult to show accumulation of LAK cells in tumour sites. The direct action of LAK cells in tumour cell killing *in vivo* is therefore hard to prove.

The potential killing of tumour cells by immune-specific mechanisms is dependent on how well tumour-specific antigens are recognized as 'non-self' by CTL. Cytokines such as IFNs and TNFs are well known to induce or enhance the expression of MHC class I molecules, and thus increase the recognition of tumour-specific antigens. These cytokines also activate CTL cytolytic functions. Cytokine-augmented CTL killing of MHC-matched tumour (or virally infected) targets can be readily demonstrated *in vitro*, but the importance of the potential tumoricidal activity of CTL *in vivo* remains an open question. CTL, and probably also NK cells, can kill tumour cells following cell-contact by a cytokine-independent mechanism. Proteins present in the cytoplasmic granules of CTL and NK cells polymerize to form 'washer-like' complexes, known as perforins, and these are inserted into the tumour cell plasma membrane (Figure 6.4). This effectively makes pores or channels in the membrane through which water, ions, and macromolecules leak out of the tumour cell and result in its death. Interestingly, the sub-unit proteins of perforins are antigenically and structurally related to certain components of the complement cascade, e.g. C9 complement. CTL may also damage tumour cells by secretion of serine proteases, enzymes which may activate lytic mechanisms such as complement cascade.

In animal tumour model systems, the antitumour effects of particular cytokines may be readily evaluated. For instance, tumour explants from cancer patients may be transplanted into T-cell deficient nude mice where the tumour cells proliferate to form nodules. Some, but not all, of these tumour cells are sensitive to the antiproliferative effects of human IFNα *in vitro*, and appear also to be sensitive to the antitumour effects of injected HuIFNα when grown as 'xenografts' in nude mice. Since HuIFNα is reasonably species specific and has little biological/pharmacological activity in mice, the antitumour effect is most likely to be mediated by the direct antiproliferative activity of HuIFNα. Nevertheless, murine IFNα/β has sometimes been demonstrated to have antitumour activity against the human xenografts. In these cases, the antitumour activity is more likely to be mediated through indirect mechanisms, e.g. NK-cell-mediated cytotoxicity, because MuIFNα/β has little biological activity in human cells. In immunocompetent mice, i.e. those having T-lymphocytes, it is probable that the antitumour activity of MuIFNα/β against murine transplantable tumours is indirectly mediated by T-lymphocytes, since it has been found that MuIFNα/β has weaker antitumour activity in T-cell defective, e.g. thymectomized–irradiated, mice.

In the human xenograft–nude mouse model, HuIFNα subtypes have been found to be more effective in causing tumoristasis than either IFNβ or IFNγ. HuIFNα is probably more potent than IFNβ for the reason that it is easier to achieve high circulating levels of IFNα than of IFNβ. The mode of action of IFNγ is different from that of IFNα since it binds to a separate cell receptor, and IFNγ may therefore be ineffective when used alone. However, positive interactions between IFNα and IFNγ, giving rise to additive or synergistic tumoristatic or tumoricidal effects, similar to those observed *in vitro*, have been demonstrated in some instances.

Besides cytotoxicity of TNFα/β to murine cell lines in culture, these cytokines have been shown to cause haemorrhagic necrosis of solid tumours arising from transplantation of certain murine tumour cells into mice. They may also cause tumoristasis of some ascitic tumours. For example, tumours such as MethA sarcoma, EL-4 leukaemia, and P815 mastocytoma are highly sensitive to injected TNFα, while AKR leukaemia shows partial sensitivity. In human tumour-model systems, such as the growth of tumour explants in nude mice, TNFα injected intravenously has been demonstrated to cause necrosis or regression of human breast carcinoma. Various other human tumour explants, hetero-transplanted into nude mice, have also been shown to regress following intratumoral injection of TNFα. Again it is clear that the antitumour effects of TNFα may be mediated via both direct and indirect mechanisms. The latter are probably responsible for the regression/necrosis of tumour cells, e.g. MethA sarcoma, which are insensitive to the cytotoxicity of TNFα *in vitro*. Besides immune-specific mechanisms, it is thought likely that TNFα produces tumour necrosis through its blood coagulating activity (Figure 6.4). TNFα has been shown to impair microcirculation in tumour blood capillaries by inducing the production of fibrin-like substances. Restriction of blood supply leading to oxygen- and nutrient-deprivation then causes autolysis of tumour cells. In addition, both TNFα and TNFβ have been shown to inhibit angiogenesis, the process of blood capillary formation, *in vitro*, and thus may antagonize the vascularization of growing tumours *in vivo* (Figure 6.4). Synergistic antitumour action has been demonstrated for combinations of TNFα and IFNγ in the transplantable human xenograft–mouse model system, suggesting that particular cytokine combinations may offer more potent anticancer therapies.

Further reading

Interferons alpha and beta

This field has been extensively reviewed, and the following books and articles are suggested for background reading and for more detailed information.

De Maeyer, E. and De Maeyer-Guignard, J. (1988) *Interferons and other Regulatory Cytokines*. John Wiley, New York.

Langer, J.A. and Pestka, S. (1985) Structure of interferons, in *Pharmacological Therapy* **27**, Pergamon Press, London, p. 371.

Lengyel, P. (1982) Biochemistry of interferons and their actions. *Annual Reviews of Biochemistry* **51**, 251.

Revel, M. (1984) The interferon system in man: nature of the interferon molecules and mode of action, in *Antiviral Drugs and Interferons: The Molecular Basis of their Activity* (Becker, Y., ed.) Martinus Nijhoff, Boston, p. 357.

Stewart, W.E. II (1978) *The Interferon System*. Springer-Verlag, Vienna.

Stringfellow, D.A. (ed.) (1980) *Interferon and Interferon Inducers: Clinical Applications. Modern Pharmacology-Toxicology* **17**. Marcel Dekker, New York.

Taylor-Papadimitriou, J. (ed.) (1985) *Interferons: Their Impact in Biology and Medi-cine*. Oxford University Press, Oxford.
Zoon, K.C. (1987) Human interferons: structure and function, in *Interferon 9* (Gres-ser, I., ed.). Academic Press, London, p. 1 (This series of annual compilations covering many aspects of interferon research is generally helpful.)

Other articles
Langer, J.A. and Pestka, S. (1988) Interferon receptors. *Immunology Today* **9**, 393.
Miyamoto, M., Fujita, T., Kimura, Y., *et al.* (1988) Regulated expression of a gene encoding a nuclear factor, IRF-1, that specifically binds to IFN-beta gene regula-tory elements. *Cell* **54**, 903.
Revel, M. and Chebath, J. (1986) Interferon-activated genes. *Trends in Biochemical Sciences* **11**, 166.
Visvanathan, K.V. and Goodbourn, S. (1989) Double-stranded RNA activates bind-ing of NF-κB to an inducible element in the human beta-interferon promoter. The *EMBO Journal* **8**, 1129.
Xanthoudakis, S., Cohen, L., and Hiscott, J. (1989) Multiple protein-DNA interac-tions within the human interferon-beta regulatory element. *Journal of Biological Chemistry* **264**, 1139.

Antiviral activity (see also under antiviral cytokines)

Hughes, T.K. and Baron, S. (1987) A large component of the antiviral activity of mouse interferon-gamma may be due to its induction of interferon-alpha. *Journal of Biological Regulators and Homeostatic Agents* **1**, 29.
Ito, M. and O'Malley, J.A. (1987) Antiviral effects of recombinant human tumour necrosis factor. *Lymphokine Research* **6**, 309.
Leuwenberg, J.F.M., Van Damme, J., Jeunhomme, G.M.A.A., and Buurman, W.A. (1987) Interferon beta 1, an intermediate in the tumour necrosis factor-alpha-induced increased MHC class I expression and an autocrine regulator of the constitutive MHC class I expression. *Journal of Experimental Medicine* **166**, 1180.
Mestan, J., Digel, W., Mittnacht, S., *et al.* (1986) Antiviral effects of recombinant tumour necrosis factor *in vitro*. *Nature* **323**, 816.
Wong, G.H.W. and Goeddel, D.V. (1986) Tumour necrosis factors alpha and beta inhibit virus replication and synergize with interferons. *Nature* **323**, 819.

Antiproliferative effects (see also under interferons alpha and -beta)

Pfeffer, L.M., Donner, D.B., and Tamm, I. (1987) Interferon-alpha down-regulates insulin receptors in lymphoblastoid (Daudi) cells: relationship to inhibition of cell proliferation. *Journal of Biological Chemistry* **262**, 3665.
Zoon, K.C., Karasaki, Y., zur Nedden, D.L., *et al.* (1986) Modulation of epidermal growth factor receptors by human alpha interferon. *Proceedings of the National Academy of Sciences USA* **83**, 8226.

Differentiation and immunomodulation (see also under interferons alpha and -beta)

Amaldi, I., Reikk, W., Berte, C., and Mach, B. (1989) Induction of HLA class II genes by IFN-gamma is transcriptional and requires a trans-acting protein. *Journal of Immunology* **142**, 999.

Blanar, M.A., Baldwin, A.S.Jr., Flavell, R.A., and Sharp, P.A. (1989) A gamma-interferon-induced factor that binds the interferon response sequence of the MHC class I molecule. *The EMBO Journal* **8**, 1139.

Burns, G.F., Begley, C.G., Mackay, I.R., *et al.* (1985) Supernatural killer cells. *Immunology Today* **6**, 370.

Dale, T.C., Ali Iman, A.M., Kerr, I.M., and Stark, G.R. (1989) Rapid activation by interferon-alpha of a latent DNA-binding protein present in the cytoplasm of untreated cells. *Proceedings of the National Academy of Sciences USA* **86**, 1203.

Rager-Zisman, B. and Bloom, B.R. (1985) Interferons and natural killer cells. *British Medical Bulletin* **41** (1), 22.

Saksela, E. (1981) Interferon and natural killer cells, in *Interferon 3* (Gresser, I., ed.) Academic Press, New York, p. 45.

Trinchieri, G. and Perussia, B. (1984) Human natural killer cells: biologic and pathologic aspects. *Laboratory Investigation* **50**, 489.

Antiviral cytokines

Askonas, B.A. and Taylor, P.M. (1987) T cell mediated immunity in virus infection. *Immunology Letters* **16**, 337.

Beresini, M.H., Lempert, M.J., and Epstein, L.B. (1988) Overlapping polypeptide induction in human fibroblasts in response to treatment with interferon-alpha, interferon-gamma, interleukin-1 alpha, interleukin-1 beta and tumour necrosis factor. *Journal of Immunology* **140**, 485.

Hammer, S.M., Gillis, J.M., Groopman, J.E., and Rose, R.M. (1986) *In vitro* modification of human immunodeficiency virus infection by granulocyte-macrophage colony-stimulating factor and gamma-interferon. *Proceedings of the National Academy of Sciences USA* **83**, 8734.

Ito, M., Baba, M., Sato, A., *et al.* (1989) Tumour necrosis factor enhances replication of human immunodeficiency virus (HIV) *in vitro*. *Biochemical and Biophysical Research Communications* **158**, 307.

Paya, C.V., Kenmotsu, N., Schoon, R.A., and Leibson, P.L. (1988) Tumour necrosis factor and lymphotoxin secretion by human natural killer cells leads to antiviral cytotoxicity. *Journal of Immunology* **141**, 1989.

Pomerantz, R.J. and Hirsch, M.S. (1987) Interferon and human immunodeficiency virus infection, in *Interferon 9* (Gresser, I., ed.) Academic Press, London, p. 113.

Rubin, B.Y., Anderson, S.L., Lunn, R.M., *et al.* (1988) Tumour necrosis factor and IFN induce a common set of proteins. *Journal of Immunology* **141**, 1180.

Samuel, C.E. (1988) Mechanisms of the antiviral action of interferons, in *Progress in Nucleic Acid Research and Molecular Biology* 35 (Cohn, W.E. and Moldave, K. eds) Academic Press, San Diego, p. 29.

Wong, G.H.W., Krowke, J.F., Stites, D.P., and Goeddel, D.V. (1988) *In vitro* anti-human immunodeficiency virus activities of tumour necrosis factor-alpha and interferon-gamma. *Journal of Immunology* **140**, 120.

Antimicrobial cytokines

Bermudez, L.E.M. and Young, L.S. (1988) Tumour necrosis factor alone or in combination with IL-2, but not IFN-gamma, is associated with macrophage killing of *Mycobacterium avium* complex. *Journal of Immunology* **140**, 3006.

Brummer, E. and Stevens, D.A. (1987) Activation of pulmonary macrophages for fungicidal activity by gamma-interferon or lymphokines. *Clinical and Experimental Immunology* **70**, 520.

Byrne, G. and Turco, J. (eds) (1988) *Interferon and Nonviral Pathogens*. Immunology Series **42** Marcel Dekker, New York.

Clark, I.A., Hunt, N.H., Butcher, G.A., and Cowden, W.B. (1987) Inhibition of murine malaria (*Plasmodium chabaudi*) *in vivo* by recombinant interferon-gamma or tumour necrosis factor, and its enhancement by butylated hydroxyanisole. *Journal of Immunology* **139**, 3493.

Esparza, I., Männel, D., Ruppel, A., et al. (1987) Interferon-gamma and lymphotoxin or tumour necrosis factor act synergistically to induce macrophage killing of tumour cells and schistosomula of *Schistosoma mansoni*. *Journal of Experimental Medicine* **166**, 589.

Flesch, I. and Kaufmann, S.H.E. (1987) Mycobacterial growth inhibition by interferon-gamma-activated bone marrow macrophages and differential susceptibility among strains of *Mycobacterium tuberculosis*. *Journal of Immunology* **138**, 4408.

Male, D., Champion, B., and Cooke, A. (1987) *Advanced Immunology*. Gower Medical Publishing, London. Chapter 15.

Mellouk, S., Maheshwari, R.K., Rhodes-Feuillette, A., et al. (1987) Inhibitory activity of interferons and interleukin 1 on the development of *Plasmodium falciparum* in human hepatocyte cultures. *Journal of Immunology* **139**, 4192.

Murray, H.W., Stern, J.J., Welte, K., et al. (1987) Experimental visceral leishmaniasis: production of interleukin 2 and interferon-gamma, tissue immune reaction and response to treatment with interleukin 2 and interferon-gamma. *Journal of Immunology* **138**, 2290.

Nakane, A., Minagawa, T. and Kato, K. (1988) Endogenous tumour necrosis factor (cachectin) is essential to host resistance against *Listeria monocytogenes* infection. *Infection and Immunity* **56**, 2563.

Passwell, J.H., Shor, R., Trau, H., et al. (1987) Antigen-stimulated lymphokines from patients with cutaneous leishmaniasis induce monocyte killing of *Leishmania major* intracellular amastigotes. *Journal of Immunology* **139**, 4208.

Schofield, L., Ferreira, A., Altszuler, R., et al. (1987) Interferon-gamma inhibits the intrahepatocytic development of malaria parasites *in vitro*. *Journal of Immunology* **139**, 2020.

Stewart, W.E. II. (1978) *The Interferon System*. Springer-Verlag, Vienna. Chapter III, p. 27.

Vergara, J., Ferreira, A., Schellekens, H., and Nussenzweig, V. (1987) Mechanism of escape of exoerythrocytic-forms (EEF) of malaria parasites from the inhibitory effects of interferon-gamma. *Journal of Immunology* **138**, 4447.

Volc-Platzer, B., Stemberger, H., Luger, T., et al. (1988) Defective intralesional interferon-gamma in patients with lepromatous leprosy. *Clinical and Experimental Immunology* **71**, 235.

Antitumour cytokines

Bock, G. and Marsh, J. (eds.) (1987) *Tumour Necrosis Factor and Related Cytotoxins*. Ciba Foundation Symposium **131**. Chapters by Palladino, M.A. et al. p. 21, Haranaka, K. et al. p. 140, and Balkwill, F.R. et al. p. 154.

Brown, T.J., Lioubin, M.N., and Marquardt, H. (1987) Purification and characterization of cytostatic lymphokines produced by activated human T lymphocytes. *Journal of Immunology* **139**, 2977.

Chen, L., Suzuki, Y., and Wheelock, E.F. (1987) Interferon-gamma synergises with tumour necrosis factor and with interleukin 1 and requires the presence of both monokines to induce antitumour cytotoxic activity in macrophages. *Journal of Immunology* **139**, 4096.

De la Maza, L.M. and Peterson, E.M. (1988) Dependence of the *in vitro* antiprolifera-tive activity of recombinant human gamma IFN on the concentration of tryp-tophan in culture media. *Cancer Research* **48**, 346.

Decker, T., Lohmann-Matthes, M.-L., and Gifford, G.E. (1987) Cell-associated tumour necrosis factor (TNF) as a killing mechanism of activated cytotoxic macrophages. *Journal of Immunology* **138**, 957.

Espevik, T., Figari, I.S., Ranges, G.E., and Palladino, M.A. (1988) Transforming growth factor-beta 1 and recombinant human tumour necrosis alpha reciprocally regulate the generation of lymphokine-activated killer cell activity. *Journal of Immunology* **140**, 2312.

Feng, G.-S., Gray, P.W., Shepard, H.M., and Taylor, M.W. (1988) Antiproliferative activity of a hybrid protein between interferon-gamma and tumour necrosis factor-beta. *Science* **241**, 1501.

Fidler, I.J. (1985) Macrophages and metastasis — a biological approach to cancer therapy. *Cancer Research* **45**, 4714.

Gershenfield, H.K. and Weissman, I.L. (1986) Cloning of a cDNA for a T-cell-specific serine protease from a cytotoxic T lymphocyte. *Science* **232**, 854.

Gresser, I. (1985) How does interferon inhibit tumour growth? in *Interferon 6* (Gresser, I., ed.) Academic Press, New York, p. 93.

Hanna, N. (1985) The role of natural killer cells in the control of tumour growth and metastasis. *Biochemica et Biophysica Acta* **780**, 213.

Heicappel, R., Naito, S., Ichinose, Y., *et al.* (1987) Cytostatic and cytolytic effects of human recombinant tumour necrosis factor on human renal cell carcinoma cell lines derived from a single surgical specimen. *Journal of Immunology* **138**, 1634.

Herbermann, R.B., Reynolds, C.W., and Ortaldo, J.R. (1986) Mechanisms of cytotoxicity by natural killer (NK) cells. *Annual Reviews of Immunology* **4**, 651.

Hoffman, H. and Wallach, D. (1987) Down regulation of receptors for tumour necrosis factor by interleukin 1 and 4-phorbol-12-myristate-13-acetate. *Journal of Immunology* **139**, 1161.

Kerr, D.J., Pragnell, I.B., Sproul, A., *et al.* (1989) The cytostatic effects of alpha-interferon may be mediated by transforming growth factor-beta. *Journal of Molecular Endocrinology* **2**, 131.

Klostergaard, J. (1987) Role of tumour necrosis factor in monocyte/macrophage tumour cytotoxicity *in vitro*. *Natural Immunity and Cell Growth Regulators* **6**, 161.

Kriegler, M., Perez, C., DeFay, K., *et al.* (1988) A novel form of TNF/cachectin is a cell surface cytotoxic transmembrane protein: ramifications for the complex physiology of TNF. *Cell* **53**, 45.

Linsley, P.S., Bolton-Hanson, M. Horn, D., *et al.* (1989) Identification and character-ization of cellular receptors for the growth regulator, oncostatin M. *Journal of Biological Chemistry* **264**, 4282.

Lobe, C., Finlay, B.B., Paranchych, W., *et al.* (1986) Novel serine protease encoded by two cytotoxic T-lymphocyte-specific genes. *Science* **232**, 858.

Moore, M. (1985) Natural immunity to tumours — theoretical predictions and biological observations. *British Journal of Cancer* **52**, 147.

Nawroth, P., Handley, D., Matsueda, G., *et al.* (1988) Tumour necrosis factor/cachectin-induced intravascular fibrin formation in MethA fibrosarcomas. *Journal of Experimental Medicine* **168**, 637.

Neale, M.L., Fiera, R.A., and Matthews, N. (1988) Involvement of phospholipase A2 activation in tumour cell killing by tumour necrosis factor. *Immunology* **64**, 81.

Nissen-Meyer, J. and Espevik, T. (1987) Effect of antisera against recombinant tumour necrosis factor and the monocyte-derived cytotoxin(s) on monocyte-mediated killing of various tumour cells. *Cellular Immunology* **109**, 384.

Ortaldo, J.R., Mason, A., and Overton, R. (1986) Lymphokine-activated killer cells:

analysis of progenitors and effectors. *Journal of Experimental Medicine* **164**, 1193.

Ostensen, M.E., Thiele, D.L., and Lipsky, P.E. (1987) Tumour necrosis factor alpha enhances cytolytic activity of human natural killer cells. *Journal of Immunology* **138**, 4185.

Ozaki, Y., Edelstein, M.P., and Duch, D.S. (1988) Induction of indoleamine 2,3-dioxygenase; a mechanism of the antitumour activity of interferon-gamma. *Proceedings of the National Academy of Sciences USA* **85**, 1242.

Price, G., Brenner, M.K., Prentice, H.G., *et al.* (1987) Cytotoxic effects of tumour necrosis factor and gamma-interferon on acute myeloid leukaemia blasts. *British Journal of Cancer* **55**, 287.

Rosenberg, S.A., Spiess, P., and Lafreniere, R. (1986) A new approach to the adoptive immunotherapy of cancer with tumour-infiltrating lymphocytes. *Science* **233**, 1318.

Rubin, B.Y., Smith, L.J., Hellermann, G.R., *et al.* (1988) Correlation between the anticellular and DNA fragmenting activities of tumour necrosis factor. *Cancer Research* **48**, 6006.

Ruddle, N.H. (1985) Lymphotoxin redux. *Immunology Today* **6**, 156.

Sato, N., Fukuda, K., Nariuchi, H., and Sagara, N. (1987) Tumour necrosis factor inhibiting angiogenesis *in vitro*. *Journal of the National Cancer Institute* **79**, 1383.

Schaub, L.B.O., Guttermann, J.U., and Grimm, E.A. (1988) Synergy of tumour necrosis factor and interleukin 2 in the activation of human cytotoxic lympho-cytes: effect of tumour necrosis factor alpha and interleukin 2 in the generation of human lymphokine-activated killer cell cytotoxicity. *Cancer Research* **48**, 788.

Schiller, J.H., Bittner, G., Storer, B., and Willson, J.K.V. (1987) Synergistic anti-tumour effects of tumour necrosis factor and gamma interferon on human colon carcinoma cell lines. *Cancer Research* **47**, 2809.

Schmid, D.S., Hornung, R., McGrath, K.M., *et al.* (1987) Target cell DNA frag-mentation is mediated by lymphotoxin and tumour necrosis factor. *Lymphokine Research* **6**, 195.

Shimomoura, K., Manda, T., Mukumoto, S., *et al.* (1988) Recombinant human tumour necrosis factor-alpha: thrombus formation is a cause of anti-tumour activity. *International Journal of Cancer* **41**, 243.

Shoyab, M., Plowman, G.D., McDonald, V.L. *et al.* (1989) Structure and function of human amphiregulin: a member of the epidermal growth factor family. *Science* **243**, 1074.

Suffys, P., Beyaert, R., van Roy, F., and Fiers, W., (1987) Reduced tumour necrosis factor-induced cytotoxicity by inhibition of the arachidonic acid metabolism. *Biochemical and Biophysical Research Communications* **149**, 735.

Tanoka, M., Kimura, K., and Yoshida, S. (1987) Inhibition of mammalian DNA polymerases by recombinant alpha-interferon and gamma-interferon. *Cancer Research* **47**, 5971.

Trotta, P.P. and Harrison, S.D. Jr. (1987) Evaluation of the antitumour activity of recombinant human gamma-interferon employing human melanoma xenografts in athymic nude mice. *Cancer Research* **47**, 5347.

Tsuruoka, N., Sugiyama, M., Tawaragi, Y., *et al.* (1988) Inhibition of *in vitro* angiogenesis by lymphotoxin and interferon-gamma. *Biochemical and Biophysic-al Research Communications* **155**, 429.

Urban, J.L., Shepard, H.M., Rothstein, J.L., *et al.* (1986) Tumour necrosis factor: a potent effector molecule for tumour cell killing by activated macrophages. *Proceedings of the National Academy of Sciences USA* **83**, 5233.

Wong, G.H.W. and Goeddel, D. (1988) Induction of manganous superoxide dis-mutase by tumour necrosis factor: possible protective mechanism. *Science* **242**, 941.

Young, J.D-E. and Cohn, Z.A. (1986) Cell-mediated killing: a common mechanism. *Cell* **46**, 641.

Zarling, J.M., Shoyab, M., Marquardt, H., *et al.* (1986) Oncostatin M: a growth regulator produced by differentiated histocytic lymphoma cells. *Proceedings of the National Academy of Sciences USA* **83**, 9739.

7

Cytokine interactions

7.1 Introduction

The response of cells to stimuli mediated by cytokines acting through their cognate receptors is proliferation and/or differentiation, the latter often being indicative of loss of proliferative capacity — usually observed as apparent growth inhibition. Superficially, proliferation and differentiation are distinct if not contradictory processes. However, from the actions of cytokines it has been seen that whether they evoke proliferation or differentiation there is a similarity both in the response elements used for signal transmission and in gene induction and expression. This suggests the existence of fundamental processes which are common to both proliferation and differentiation, and this is not so surprising given that in either case the responding cell is required to 're-shape' its metabolism and structure accordingly.

The first part of this chapter (Sections 7.1–7.5) addresses the molecular interactions occasioned by cytokine stimulation in the light of new facts, which are emerging all the time, and attempts to place into perspective the several 'bits' of a cell's response. New information about novel cytokines, e.g. amphiregulin, and about the elucidation of the structures of receptors for cytokines previously discussed, e.g. EPO-R and IL-2R, will also be included. Further, putative interactions at the cellular level regarding the regulation of certain aspects of immune function, e.g. the allergic response, and cellular development not so far covered in the preceding chapters will be discussed. Section 7.6 deals with interactions among cytokines and other mediators in the regulation of tissue growth and organ function, mentioning examples of how cytokine activities may relate to the control of other physiological systems, e.g. the 'neuroendocrine' system.

7.2   Competence/progression factors revisited

In Chapter 2, the theory of competence and progression relating to growth factors, their receptors, and oncoproteins was outlined. Competence factors were considered to be elements of cell activation pathways which committed cells to a series of stimulatable, contingent events. For example, they were necessary, but not sufficient, for a cell to proceed from G_0 (quiescent stage) to S-phase (DNA synthesis) of the cell cycle. Secondarily acting factors, known as progression factors, were required to complement the competence-factor-dependent mechanisms and allow the 'predetermined' contingent events to ensue. Now that many more cytokines have been described, is it possible to fit them into the roles of competence and progression factors? Regrettably, there appears to be no easy answer and any proposed solution will remain open to question. Nevertheless, it may be possible to address the question, if only in a rather imperfect way, by considering which cytokines are mainly responsible for activation/differentiation (competence) and which are involved in proliferation/differentiation (progression). On this basis, cytokines such as IL-1, IL-4, IL-6, IFNγ, etc. (Table 7.1) resemble competence factors, whereas other cytokines, such as CSFs, IL-2, IL-3, IL-5, etc. are more like progression factors. The competence class of cytokines have often been shown to act as co-stimulants of cellular responses. For instance, IL-1 appears to

1   augment antigen-activation of T-lymphocytes, and
2   potentiate the proliferation of haemopoietic progenitor cells.

IL-4 and IFNγ may fulfil similar roles in B-cell activation. In the absence of further stimuli, the end-result of 'competence' cytokine-activation may be differentiation without proliferation, e.g. IL-4 increases the expression of a number of cell surface markers and IgM in resting B-lymphocytes (Chapter 4). Further, competence cytokines have often also been found to induce other cytokines, e.g. IL-1 induction of

a   PDGF in fibroblasts,
b   GM-CSF in endothelial cells, and
c   IL-2 in T-lymphocytes.

On the other hand, cytokines of the 'progression' category appear to be more closely associated with the proliferative response of committed cells, e.g. IL-2 in activated T-lymphocytes, GM-CSF in myeloid cell precursors, EPO in erythroblasts, etc. However, 'progression' cytokines may also induce differentiation, e.g. IL-3 and CSFs in haemopoietic cell lineages, and this they may do in cells of little or no proliferative capacity such as mature macrophages and granulocytes. The rules for categorizing cytokines into competence and progression factors appear to break down totally when tumour cells are considered. For instance, examples of tumour cell lines dependent on IL-1, IL-4, or IL-6 (competence cytokines) as growth factors exist, besides those dependent on IL-2, IL-3, IL-5, EPO, or GM-CSF (progression cyto-

Table 7.1   Competence and progression categories of cytokines

Competence (activation/ differentiation) factors	Progression (proliferation/ differentiation) factors
PDGF	EGF/TGFα
TGFβ family	FGF
IL-1	NGF
IL-4	IGF-I, -II
IL-6	IL-2
IL-7	IL-3
IL-8	IL-5
IFNα/β	G-CSF
IFNγ	M-CSF
TNFα/β	GM-CSF
	EPO

kines) for proliferation. In other cases, cytokines from either category may have antiproliferative effects, e.g. IL-1 in the A375 melanoma cell line or IL-3 in murine WEHI-3B (D$^+$) myelomonocytic leukaemia cells, although there are possibly greater numbers of 'antiproliferative cytokines' in the 'competence' category (Table 7.1).

Obviously, it is rather difficult to generalize, given the rather complex biology of most cytokines, as to which category of factors, competence or progression, a particular cytokine belongs. It is possibly best to consider this on a case-to-case basis, i.e. in individual cytokine–cell systems. Even then, it may be impossible to predict the predominant biological activities of individual cytokines in any particular cell line. Part of the problem may lie in the fact that cells grown or maintained in culture for *in vitro* experimental investigations have usually been preselected on the basis of survival, either deliberately or by serendipitous routes, and are thus set up to meet specific, desirable goals following interventional manipulation, including the addition of particular cytokines. Thus, the end result, the observable or measurable cell response, will be determined by how far manipulative stimulation complements, enhances, or inhibits the underlying levels of cellular metabolic processes that are already present in such cells.

7.3   Amphiregulin — a bifunctional growth-modulating cytokine

The recent molecular and biological characterization of a novel cytokine of the EGF family named amphiregulin (AR) serves to illustrate how dependent cytokine-mediated cellular responses are on cell phenotype. AR was first isolated from the MCF-7 human breast carcinoma cell line. Its subsequent molecular cloning has revealed it to be a novel protein, but one which shows

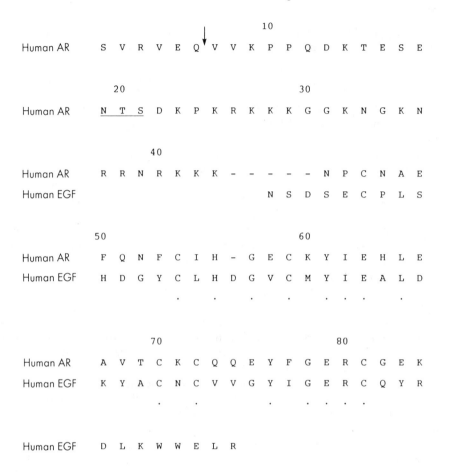

Figure 7.1 Primary structure of amphiregulin (AR) — comparison with EGF. The underlined sequence is a potential N-glycosylation site; the vertical arrow indicates the beginning of the truncated form of AR.

strong homology to EGF and TGFα, especially in the C-terminal region. Two forms of AR have been predicted — a truncated form containing 78 amino acids and a slightly larger form having an additional six N-terminal amino acids. The N-terminal region is distinctly hydrophilic, with several lysine, arginine and asparagine residues; the C-terminal half of the molecule resembles the structures of EGF and TGFα, and the positions of the three intrachain disulphide bonds via six cysteine residues are precisely conserved (Figure 7.1).

AR can bind to the EGF-receptor, EGF-R, but appears to have a lower affinity for this than either EGF or TGFα. On this basis, it was predicted that AR would stimulate similar proliferative responses to EGF/TGFα and indeed this has been found to be the case in some, but not all, cell systems tested. For example, AR has been shown to fully supplant the requirement for EGF/TGFα in the proliferation of a murine keratinocyte cell line, Balb/MK. In contrast, while EGF/TGFα induce the anchorage-independent growth of rat kidney cells, NRK-SA6, in the presence of TGFβ, AR was found to be inactive in stimulating colony formation in soft agar under the same conditions. In further apparent contrast, AR exerted an antiproliferative effect in certain human tumour cell lines, including the A431 epidermoid carcinoma and various breast and ovarian carcinoma cell lines, although it should be pointed out that EGF has been reported to have inhibitory effects in such cells as well. Thus, AR can behave as a growth factor in one case, as a cytokine with no observable effect in another, and as an antiproliferative agent in yet another, highlighting the fact that the nature of cellular responses frequently has more to do with cells than cytokines.

Conceptually, it is simple to envisage a set of cytokine-inducible genes that coordinate and account for modified metabolic processes, and ultimately for microsopically observable changes in cytoskeletal components and cell size together with measurable changes in cell function. What is less obvious, and probably more difficult to comprehend, is the nature of the discriminatory 'apparatus' that a cell has to interpret cytokine-generated signals into a proliferative response, or a differentiation response, or in some cases a combination of both responses. In this respect, it is suggested that the following may be relevant: the extent of gene and enzyme activation and the levels of gene products and cellular metabolites generated in response to cytokine stimulation, itself a variable process dependent upon the availability of cytokines and their receptors, probably play decisive roles in whether proliferation or differentiation or cell growth inhibition ensues. This presumed rather delicate balance of inducible gene products, activatable enzymes, and their metabolites probably reflects a particular 'state' of a cell. This state is related to its phenotype, ontogenic history (stage of development) and cycle phase. But from among inducible gene products, activatable enzymes, and their metabolites, from among measurable changes in ion fluxes, cyclic nucleotide- and phosphoinositide-derived second messengers, kinase and phosphatase activities, enzymes controlling energy metabolism, oncoproteins, etc., is it possible to ascertain what controls particular cellular responses? If this could be done, then perhaps more effective treatment of cancers could be developed, for example. While our understanding of 'discriminatory apparatus' at the molecular level remains fragmented, knowledge of the structure and functioning of cytokine receptors, together with that of downstream signalling pathways and the processes connected with gene induction, is fast accruing. It is to be hoped that this will lead us away from 'black boxes' and towards a more enlightened appreciation of molecular events regulating cellular responses.

7.4   Cytokine receptors: novel structures and new insights

Even in the few months that have passed since the writing of this book was begun, at least half a dozen more cytokine receptors have been molecularly cloned. These include a second novel receptor for PDGF, the receptor for EPO, the medium-affinity IL-2R, the p70 IL-2Rβ, a receptor for bFGF, and one for GM-CSF. The first four of these receptors are described below.

A novel receptor for PDGF

In Chapter 2 (p. 48) mention was made of the observation that the three PDGF isoforms, while binding to the well-characterized tyrosine kinase containing PDGF-R, may also differentially bind to another distinct class of receptors. The recent isolation of a 'novel PDGF receptor' that bound the PDGF-AA homodimer better than PDGF-BB, to which the 'established PDGF-R' responds best, confirms receptor heterogeneity for PDGF isoforms. The new PDGF-R, for which the term α-PDGF-R has been proposed since it binds the PDGF-AA isoform preferentially (the PDGF-BB binding receptor thus becoming β-PDGF-R), has been molecularly cloned and its gene located to the long arm of chromosome 4. In distinction, the β-PDGF-R gene has been assigned to the long arm of chromosome 5, together with other cytokine- and cytokine-receptor genes. The α-PDGF-R cDNA predicts a polypeptide containing 1065 amino acids preceded by an N-terminal 24 amino acid signal sequence. The inferred structure is similar to that of β-PDGF-R with which it shares 31 per cent overall sequence homology (Figure 7.2). In particular, the intracellular domain is divided into two tyrosine kinase moieties, of 85 and 75 per cent homology respectively with those of β-PDGF-R, intersected by a interkinase region (kinase insert) with 27 per cent homology to the same region in β-PDGF-R. The extracellular domain of about 500 amino acids also exhibits a similarity in structure to the extracellular domains of β-PDGF-R, c-KIT and M-CSF-R. For instance, spacing of 10 cysteines is the same as in β-PDGF-R, resembling in both cases that found in members of the immunoglobulin (Ig) superfamily (Figure 7.2). It is expected that the extracellular domain of α-PDGF-R is heavily glycosylated because it contains eight potential N-linked glycosylation sites.

Most normal cell types, e.g. fibroblasts, appear to contain mRNA transcripts for both α and β-PDGF-R. In contrast, tumour cell lines were found to express either α-PDGF-R or β-PDGF-R transcripts, but not both. Both types of receptors probably transduce signals (see p. 225) across the plasma membrane in a similar way, leading to a mitogenic response. However, while both PDGF-BB and PDGF-AB isoforms triggered tyrosine kinase-mediated autophosphorylation in each receptor, PDGF-AA was only effective in this respect in α-PDGF-R. It is not yet known whether this receptor discrimination among different PDGF isoforms has any physiological significance.

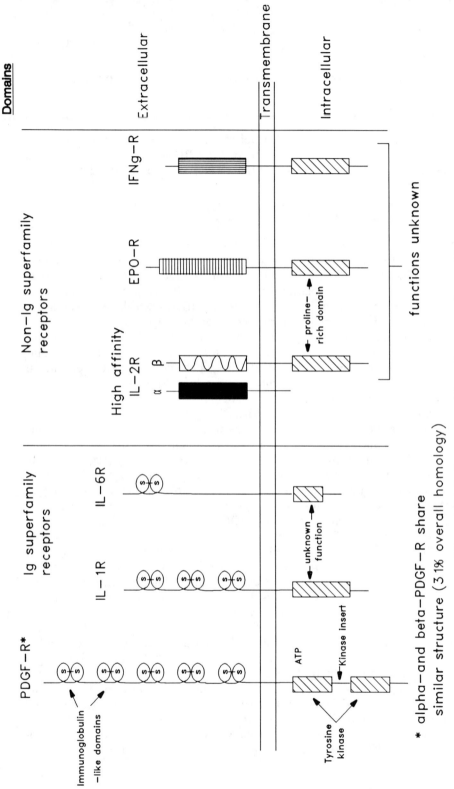

Figure 7.2 Basic structures of novel receptors for cytokines.

The basic fibroblast growth factor receptor

A putative receptor for bFGF has recently been molecularly cloned from a chick embryo cDNA library. The deduced amino acid sequence indicates a receptor polypeptide of 91.7 kDa. The N-terminal extracellular portion has three immunoglobulin-like domains and is similar to IL-1R in this respect. It is likely that the extracellular domain is heavily glycosylated as there are eleven possible N-linked glycosylation sites. Addition of N-and O-linked oligosaccharides probably accounts for the observed 130 kDa size of the bFGF-R glycoprotein. The amino acid sequence of bFGF-R is around 25–30 per cent homologous with that of IL-1R, but unlike the latter it includes an intracellular tyrosine kinase domain. Thus, the basic structure of bFGF-R strongly resembles that of PDGF-R (Figure 7.2), with the tyrosine kinase domain being intersected by a kinase insert region. The human counterpart of chicken bFGF-R is probably encoded by a gene known as *flg* (*fms*-like gene) and shows a high degree of homology with chicken bFGF-R.

The erythropoietin receptor

The EPO receptor (EPO-R)-cDNA was isolated from a cDNA expression library derived from murine erythroleukaemia (MEL) cells by screening monkey COS cell transfectants for binding of ^{125}I-EPO. From the nucleotide sequence of EPO-R-cDNA, an inferred amino acid sequence of the complete receptor polypeptide was obtained. This was found to contain a 24 amino acid N-terminal signal sequence followed by a 483 amino acid mature receptor protein. A hydropathy plot predicted a 23 amino acid hydrophobic region in roughly the middle of the receptor polypeptide which probably corresponds to the transmembrane segment. The extracellular domain is probably extensively O-glycosylated through serine and threonine residues which form a high percentage of the total amino acid content, although rather surprisingly there is only one potential N-linked glycosylation site in this domain. This glycosylation probably accounts for the discrepancy in molecular weight between the native receptor (85–100 kDa) identified by chemical cross-linking and the 55 kDa predicted for the non-glycosylated receptor polypeptide. No striking homology with the sequences of other known receptors has been found when the EPO-R sequence was compared with data in gene banks, nor does the N-terminal extracellular domain, which presumably contains the EPO-binding site, have any characteristics of receptors in the immunoglobulin (Ig) superfamily. Nor does the relatively large (234 amino acid) intracellular domain, which is the putative signal transducing element, have any homology with the catalytic domain of any cytokine receptor known to be a tyrosine kinase (Figure 7.2).

It is not yet clear whether the cloned EPO-R is solely responsible for EPO-mediated responses. As in many other instances of cytokine receptors, cells appear to have high- and low-affinity binding sites for EPO. This may reflect differing levels of post-translational modification of EPO-R, or the requirement for receptor association, e.g. dimerization, or the requirement of a further plasma membrane component to provide high-affinity binding sites. Rather interestingly, EPO has no apparent effect in MEL cells, despite the presence of high numbers of EPO-R, and it has been suggested that the Friend leukaemia virus (a retrovirus) present in these cells stimulates a proliferative response which by-passes the EPO-R.

The p70 interleukin-2 beta receptor

Binding studies with radiolabelled IL-2 established that there were different classes of binding sites with variable affinity for IL-2. Low-affinity binding sites were correlated to the presence of a p55 receptor protein, known to be synonymous with the Tac antigen, whereas medium-affinity binding sites were associated with the presence of a higher molecular weight p70 receptor. It is widely believed that p55 (IL-2Rα) and p70 (IR-2Rβ) combine to form a heterodimeric high-affinity binding site, although evidence to support this idea was missing until the recent molecular cloning of p70. The isolation of a cDNA clone for p70 stemmed from an expression cloning strategy in which cDNAs from a library derived from the human leukaemic cell line YT were transfected into monkey COS cells and expression of p70 identified by binding of specific monoclonal antibodies against p70. Nucleotide sequencing of p70 cDNAs has revealed that the receptor polypeptide contains 551 amino acids, a 26 amino acid signal sequence preceding the mature receptor of 525 amino acids. The latter consists of a 214 amino acid N-terminal extracellular domain, a 25 hydrophobic amino acid transmembrane section and a cytoplasmic domain of 286 amino acids (Figure 7.2). The amino acid sequence of p70 shows no significant homology to the sequences of other known proteins, nor does the sequence of the extracellular domain predict any similarity to members of the Ig superfamily (p55 Tac also does not belong to the Ig superfamily). The intracellular domain of p70 is far greater in size than the 13 amino acid 'tail' of p55, and while it is predicted that this probably has catalytic activity, there do not appear to be any consensus sequences typical of tyrosine kinases. Possibly it does have a kinase activity, but this remains to be tested. This domain also contains an unusually high percentage (14.7 per cent) of proline residues, a characteristic it shares with the cytoplasmic domain of EPO-R (13.7 per cent prolines), and thus the signal transducing mechanism of the two receptors may be similar. (A 'proline-rich' structure is also present in the cytoplasmic domain of the CD2 antigen present in the T-cell membrane.) The extracellular domain of p70 has four potential sites for N-linked glycosylation, and attachment of oligosaccharides in the native p70 glycoprotein probably accounts for the higher molecular weight (70–75 kDa) compared with the 58 kDa size predicted from the amino acid content alone.

p70 has been demonstrated to be present constitutively in certain cell lines such as the 'NK cell-like' YT and MT-2 leukaemic cell lines and the HTLV-1 transformed T-cell line, HUT102. It is absent in other leukaemic cell lines, e.g. Jurkat and U-937, and in unstimulated peripheral blood T-lymphocytes.

Following mitogen stimulation, p70 is transiently expressed in T-lympho-cytes, independently of p55 Tac. Transfection experiments with p70 and p55 cDNAs have confirmed that alone

a   expression of p70 confers the presence of medium-affinity binding sites,
b   expression of p55 confers the presence of low-affinity binding sites, but together
c   co-expression of p70 and p55 confers the presence of high and low affinity binding sites.

Treatment of cells expressing both p70 and p55 with monoclonal antibody against p70 abolished the presence only of high-affinity binding, strongly suggesting that p70.p55 heterodimers form high-affinity IL-2R complexes (Figure 7.2). Both the intermediate-affinity p70 receptors and the high-affinity p70.p55 heterodimeric receptors are capable of being internalized, whereas low-affinity p55 Tac, which has a very short cytoplasmic region, cannot be. This demonstrates that cytokine–receptor complexes can only be internalized if the receptor, or a component thereof, has an intact intracellu-lar domain. Despite the new knowledge of the structure of IL-2R, little is known as yet about the signal transmission pathway downstream from the receptor, except that it appears not to involve any known second-messenger system. It is virtually certain that the availability of p70 and the ability to produce mutant receptor proteins of it will provide exciting new insights into both the structure of the IL-2 binding site and the mechanism of signal transduction.

Other receptors

The molecular cloning of further cytokine receptors, e.g. IL-4R, GM-CSF-R, has recently been achieved. That of others is undoubtedly being tackled. Specific monoclonal antibodies have been raised against the IL-3- and IL-5-receptors, suggesting that cloning of these cannot be far away. In the case of murine IL-3R, one monoclonal antibody (F9) has been shown to partly mimic the activity of IL-3. In other words, this monoclonal antibody binds to the extracellular domain of IL-3R at or near the IL-3 binding site to trigger intracellular phosphorylation of various substrates usually associated with IL-3-mediated activation. F9 also competed with the binding of IL-3 to putative receptors of MW 130, 110, and 72 kDa, the species of highest molecular weight being similar in size to a 140 kDa tyrosine phosphoprotein, previously shown to bind IL-3 (see Chapter 3). Possibly the species of lower molecular weight are breakdown products of the 140 kDa phosphoprotein. It appears likely that IL-3R has (or is coupled to another membrane protein having) tyrosine kinase activity, since the IL-3 inducible proliferation of IL-3-dependent leukaemic cell lines may be subverted by the introduction of tyrosine kinase oncoproteins to yield IL-3 independent cell lines.

Although the IL-1R has no apparent integral kinase, the recent character-ization of an IL-1-induced tyrosine phosphoprotein of 41 kDa in the plasma membranes of the human tumour cell line K562, suggests that IL-1R is functionally linked to a protein–tyrosine kinase. It is also becoming increasingly clear that several other cytokine receptors require accessory membrane proteins for signal transduction to occur. For example, IL-6 binding to IL-6R probably triggers an association between IL-6R and a further membrane glycoprotein, gp130, to enable signal transduction to take place. It is likely that a similar receptor-accessory glycoprotein complex also exists for IFN gamma signalling since a second gene product, specified by a gene on human chromosome 21, is required for IFNg-R to be functional (see p. 149). The recent cloning of an IFNa/b-R also favours this model of signal transduction.

PDGF-R signal transduction

Most of the recent information on the mechanism of signal transduction has come from tyrosine kinase receptors, e.g. EGF-R, where it has been possible to introduce site-specific mutations in order to study receptor activation and function (see Chapter 2). The β-PDGF-R (see p. 221) is such a tyrosine kinase receptor and, subsequent to its molecular cloning, it has been possible to investigate the effect of mutations in its extra- and intracellular domains. The extracellular PDGF-binding domain of β-PDGF-R has a structure which consists of five Ig-like sections that classifies it as belonging to the Ig superfamily. (The M-CSF-R (c-FMS) and c-KIT oncoprotein, a putative cytokine receptor whose cognate ligand remains unidentified, have a similar pattern of Ig-like domain organization to β-PDGF-R.) Relatively little is known about how PDGF binding to the extracellular domain binding site of β-PDGF-R effects the process of signal transmission across the membrane. Most current hypotheses favour a mechanically induced alteration whereby the β-PDGF-R molecule is displaced perpendicularly to the plane of the plasma membrane, thereby leading to a perturbation of juxtaposed membrane components. Possibly dimerization of β-PDGF-R molecules is involved in this step. Replacement of the short transmembrane region of β-PDGF-R by that of the *neu* gene oncoprotein, a tyrosine kinase receptor related to EGF-R, has been found to prevent signal transmission, even though this modified receptor bound PDGF with equal affinity to normal β-PDGF-R. This suggests that the transmembrane region is not there simply to anchor the receptor, but is a necessary functional element within the receptor molecule. Possibly, the transmembrane region provides essential steric interactions with other membrane components, or alternatively controls the orientation of the extracellular and intracellular domains with respect to one another such that replacement with structurally distinct transmembrane segments results in non-functioning of the receptor.

Other mutations and rearrangements within the cytoplasmic tyrosine kinase domain also abolish or reduce signal transduction. For example, mutation of the ATP binding site in the first tyrosine kinase region (Figure 7.2) leads to loss of function, as also does removal of 97 amino acids on the

C-terminal side of the second tyrosine kinase region. Most interestingly, removal of the kinase insert region between the first and second tyrosine kinase domains, while destroying PDGF-induced mitogenic activity, did not prevent most of the other responses induced by PDGF, including increased phosphoinositide turnover, increased intracellular Ca^{2+} and pH, and auto-phosphorylation, from occurring. This suggests that the latter are not sufficient for the mitogenic effect of PDGF, and indicates that the kinase insert region plays a specific role in signal transduction, possibly determining the substrate specificity of the tyrosine kinase. For instance, it has recently been shown that β-PDGF-R physically associates with a phosphoinositide kinase (PIK), which may catalyse the generation of a novel class of phosphoinositide intermediates, e.g. inositol polyphosphates, acting as second messengers

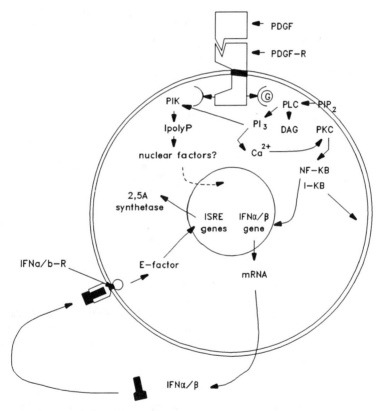

Figure 7.3 Proposed signalling pathways with involvement of nuclear transcription factors. Abbreviations: PDGF, platelet-derived growth factor; PDGF-R, PDGF receptor; PLC, phospholipase C; PKC, protein kinase C; PIK, phosphoinositide kinase; PIP_2, phosphatidylinositol 4,5-bisphosphate; PI_3, inositol 1,4,5 triphosphate; DAG, diacylglycerol; IpolyP, inositol polyphosphates; G, G-protein; NF-κB, nuclear factor κB; I-κB, cytosolic inhibitor protein of NF-κB; ISRE, IFN-stimulated regulatory elements.

necessary for the mitogenic response; loss of the tyrosine kinase insert region may abrogate this interaction (Figure 7.3). However, deletion of the kinase insert does not inhibit PDGF-induced hydrolysis of phosphatidylinositol, indicating that activation of phospholipase C (PLC) activity is unaffected.

The above findings strongly indicate that the integrity of β-PDGF-R and the activation of its tyrosine kinase are crucial for signal transduction into the cytoplasm. However, it is difficult to proceed further along the signal transmission pathway since the identity of the substrates of β-PDGF-R tyrosine kinase are as yet unknown. Possibly, PIK is one substrate, and there is some suggestion that c-RAF, a membrane serine/threonine kinase is another. Involvement of PLC in the breakdown of phosphatidylinositol 4,5-bisphosphate (PIP_2) appears to be critical, but it is not known how β-PDGF-R tyrosine kinase activity modulates PLC activity (Figure 7.3). PLC itself is now known to reside in at least four isoenzymes varying in size and structure, and activity may be controlled by interactions with various members of the large G-protein family. Here at least there may be possibilities for discrimination of signals, in that the PLC isoenzymes and G-proteins appear to be tissue specific, and thus different combinations may regulate signal transmission in different cells.

Signal transmission pathways: new information

Regulation of PLC activity is likely to be complex, but it has been recently shown that antibody against PIP_2 inhibits oncogene-induced mitogenesis, e.g. in ras-, src-, or erbB-transformed cells. This then indicates that PIP_2 breakdown mediated by PLC is in the chain of events leading to mitogenesis in oncogene-transformed cells. Of further interest here has been the discovery that certain structures in the non-catalytic domain of the PLCγ isoenzyme, which may regulate activity, are also found in certain oncoproteins, e.g. the SRC receptorless tyrosine kinase and the CRK oncoprotein, which may be a defective form of a receptorless tyrosine kinase. Both the tyrosine kinase-containing SRC and the defective CRK without tyrosine kinase activity transform cells, and it has been suggested that their PLC-like structures titrate out elements that negatively regulate PLCγ activity. Going back to the β-PDGF-R signal transmission pathway, it is therefore tempting to speculate that activation of PLC occurs by a process which inactivates negative control elements, the precise details of which remain obscure, leading to PIP_2 hydrolysis. The metabolism of the IP_3 so generated by the β-PDGF-R-activated PIK then leads to the production of inositol polyphosphates, speculated to be second messengers important in the signal transmission pathway culminating in DNA synthesis and mitogenesis (Figure 7.3).

While the early molecular events following cytokine stimulation are now, in some cases, beginning to make sense in terms of signal transmission, intermediate events before the induction of nuclear genes are still enigmatic. It is widely assumed that these involve activated protein kinases and phosphatases and thus much depends on whether the target proteins of the proposed phosphorylation cascade can be identified. PDGF is now known to induce the phosphorylation of a nuclear 64 kDa protein within 30 minutes of stimulation, but this may represent the end-link in a chain of phosphorylation–dephosphorylation reactions involving several cytoplasmic proteins. Clearly these reactions take place in the absence of new protein synthesis. One of these reactions appears to be the dissociation of the nuclear transcription factor NF-$\varkappa$B from a cytosolic inhibitor protein (I-$\varkappa$B) and translocation of NF-$\varkappa$B into the nucleus (Figure 7.3). The 'activation' of latent NF-$\varkappa$B is inducible by many types of proliferation-inducing agents such as phorbolesters, LPS, TNFα, etc. In addition, IFNα, a differentiating or antiproliferative cytokine, appears to rapidly activate a latent DNA-binding protein (E-factor) present in the cytoplasm, which subsequently migrates to the nucleus where it binds to IFN-stimulated regulatory elements (ISREs), present in the 5' flanking regions of IFN-inducible genes, to initiate transcription (Figure 7.3). However, it is probable that the signal transmission pathways for NF-$\varkappa$B and E-factor activation are separate, since it has recently been shown that IFN-induced 2,5A-synthetase occurs by a pathway not involving the phorbol ester/diacylglycerol/PKC activation route, as is necessary for NF-$\varkappa$B (Figure 7.3). Thus, cellular responses involving new protein synthesis are probably controlled by the gene-specificity of latent DNA-binding nuclear transcription factors that lie in particular signal transmission pathways. Ultimately, therefore, whether proliferation of differentiation (i.e. the qualitative nature of the response) follows cytokine stimulation may depend upon which signal transmission pathways are activated and the nuclear transcription factors they contain as much as the quantitative balance of activatable enzymes and their metabolites, which may govern more the strength of the response (see p. 220). It must also be assumed that while individual signal transmission pathways may operate independently, there can be interaction among different pathways at various points, and that the eventual cellular response depends on the extent of cooperation or restraint among participating regulatory circuits. It will be the goal of future research to unravel this complex circuitry at the molecular level.

7.5   Further cellular interactions

Allergic responses

The main purpose of the immune system appears to be the discrimination of that which is foreign, 'non-self', from that which is self. This is largely achieved by specific leukocytes, the T_H lymphocytes that recognize foreign antigens in combination with MHC molecules expressed on presenting cells such as macrophages. The process of presentation and T_H cell activation may be viewed as the induction phase of the immune response (Figure 7.4). Activated T_H cells produce a package of several cytokines that act on other

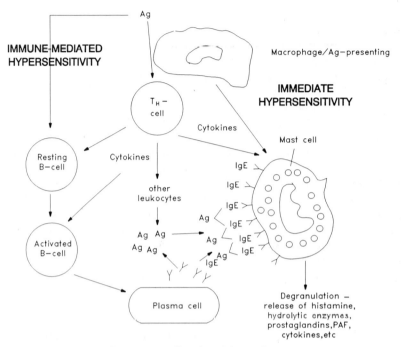

Figure 7.4   Immune-mediated and immediate hypersensitivity.

leukocytes, e.g. B-lymphocytes, macrophages, or granulocytes, to stimulate immunological function such as antibody production. These activated leukocytes provide the effector arm of the immune response, in which the foreign antigens are destroyed and eliminated. They also produce a number of cytokines which may amplify defensive effector mechanisms and which probably play complex biological roles in the control of immunocyte proliferation and differentiation, together with profound local and systemic effects in many cells throughout the body.

Normally, T_H cells can affect a further tier of discrimination in recognizing foreign antigens in that potentially harmful substances can be distinguished from harmless ones. Where this system breaks down, harmless substances are mistaken for harmful ones and recognized as foreign antigens to provoke the kind of immune response detailed in the preceding paragraph. This is why some people develop what is known as an allergy to particular, normally harmless, substances. For example, following skin contact with the substance they are allergic to, they develop a rash. Commonly, the rash may take about one to two days to develop, and this is an example of inflammation due to a delayed hypersensitivity (DH) reaction (Figure 7.4) (see pp. 168–70). There is, however, another kind of allergic reaction which occurs rapidly following contact with the 'allergen', and may have more dramatic consequences for the afflicted person. This 'immediate hypersensitivity' or anaphylactic response is not mediated by macrophages and T-cells as in the DH reactions, but by antibody and specifically by immunoglobulin type E (IgE). The latter is normally found in very small amounts, and has a fairly limited role in host defence against invasive parasites. For reasons that are still not understood, in the allergic person the allergen triggers an immune response which leads to transformation and activation of those B-lymphocytes that produce IgE. The presence of IgE alone is, however, not sufficient to cause immediate hypersensitivity. Mast cells, which are a type of basophilic granulocyte and are found widely distributed in connective tissues throughout the body, have high numbers of receptors (100 000–500 000 per cell) for IgE on their cell surface. In the allergic person, mast cells will be coated with IgE molecules specific for the sensitizing allergen, and on binding with the allergen from the circulation these cells degranulate releasing large quantities of pre-formed chemicals, e.g. vasoactive amines, chemotactic factors and hydrolytic enzymes such as neutral proteases and acid hydrolases (Figure 7.4). In addition, mast cells secondarily produce arachidonic acid metabolites, e.g. PAF, prostaglandins, and leukotrienes, which are also known to mediate inflammatory reactions.

From the known biological activities of cytokines, there are several that have potential roles in regulating allergic responses. Activated T_H lymphocytes produce IL-2, -3, -4, -5, and IFNγ all of which in the mouse, at least, may stimulate B-lymphocyte proliferation, differentiation, and antibody production. IL-4 in particular has been associated with B-cell isotype switching to IgE production. IFNγ may antagonize this function and possibly the relative amounts of these two cytokines controls IgE production. Perhaps, an imbalance in the activation or numbers of suppressor–inducer T_H1 (IL-2 and IFNγ producer) and helper–inducer T_H2 (IL-4 and IL-5 producer) classes of T_H lymphocytes leads to elevated IgE production in response to allergen. Additionally, IL-3 and IL-4 have been shown to have growth promoting activity in murine mast cells. However, the role(s) of IL-3 or IL-4 in human mast cell proliferation and differentiation is less well defined. A role for NGF in rat mast cell growth and degranulation has also been posited (see p. 58).

Besides the well-known degranulation response and synthesis of arachidonic acid metabolites, mast cells are probably also able to produce potentially inflammatory cytokines such as TNFα. These could also contribute to some of the symptoms associated with allergic reactions.

Upper respiratory tract infections may precipitate allergic reactions, e.g. in bronchial asthma. Viral infections are known to stimulate the production of IFNα/β, and the latter has been shown to enhance histamine release by basophils, suggesting another cytokine-mediated interaction that may exacerbate the allergic response. However, the involvement of IFNα/β in mediating histamine release during allergic responses is apparently contradicted by a recent report that IFNα/β inhibits IgE-dependent histamine release from rat mast cells. The earlier studies were carried out with rather impure basophil preparations, and it is suggested that the presence of other leukocytes in these probably affected the outcome with IFNα/β treatment.

7.6   Normal tissue growth and remodelling

Regulation of liver growth

The main liver cells, the hepatocytes, stop dividing once the liver has reached a certain size following fetal and postnatal development. While the majority of hepatocytes then remain quiescent for the duration of adult life, liver injury or infection may provoke a rapid compensatory response in which hepatocytes proliferate to restore the organ to its normal mass. This may be demonstrated experimentally in rats, when the liver is regenerated to its original size following partial hepatectomy. Thus, hepatocytes appear to retain the capacity to respond to proliferation-inducing signals and when the liver is restored to full size to become quiescent once more. How is this process regulated? Firstly, since liver regeneration starts within a few hours of partial hepatectomy, it is clear that hepatocytes must 'sense' tissue loss. Possibly they respond to the increased metabolic load placed on the reduced liver. Alternatively, monocytes, granulocytes, and platelets recruited from the circulation to the site of tissue injury provide the necessary growth factors, e.g. PDGF or IL-1, to 'prime' hepatocytes for mitogenesis. It is harder to explain why hepatocytes at sites of necrosis caused by viral infection or chemicals respond in a similar way. In this case, changes in the local microenvironment, e.g. cell contacts and matrices, have been suggested to provide the initiating stimuli.

Once primed, quiescent hepatocytes move out of the G_0 cell cycle phase into G_1 and this is associated with increased proto-oncogene expression. Both c-*fos* and c-*myc* transcripts are found in abundance at this stage. 'Competent' hepatocytes may then progress to S-phase and DNA-synthesis if they are triggered by appropriate growth factor stimulation. It is speculated that this progression step is activated by an autocrine circuit involving TGFα as a mitogenic growth factor. The amount of TGFα mRNA has been shown to increase significantly from about 12 hours after partial hepatectomy, coinciding with the major wave of hepatocyte DNA synthesis, although the numbers of hepatocyte EGF-R, to which TGFα binds, decline in regenerating liver. Internalization and/or down-regulation of EGF-R may, however, be in response to TGFα binding, and therefore it is still possible that TGFα acts as an autocrine growth stimulator of hepatocytes. Other serum growth factors and hormones, such as norepinephrine or angiotensin, may also be involved in both priming and progression stages of liver regeneration.

The inhibition of hepatocyte proliferation may also be regulated by cytokines. In particular, it has been found that TGFβ, a dimeric protein completely unrelated to TGFα, is present in increasing amounts as the regenerative process comes to a halt. In this case, it has been suggested that TGFβ is more likely to originate from cell types other than hepatocytes, for instance endothelial cells or leukocytes, and thus acts in a paracrine fashion on hepatocytes. TGFβ has been shown to inhibit EGF-induced DNA synthesis in cultured hepatocytes. Whether this direct antiproliferative effect of TGFβ applies *in vivo*, or whether other TGFβ-mediated responses such as increased extracellular matrix synthesis are more important in causing the eventual cessation of hepatocyte proliferation, remains an open question.

Remodelling of normal tissue and bone

Throughout life, many cell types go through an 'ageing' process in which they ultimately become senescent and useless to the organism. The removal of such cells, e.g. senescent erythrocytes, is dependent upon their recognition and engulfment by mononuclear phagocytes. Recognition of senescent cells appears to depend partly upon the formation of advanced glycosylation end-products (AGEs), which are the result of accumulative non-enzymatic reactions of cellular proteins with glucose with time. Macrophages recognize cells with AGEs and respond in a similar way to LPS stimulation, i.e. they become functionally activated and release a number of cytokines, including TNFα and IL-1β. The latter two cytokines have overlapping biological activities, some of which are consistent with a potential role in the co-ordinated removal and replacement of senescent extracellular matrix components, and thus in tissue remodelling. For example, both TNFα and IL-1 stimulate mesenchymal cells to produce matrix-degrading enzymes such as collagenase and transin (stromelysin). Such mesenchymal cells can also produce TGFβ which may act as an autocrine factor to down-regulate degradative processes. At the same time, TNFα and IL-1 could stimulate the proliferation of fibroblasts and possibly other cells either directly, or indirectly, through secretion of growth factors, e.g. PDGF-AA, synthesized in response to these cytokines. In diabetes, where the process of AGE formation is accelerated by high circulating levels of glucose, certain tissues exhibit high proliferative phases resulting in abnormal tissue deposition, and this may be caused by imbalances in cytokine release. Similar high levels of fibrotic tissue may occur in old people where AGEs have accumulated as a function of time.

Bone remodelling offers a good example where both local and systemic mediators interact to regulate bone formation and bone resorption closely. Bone is a heterogeneous collection of cell types, many of which interface with other tissues, e.g. cartilage and bone marrow. It is likely that several cytokines are produced locally in bone matrices, although the identity of cell types secreting particular cytokines is difficult to ascertain. In addition, other cytokines may be present via the circulation from distant sources or from infiltrating leukocytes.

Isoforms of TGFβ and the more recently discovered bone morphogenetic proteins, BMP-2A and -3 (see pp. 50–6) are found in high concentrations in bone extracts, suggesting that they play a role in bone formation, e.g. by stimulating cell replication and differentiated function. Their interactions with osteotropic hormones such as parathormone and calcitonin, which control Ca^{2+} and phosphate metabolism, may also contribute to homeostatic mechanisms regulating, for example, the polymerization–depolymerization of proteoglycan aggregates present in the less dense areas of bone. Parathormone may also directly stimulate bone cells to activate membrane-bound adenylate cyclase and to increase Ca^{2+} influx and thereby activate the cellular systems involved in bone resorption, e.g. inhibition of collagen synthesis by osteoblasts. Such an effect may be mediated by cytokines such as TNFα which has been shown to inhibit osteoblastic collagen synthesis and to increase collagenase secretion by synovial cells. IL-1α/β also represent cytokines potent in the induction of bone resorption, acting indirectly through osteoblasts, perhaps by inducing TNF secretion, to activate osteoclastic-resorption. In addition, both TNF and IL-1 stimulate cartilage resorption and inhibit synthesis of proteoglycan, the essential matrix component of cartilage. Interestingly, such effects of TNF and IL-1, which can be demonstrated in bone cell systems, *in vitro*, require relatively high concentrations of these cytokines. Low cytokine (TNF or IL-1) concentrations, in contrast, may promote osteoblastic cell proliferation and transiently stimulate collagen synthesis. All this suggests that the roles of TNF and IL-1 in bone remodelling may vary according to their local concentrations in bone matrices from being part of the physiological activating processes required for coupling synthetic and degradative mechanisms to that of potentially pathological agents causing osteolysis and cartilage destruction.

Other cytokines such as FGFs and IGF-1 acting as growth factors may be involved in stimulating pre-osteoblast proliferation, resulting in an enlarged population of osteoblasts capable of producing bone matrices. Bone cell cultures do not, however, secrete FGFs, and thus their occurrence in bone extracts suggests they are either not exported due to the lack of a signal sequence (see p. 45) or are produced elsewhere in the body and migrate to bone matrices via the circulation. The role of FGFs in stimulating the vascularization of bone tissues is probably of equal or more importance in bone development and repair (see below).

Vascularization and angiogenic factors

The formation of new blood vessels leading to vascularization of tissues is under the control of 'angiogenic' factors. The growth of blood capillaries depends on the activities and proliferation of vascular endothelial cells. To produce new capillary growth, the basement membrane has first to be enzymatically degraded. This is followed by endothelial cell locomotion and proliferation. The heparin-binding cytokines, acidic and basic FGF (pp. 44–7), appear to be among angiogenic factors providing mitogenic stimuli to endothelial cells. Both aFGF and bFGF in nanogram amounts have been shown to stimulate angiogenesis *in vitro* and *in vivo*. In adults, angiogenesis occurs at a relatively slow rate in most tissues and therefore the question is how the activities of potent mitogenic cytokines such as FGFs are regulated. Part of the answer is probably due to the low rate of secretion of FGFs, which is a result of their lack of a signal sequence. FGFs may therefore only be released in physiological amounts in special circumstances, e.g. during ovulation in females, or following tissue damage. They may also be important in the neovascularization of solid tumours. Their molecular relationship with *int-2, hst*, and *fgf-5* proto-oncogene products (see pp. 45, 46) suggests that the latter, which may be secreted by tumour cells, may also be involved in tumour vascularization. For example, Kaposi's sarcoma, associated with AIDS, is usually classified as an angiogenic tumour.

TGFα has also been demonstrated to be a potent angiogenic factor; it appears to have a ten-fold greater activity that EGF in this respect. However, it is difficult to assess whether TGFα has a physiological role in angiogenesis. Nevertheless, in psoriasis, a skin disease often characterized by blood capillary elongation and epidermal hyperplasia with acute or chronic inflammation, TGFα mRNA and protein are found in much higher amounts in lesional psoriatic epidermis than in normal skin suggesting that TGFα has a pathophysiological role. On the other hand, TGFβ, whose activity may retard that of TGFα, is not increased in psoriatic lesions.

A further angiogenic factor is a protein designated angiogenin. This is a highly basic protein with a molecular weight of 14 400 which shares approximately 35 per cent structural homology with a family of pancreatic ribonucleases. Whether the ribonucleolytic activity of angiogenin has anything to do with its angiogenic activity remains an open question. Further, the target cell for angiogenin is unknown, and thus its mode of action is obscure. Possibly the action of angiogenin is indirect, causing the release of growth factors or chemoattractants for instance.

It is likely that other soluble factors, besides angiogenin, FGFs, and TGFα are involved directly or indirectly in the process of angiogenesis. For instance, the directional locomotion of endothelial cells is probably controlled by a number of chemotactic factors. Lipid-like substances such as prostaglandins also appear to be angiogenic. IFNs are anti-angiogenic. In the presence of heparin, steroids inhibit angiogenesis. Clearly, the modulation of angiogenesis is complex; understanding the biological pathways involved requires more research, but might possibly lead to therapeutic approaches for 'angiogenic diseases', i.e. those involving aberrant neovascularization.

Tumour progression

In earlier chapters, the potential role of cytokines as autocrine growth factors for tumour cell proliferation has been mentioned several times. The simple equation of elevated expression of growth factor and/or its receptor equalling abnormal mitogenic response was proposed to explain excessive tumour cell proliferation. However, growth-factor-dependent proliferation is probably an intermediate stage of neoplastic transformation. For example, many leukaemic cells progress from a growth-factor-dependent stage to a growth-factor-independent stage. Invariably, tumour progression, particularly in solid tumours, is much more complex than this. Why for instance do tumour cells often become more 'aggressive', more 'malignant' in their behaviour and characteristics as time elapses? What controls the capacity of tumour cells to metastasize and spread to various anatomical sites throughout the body? How does the growing tumour subvert the metabolism and growth of tissues surrounding it to its own needs?

Clearly, tumour progression is a multifactorial, time-dependent process. Throughout its life history, a tumour, starting with the escape of a normal cell from local growth control mechanisms, must maintain a series of morphological and metabolic alterations that provide its component cells with a selective advantage over normal cell replication, and the ability to evade host defence mechanisms. This is often reflected by the heterogeneity of tumour cells contained in a single tumour where some cells have progressed further towards the malignant state than others. In many cases, tumour cells appear to de-differentiate with loss of specialized organelles for specific normal cell functions, leading to the outgrowth of malignant cell populations with 'embryonic' or 'stem cell' characteristics. Tumour progression is often preceeded or accompanied by 'genetic lability' where breaks occur in chromosomes followed by translocation events, or where genetic instability is induced by oncogenic viruses, radiation, or carcinogenic chemicals.

A large number of host factors are important in modulating tumour progression, and the wide biological activities of cytokines suggests that they may play pivotal roles in many, if not all stages, of tumour development. There is enormous potential for cytokines to modulate tumour cell proliferation (see for example, Section 6.5), and this relates not only to the induction of the mitogenic response, but also to expression of catabolic enzymes, oncogenes, and cell-surface adhesion molecules, to alterations in cytoskeletal components and membrane phospholipid/glycosphingolipid composition, and to the secretion of factors regulating environmental conditions. For instance, certain cytokines e.g. TNF and IL-1, induce the synthesis of degradative enzymes which break down the extracellular matrix or lead to the resorption of connective tissues. Others, e.g. FGFs and TGFα, are probably involved in neovascularization of tumours. Obviously, immunoregulatory cytokines, e.g. IL-2 and IFNγ, which control the activities of leukocytes, will be important for immune surveillance and tumoricidal mechanisms. Nevertheless, despite some 30 years or more of progress in the isolation and characterization of cytokines, and the overwhelming circumstantial evidence implicating the relevance of their activities in tumour cell growth and tumour progression, the precise details of their interactive tumour-modulating mechanisms in individual tumour types remain unknown. As L. Foulds concluded in 1957 at the very beginning of cytokine isolations, 'It is possible, as long suspected by some, that the characters that most decisively govern the outcome of neoplasia and its response to treatment are as yet unknown'. It may be now that some of these 'characters' have been identified, but much more information concerning how they interact during tumour progression is required before the above statement can be finally 'laid to rest'.

Cytokine interactions with other physiological systems

Cytokines by their very nature are similar to, and may have overlapping functions with, polypeptide hormones that mediate specific actions within the endocrine system. EPO, produced in the kidney and stimulating the production of erythrocytes in the bone marrow, is probably more a hormone than a cytokine. Other mediators, e.g. inhibins and Müllerian inhibitory substance (MIS) of the 'TGFβ superfamily', are also widely recognized as hormones, as are insulin and IGF-I and -II. Cachectin, a hormone that inhibits lipoprotein lipase activity in adipocytes, is now known to be identical to TNFα. Endogenous pyrogen (EP) has been identified with IL-1. Other examples of cytokines acting as hormones and vice versa are being discovered. For instance, the prevention of corpus luteum regression, essential to maintain progesterone secretion and thus endometrial gland secretion and the establishment of pregnancy, is mediated in sheep by ovine trophoblastic anti-luteolytic protein (oTP-1). Studies based on amino acid sequencing and receptor-binding assays have shown significant homology (45–70 per cent) between oTP-1 and human, bovine, pig, mouse, or rat subtypes of IFNα, particularly bovine IFNα-II, suggesting that oTP-1 is probably a member of the IFNα family. Furthermore, oTP-1 has been demonstrated to possess antiviral and antiproliferative properties. IFNα/oTP-1 protein(s) may play a similar role in human pregnancies. HuIFNα has been found in amniotic fluid during the first trimester, and perhaps more significantly HuIFNα has been localized to the syncytiotrophoblast, the interface between the fetus and the maternal placenta, where its biological actions may be expected to be most effective.

Several other cytokines have been found in the 'feto-placental unit'. IL-2 transcripts, for example, have been shown to be expressed in the syncytio-trophoblast suggesting that IL-2 may have some role, perhaps mediating immune interactions between the fetal allograft and the maternal host, during pregnancy. Such expression of the IL-2 gene in non-T cells also calls into question whether IL-2 is exclusively synthesized by activated T_H-lymphocytes. M-CSF has been reported to be produced by uterine luminal and glandular secretory epithelial cells, and IL-1 by purified cytotrophoblasts. Additionally, GM-CSF and TGFβ have been found in placental tissue. All of these cytokines may be envisaged to play physiological roles in the maintenance and protection of the feto-placental unit.

There is recent evidence that TNF can increase liver uptake of amino acids and stimulate glucagon release. This not only strengthens the link between the immune and endocrine systems, but also suggests that TNF may be important for the integration of catabolic changes such as suppression of lipid synthesis in fat cells or breakdown of skeletal muscle, and anabolic changes such as synthesis of acute phase proteins or wound healing that occur during acute stress, injury, or infection. IFNγ also appears to have significant effects of the endocrine system. For example, IFNγ injected into cancer patients was shown to increase adrenocorticotropic hormone (ACTH), cortisol, and growth hormone levels within a few hours of administration. IL-1 (and TNF) has been shown to decrease secretion of thyroid hormones, T_4 and T_3, from the thyroid gland of mice, probably by directly inhibiting the action of thyrotropin (TSH). Indeed, there are many more examples where cyto-

Table 7.2   Cytokines, hormones, neuropeptides — interactions

Mediator substance	Effects
IFNα/β	Adrenal steroids ↗
	Melanin synthesis ↗
	Iodine uptake in thyroid ↗
IFNγ	ACTH ↗
	Cortisol ↗
	Growth hormone ↗
IL-1	Fever induction
	Pituitary ACTH and endorphins ↗
	Glucocorticoids ↗
	β-endorphin ↗
	Thyroid hormones, T_4 and T_3 ↙
TNF (cachectin)	Glucagon ↗
	Fever induction
ACTH	IFNγ synthesis ↙
	IFNγ-mediated macrophage activation ↙
	Ig synthesis ↙
Human chorionic gonadotrophin (HCG)	CTL, NK cell activation ↙
	T-cell proliferation ↙
Somatostatin	Histamine and leukotriene release from basophils ↙
	T-cell proliferation ↙
Substance P	TNF and IL-1 secretion by macrophages ↗
	T-cell proliferation ↗
Arginine vasopressin and oxytocin	IFNγ synthesis ↗
β-Endorphin and morphine	IFNγ synthesis ↙
α-Endorphin and enkephalins	Ig synthesis and secretion ↙
Glucocorticoids	Macrophage activation ↙
	Production and action of IL-1 and other cytokines ↙

kines have been reported as having profound effects on the endocrine system, and particularly within the pituitary– adrenal axis (see Table 7.2). However, these interactions are not completely one-sided. It is becoming increasingly clear that many hormones have actions on leukocytes within the immune system. ACTH, for example, suppresses IFNγ synthesis and IFNγ-mediated activation of macrophages. Human chorionic gonadotropin suppresses activity of CTL and NK cells and proliferation of T-cells, actions which are probably important in protecting the fetus from 'immune' rejection during pregnancy. Arginine–vasopressin or oxytocin appear to replace the IL-2 requirement of T-cells for IFNγ synthesis *in vitro*, and may be yet another example of 'endocrine–immune' interaction.

Hormonal substances produced in the peripheral and central nervous systems have also been demonstrated to affect the functioning of the immune system. For example, somatostatin suppresses T-cell proliferation, whereas the neuropeptide substance P augments T-cell proliferation. Interestingly, substance P has been shown to be a potent inducer of TNFα and IL-1 secretion in macrophages, and these cytokines may contribute to its activity in T-cells. Opiates, such as β-endorphin, which are produced in increased amount during stress, inhibit the production of IFNγ by human PBL in culture. α-Endorphin and enkephalins suppress Ig synthesis and secretion. Such activities may be of relevance to immunosuppression in opiate addiction and its consequences in relation to the pathogenesis of opportunistic infections in AIDS.

In summary, cytokines, present locally or systemically in the circulation, appear to mediate a number of hormone-like activities, and may interact with 'classical' hormones in certain endocrine functions. The reverse of this, where 'classical' hormones together with neuropeptides affect the synthesis of cytokines and modulate their activities, has already been demonstrated in numerous instances. An overlap in the integrated regulation of the immune, endocrine, and nervous systems among cytokines, 'classical' hormones, and neuropeptides therefore seems likely, and this may be particularly relevant in periods of stress or injury.

Further reading

Molecular and cellular interactions

Briskin, M., Kuwabara, M.D., Sigman, D.S., and Wall, R. (1988) Induction of κ transcription by interferon-gamma without activation of NF-κB. *Science* **242**, 1036.

Cozzolino, F., Rubartelli, A, Aldinucci, D. *et al.* (1989) Interleukin-1 as an autocrine growth factor for acute myeloid leukaemia cells. *Proceedings of the National Academy of Sciences USA* **86**, 2369.

Dale, T.C., Ali Imam, A.M., Kerr, I.M., and Stark, G.R. (1989) Rapid activation by interferon alpha of a latent DNA-binding protein present in the cytoplasm of untreated cells. *Proceedings of the National Academy of Sciences USA* **86**, 1203.

D'Andrea, A.D., Lodish, H.F., and Wong, G.G. (1989) Expression cloning of the murine erythropoietin receptor. *Cell* **57**, 277.

Daniel, T.O. and Fen, Z. (1988) Distinct pathways mediate transcriptional regulation of platelet derived growth factor B/c-*cis* expression. *Journal of Biological Chemistry* **263**, 19815.

Dinarello, C.A., Clark, B.D., Puren, J., *et al.* (1989) The interleukin-1 receptor. *Immunology Today* **10**, 49.

Fukami, K., Matsuoka, K., Nakanishi, O., *et al.* (1988) Antibody to phosphatidylinositol 4,5-bisphosphate inhibits oncogene-induced mitogenesis. *Proceedings of the National Academy of Sciences USA* **85**, 9057.

Gearing, D.P., King, J.A., Gough, N.M. and Nicola, N.A. (1989) Expression cloning of a receptor for human granulocyte-macrophage colony-stimulating factor. *The EMBO Journal* **8**, 3667.

Hatakayama, M., Tsudo, M., Minamoto, S., *et al.* (1989) Interleukin-2 receptor beta chain gene: generation of three receptor forms by cloned human alpha and beta chain cDNAs. *Science* **244**, 551.

Isfort, R., Huhn, R.D., Frackelton, A.R., and Ihle, J.N. (1988) Stimulation of factor-dependent myeloid cell lines with interleukin-3 induces tyrosine phosphorylation of several cellular substrates. *Journal of Biological Chemistry* **263**, 19203.

Kaczmarek, K. (1986) Protooncogene expression during the cell cycle. *Laboratory Investigation* **54**, 365.

Kitamura, T., Tojo, A., Kuwaki, T., *et al.* (1989) Identification and analysis of human erythropoietin receptors on a factor-dependent cell line, TF-1. *Blood* **73**, 375.

Lee, P.L., Johnson, D.E., Cousens, L.S. *et al.* (1989) Purification and complementary DNA cloning of a receptor for basic fibroblast growth factor. *Science*, **245**, 57.

Lenardo, M.J., Fan, C-M., Maniatis, T., and Baltimore, D. (1989) The involvement of NF-κB in beta-interferon gene regulation reveals its role as widely inducible mediator of signal transduction. *Cell* **57**, 287.

Matsui, T., Heidaran, M., Miki, T., *et al.* (1989) Isolation of a novel receptor cDNA establishes the existence of two PDGF receptor genes. *Science* **243**, 800.

Mita, S., Tominaga, A., Hitoshi, Y., *et al.* (1989) Characterization of high-affinity receptors for interleukin 5 on interleukin 5-dependent cell lines. *Proceedings of the National Academy of Sciences USA* **86**, 2311.

Morrison, D.K., Kaplan, D.R., Rapp, U., and Roberts, T.M. (1988) Signal transduction from membrane to cytoplasm: growth factors and membrane-bound oncogene products increase Raf-1 phosphorylation and associated protein kinase activity. *Proceedings of the National Academy of Sciences USA* **45**, 8855.

Mosley, B., Beckmann, M.P., March, C.J. *et al.* (1989) The murine interleukin-4 receptor: molecular cloning and characterization of secreted and membrane bound forms. *Cell* **59**, 335.

Rhee, S.G., Suh, P-G., S-H., and Lee, S.Y. (1989) Studies of inositol phospholipid-specific phospholipase C. *Science* **244**, 546.

Rolink, A.G., Melchers, F., and Palacios, R. (1989) Monoclonal antibodies reactive with the mouse interleukin 5 receptor. *Journal of Experimental Medicine* **169**, 1693.

Sawyer, S.T. (1989) The two proteins of the erythropoietin receptor are structurally similar. *Journal of Biological Chemistry* **264**, 13343.

Schreurs, J., Sugawara, M., Arai, K.-I., *et al.* (1989) A monoclonal antibody with IL-3-like activity blocks IL-3 binding and stimulates tyrosine phosphorylation. *Journal of Immunology* **142**, 819.

Shawver, L.K., Pierce, G.F., Kawahara, R.S., and Deuel, T.F. (1989) Platelet-derived growth factor induces phosphorylation of a 64 kDa nuclear protein. *Journal of Biological Chemistry* **264**, 1046.

Shoyab, M., McDonald, V.L., Bradley, J.G., and Todaro, G.J. (1988) Amphiregulin: a bifunctional growth-modulating glycoprotein produced by the phorbol 12-myristate 13-acetate-treated human breast adenocarcinoma cell line MCF-7. *Proceedings of the National Academy of Sciences USA* **85**, 6528.

Shoyab, M., Plowman, G.D., McDonald, V.L., *et al.* (1989) Structure and function of human amphiregulin: a member of the epidermal growth factor family. *Science* **243**, 1074.

Steffen, M., Abboud, M., Potter, G.K., *et al.* (1989) Presence of tumour necrosis factor or a related factor in human basophil/mast cells. *Immunology* **66**, 445.

Swieter, M., Ghali, W.A., Rimmer, C., and Befus, D. (1989) Interferon-alpha/beta inhibits IgE-dependent histamine release from rat mast cells. *Immunology* **66**, 606.

Toga, T., Hibi, M., Hirata, Y. *et al.* (1989) Interleukin-6 triggers the association of its receptor with a possible signal transducer, gp130. *Cell* **58**, 573.

Tigges, M.A., Casey, L.S., and Koshland, M.E. (1989) Mechanism of interleukin-2 signalling: mediation of different outcomes by a single receptor and transduction pathway. *Science* **243**, 781.

Uzé, G., Lutfalla, G., and Gresser, I. (1990) Genetic bransfer of a functional human interferon alpha receptor into mouse cells: cloning and expression of its cDNA. *Cell* **60**, 225.

Williams, L.T. (1989) Signal transduction by the platelet-derived growth factor receptor. *Science* **243**, 1564.

Wickremasinghe, R.G., Mire-Sluis, A.R., and Hoffbrand, A.V. (1988) Biochemical mechanisms of transduction of signals for proliferation and differentiation in normal and malignant haemopoietic cells, in *Recent Advances in Haematology* **5** (Hoffbrand, A.V., ed.) Churchill Livingstone, Edinburgh, p.19.

Yan, C., Sehgal, P.B., and Tamm, I. (1989) Signal transduction pathways in the induction of 2′,5′-oligoadenylate synthetase gene expression by interferon alpha/ beta. *Proceedings of the National Academy of Sciences USA* **86**, 2243.

Tissues, organs, and physiological systems

Blalock, J.E. (1989) A molecular basis for bidirectional communication between the immune and neuroendocrine systems. *Physiological Reviews* **69**, 1.

Boehm, K.D., Kelly M.F., Ilan, J., and Ilan, J. (1989) The interleukin-2 gene is expressed in the syncytiotrophoblast of human placenta. *Proceedings of the National Academy of Sciences USA* **86**, 656.

Canalis, E., McCarthy, T., and Centrella, M. (1988) Growth factors and the regulation of bone remodeling. *Journal of Clinical Investigation* **81**, 277.

Elder, J.T., Fisher, G.J., Lindquist, P.B., *et al.* (1989) Overexpression of transforming growth factor alpha in psoriatic epidermis. *Science* **243**, 811.

Fausto, N. and Mead, J.E. (1989) Regulation of liver growth: protooncogenes and transforming growth factors. *Laboratory Investigation* **60**, 4.

Folkman, J. and Klagsburn, M. (1987) Angiogenic factors. *Science* **235**, 442.

Foulds, L. (1957) Tumour progression. *Cancer Research* **17**, 355.

Fuji, T., Sato, K., Ozawa, M. *et al.* (1989) Effect of interleukin-1 on thyroid hormone metabolism in mice. *Endocrinology* **124**, 167.

Goldstein, D., Gockerman, J., Krishnan, R., *et al.* (1987) Effects of gamma-interferon on the endocrine system: results from a phase I study. *Cancer Research* **47**, 6397.

Hakomori, S. (1984) Glycosphingolipids as differentiation-dependent, tumour-associated markers and regulators of cell proliferation. *Trends in Biochemical Sciences* **9**, 453.

Hansen, T.R., Imakawa, K., Polites, H.G., *et al.* (1988) Interferon RNA of embryonic origin is expressed transiently during early pregnancy in the ewe. *Journal of Biological Chemistry* **263**, 12801.

Howatson, A.G., Farquharson, M., Meager, A., *et al.* (1988) Localization of alpha-interferon in the human feto-placental unit. *Journal of Endocrinology* **119**, 531.

Lebon, P., Girard, S., Thépot, F., and Chany, C. (1982) The presence of alpha-IFN in human amniotic fluid. *Journal of General Virology* **59**, 393.

Nowell, P.C. (1986) Mechanisms of tumour progression. *Cancer Research* **46**, 2203.

Peterson, P.K., Sharp, B., Gekker, G., *et al.* (1987) Opioid-mediated suppression of interferon gamma production by cultured peripheral blood mononuclear cells. *Journal of Clinical Investigation* **80**, 824.

Pontzer, C.H., Torres, B.A., Vallet, J.L., *et al.* (1988) Antiviral activity of the pregnancy recognition hormone ovine trophoblast protein-1. *Biochemical and Biophysical Research Communications* **152**, 801.

Sidky, Y.A. and Borden, E.C. (1987) Inhibition of angiogenesis by interferons: effects on tumour- and lymphocyte-induced vascular responses. *Cancer Research* **47**, 5155.

Vlassara, H., Brownlee, M., Manogue, K.R., *et al.* (1988) Cachectin/TNF and IL-1 induced by glucose-modified proteins: role in normal tissue remodeling. *Science* **240**, 1546.

Warren, R.S., Donner, D.B., Starnes, H.F.Jr, and Brennan, M.F. (1987) Modulation of endogenous hormone action by recombinant human tumour necrosis factor. *Proceedings of the National Academy of Sciences USA* **84**, 8619.

Cytokines and pathology

8.1 Introduction

Cytokines through their diverse biological activities have the capacity to modulate cellular metabolism and behaviour, and thus maintain homeostatic mechanisms required for the well-being of the organism. On the reverse side, any imbalance in the production and action of cytokines, and/or their receptors and cellular response elements, may disturb homeostatic processes and have pathological consequences. Cytokines may thus be viewed as 'two-edged swords', benefitting the organism when their production and action(s) are regulated normally, but threatening the well-being of the organism when these are abnormal. Putative pathophysiological roles for many cytokines have already been instanced in the text of previous chapters. Some cytokines, e.g. TNFs, IL-1s, IL-6, and IFNγ, have been implicated in causing inflammatory reactions and acute-phase responses; they may also trigger tissue degradation and resorption. Release of vasoactive peptides and prostaglandins leading to hypotension and shock may be attributed to the actions of certain cytokines, e.g. TNFα. Others may be responsible for stimulating hyperplasia, e.g. TGFα in psoriatic lesions, or the deposition of aberrant fibrous layers of tissue. Many cytokines, e.g. PDGF-BB, TGFα, IL-1–6, TNF, have been linked to autocrine or paracrine stimulation of tumour cell proliferation. In contrast, lack of certain cytokine activities may predispose the host to infection by viruses, bacteria and other opportunistic parasites. Their absence may enable enhanced tumour growth and lead to some auto-immune diseases.

There are three major ways in which the role of cytokines in pathology have been studied. First, the levels of particular cytokines in certain disease situations can be measured, and if elevated, or depressed, correlated with symptoms. Second, but only in experimental animals, neutralizing antibodies to a particular cytokine can be administered, and the consequences in terms of disease susceptibility and/or progression investigated. Third, individual cytokines can be injected into animals, or patients in the course of clinical trials, and their pathological or toxic effects evaluated. In addition, associations between host genotype, e.g. human HLA class I and class II haplotypes, and cytokine production in relation to disease susceptibility may be explored. This chapter reviews the information so far accrued on cytokine levels in diseased states, together with experimental data obtained from animal and human patient studies where exogenous cytokines or their respective neutralizing antibodies have been injected. The associations and putative roles of cytokines in pathological conditions will be discussed.

8.2   Elevated cytokine levels in disease

Measurement of cytokines

Since all cytokines are extremely biologically active, often exerting their effects in picomolar amounts, they may be readily measured in specific biological assays (bioassays) in which an 'endpoint' can be objectively determined. Most current bioassays for cytokines are carried out *in vitro* using selected, sensitive human or other mammalian cell lines. The parameters most easily assessed are those associated with cell proliferation or cell growth inhibition. For example, cell lines sensitive to and dependent upon a particular cytokine, e.g. IL-2, for growth and replication are especially valuable for bioassays. In other instances, a cytokine may induce a strong antiproliferative response, or even a cytolytic outcome, in susceptible cells, particularly certain established tumour cell lines. For example, TNF is cytotoxic to murine L-929 cells, its cytotoxity being markedly enhanced by inhibitors of macromolecular synthesis, and thus cytotoxic activity can be related to cell survival; one unit of activity is usually defined as that amount of TNF which reduces cell survival by 50 per cent. IFNs represent a special class of cytokines because of their capacity to induce antiviral effects. Bioassays for IFNs are therefore designed to measure the inhibition of replication of certain cytopathogenic viruses. In all cases, since bioassays are quite variable in their sensitivity and performance, it is necessary to use reference preparations of cytokines to calibrate them and to be able to express results in a uniform, 'reference' unitage. For many many cytokines, international reference preparations (IRP) or international standards (IS) are already available and may be obtained from World Health Organization holding centres, e.g. the UK National Institute for Biological Standards and Control and the USA National Institutes of Health (Table 8.1).

Besides bioassays, the widespread development of monoclonal antibodies (moabs) against different individual cytokines has led to the construction of immunoassays for the quantification of several cytokines. Immunoassays measure immunochemical reactivity of cytokines, dependent upon epitope

Table 8.1 International, national, and interim cytokine reference preparations

Code no.	Cytokine	Status	Holding institute
69/19	IFN, human leukocyte, α	1st IRP	NIBSC, UK
Ga23–901–532	IFN, human lymphoblastoid (Namalwa)	1st IS	NIH, USA
Gxa01–901–535	IFN, human recombinant IFNα 2a	1st IS	NIH, USA
82/576	IFN, human recombinant IFNα 2b	1st IS	NIBSC, UK
83/514	IFN, human recombinant IFNα 1	1st IS	NIBSC, UK
Gb23–902–531	IFN, human fibroblast, β	2nd IS	NIH, USA
Gxb01–901–535	IFN, human recombinant IFNβ (Ser^{17})	1st IRR	NIH, USA
Gg23–901–530	IFN, human leukocyte, γ	1st IS	NIH, USA
82/587	IFN, human leukocyte, γ	1st Br. Std.	NIBSC, UK
86/632	IL-1α, human recombinant	1st IS	NIBSC, UK
86/680	IL-1β, human recombinant	1st IS	NIBSC, UK
86/504	IL-2, human lymphoblastoid (Jurkat)	1st IS	NIBSC, UK
88/680	IL-3, human recombinant	Interim	NIBSC, UK
88/656	IL-4, human recombinant	Interim	NIBSC, UK
88/514	IL-6, human recombinant	Interim	NIBSC, UK
89/520	IL-8, human recombinant	Interim	NIBSC, UK
88/502	G-CSF, human recombinant	Interim	NIBSC, UK
88/646	GM-CSF, human recombinant	Interim	NIBSC, UK
89/512	M-CSF, human recombinant	Interim	NIBSC, UK
87/650	TNFα, human recombinant	Interim	NIBSC, UK
J-PS5K01	TNFα, human recombinant	1st Japanese Std	Japan NIH, Tokyo
89/514	TGFβ1, human recombinant	Interim	NIBSC, UK

Abbreviations: IS, International Standard; IRP, International Reference Preparation; IRR, International Reference Reagent; Br. Std, British Standard; NIH, National Institute of Health; NIBSC, National Institute for Biological Standards and Control. Interim standards are also available through the Biological Response Modifiers Program, National Cancer Institute, Frederick, Md, USA.

recognition by the moabs employed, but this may be expressed in biological activity units by calibration with appropriate IRP, IS, or other relevant reference preparations. The sensitivity, specificity, and reproducibility of immunoassays may be superior to traditional bioassays in many instances, and they also have the advantage that they are quick to perform. Immuno-assays can usually be carried out in four to eight hours, whereas bioassays take at least two days to complete.

It is beyond the scope of this chapter to give details of bioassays and immunoassays for individual cytokines, and the reader is referred to other texts (see Further reading, pp. 258–62) for more information. It should however be pointed out that the precise determination of cytokine activity in either bioassays or immunoassays is not without problems. For example, it is often difficult to exclude false positives and negatives, and this applies especially to estimations of cytokine activity in biological fluids, such as serum or plasma, where the overall biochemical composition is decidedly complex. This should be borne in mind when reading the following section where several examples of raised cytokine levels are described, but where such levels may be close to the detection limit of the assays employed. Further, it is frequently the case that cytokine activity is determined only in immunoassay and cannot for reasons connected with the nature of the biological fluid, e.g. high viscosity, be determined in a bioassay. It is therefore not possible to prove that the cytokine is biologically active. Denatured or inactivated cytokine may still retain immunoreactivity and thus generate a positive signal in an immunoassay, for example. In addition, certain non-cytokine substances may non-specifically bind to moabs to generate false positives in immunoassays.

Cytokines in acute illnesses

Many viruses induce the synthesis and secretion of IFNα/β, and this has been readily demonstrated at sites of viral replication *in vivo*. For example, washings from the nasopharyngeal passages can contain high levels of IFNα/β during common cold (rhinovirus) and influenza infections. Fluids taken from cold sores (vesicles) caused by herpes simplex viruses can be shown to contain high IFN levels, a mixture of IFNα/β, and γ. In some acute viral infections, such as infuenza and measles, IFNs can be found in the circulation; they are normally undetectable in serum or plasma, meaning they are absent or present at vanishingly low concentrations, in uninfected healthy individuals. Fever-inducing viruses such as Dengue virus lead to the secretion of IFNα/β and IFNγ in large amounts at certain stages following infection. IFNα/β is usually produced at acute stages of infection, being associated with maximum virus shedding and NK cell activity, whereas IFNγ is produced at a relatively later stage, being associated with the presence of activated T-cells. Elevated IFN levels in the circulation can often be correlated with the occurrence of fever and other symptoms of general malaise, e.g. headache, achiness, chills, rigors, etc. It is virtually certain that IFNα/β, and possibly IFNγ, themselves are responsible for such symptoms, since high-dosage formulations of IFNs given to patients in clinical trials produce side-effects which are very similar to symptoms occurring during viral infections. For example, it is clear that IFNα has pyrogenic properties, and thus induces fever.

Some viruses spread beyond their initial sites of infection and may cause CNS disease. For example, mumps virus may cause meningitis, and herpes and rubella viruses, encephalitis. In these cases, IFNα/β and IFNγ can often be detected in high levels in cerebrospinal fluid (CSpF). While IFNs are generally believed to play important roles in recovery from acute viral infections in general, it is possible that their presence in high localized concentrations, as in viral encephalitis, has pathological and potentially lethal consequences. For example, mice infected with lymphocytic choriomeningitis virus (LCMV) develop a fatal encephalitis which is directly associated with T-cell-mediated pathology and the presence of very high levels of IFNγ in CSpF. Nude mice which lack T-cells do not progress to encephalitis following LCMV infection, but remain persistently infected. A similar situation applies to influenza infection in mice, although here virus replication remains mainly confined to the lungs. In infected, immunocompetent mice, activated T-cells infiltrate the lungs and release IFNγ, which can be detected in lung lavage fluids, and this is followed by a decrease in influenza virus titre in the lungs and resolution of the infection, whereas in nude mice the virus is not cleared. However, in the case of infection with respiratory syncytial virus (RESV), which is the most common cause of lower respiratory tract disease in human infants, the cell-mediated response may lead to bronchiolitis. Paradoxically, prior vaccination of children with an inactivated RESV vaccine predisposed the children to a much more severe illness, requiring hospitalization, when they were naturally re-infected with RESV. This has suggested that vaccination with RESV, while inducing virus neutralizing antibodies, also induced delayed type hypersensitivity (DH) such that cell-mediated responses were exaggerated on re-infection. Increased release of IFNs and other cytokines during these responses possibly contribute to the severer symptoms manifested in RESV-vaccinated children. Similar DH reactions were found for an early inactivated measles vaccine. Moreover, it is suggested that cell-mediated mechanisms underlie the severe complications, including haemorrhagic manifestations and shock, associated with secondary dengue virus infection. The following hypothetical scheme may explain this: primary dengue infection, which takes place in monocytes, leads to antibody formation and sensitized T-lymphocytes. Secondary infection with a different Dengue virus serotype causes rapid T-cell activation in cross-reactive T-cells and high IFNγ secretion resulting in monocyte- and granulocyte-priming, enhanced Ig-FcR expression and binding of dengue-specific antibodies. These 'armed' cells respond on contact with viral antigens by releasing large quantities of inflammatory and vasoactive mediators, hydrolytic enzymes and cytokines. In addition, the IFNγ-augmented Ig-FcR expression in monocytes may aid reinfection of such monocytes by dengue virus–antibody complexes.

In most instances, while the presence of IFNs is clearly associated with acute viral or other infections, it is not possible to ascertain how much they contribute either to protective or pathological effects. Nevertheless, some insights into the 'biological' roles of IFNs *in vivo* have been gained by the use of neutralizing anti-IFN antibodies. For example, as has been mentioned previously, injected neutralizing antibodies to MuIFNα/β predispose mice to more severe and often lethal disease when they are subsequently infected with various viruses, e.g. encephalomyocarditis virus (EMCV). On the other hand, the repeated administration of MuIFNα/β to mice has been shown to reduce the mortality of infections due to EMCV. However, the mouse 'model' of infection and IFN/anti-IFN treatment is not without defects, e.g. the routes of application of virus and IFN/anti-IFN are not completely natural, and thus such results still require cautious interpretation. The availability of anti-IFNγ and its use in a number of studies in mouse models of human disease is begining to yield intriguing results, but since these relate more to inflammation and autoimmune reactions they will be discussed in the next section.

While elevated levels of IFNs often accompany viral infections, they may also be found in the sera of patients and animals with bacterial infections. However, more emphasis and interest has recently been placed on the finding that raised serum levels of TNFα, IL-1, and IL-6 are present during infection with particular types of bacteria and parasites. Bacteria causing meningitis and septicaemia appear to induce TNFα secretion, and this is probably through interaction of macrophages with the LPS components of the cell walls of such Gram-negative bacteria. Indeed, it is clear that injection of isolated bacterial endotoxins (LPS), for example from E.coli, into rabbits or human volunteers leads to a rapid induction of TNFα release into the bloodstream. Levels of a few hundred to a few thousand picograms of TNFα per millilitre of serum have been reported in cases of meningococcal meningitis and Gram-negative septicaemia, and in volunteers receiving LPS; in rabbits the levels can be much higher. In both meningitis and sepsis there may be severe complications, including hypotension, fever, metabolic acidosis, disseminated intravascular coagulation, respiratory failure, and these sometimes lead to fatal consequences. That TNFα alone, or in combination with other inflammatory cytokines, is responsible for mediating such pathophysiological changes and injurious effects, e.g. bowel lesions and kidney necrosis, is being intensively investigated.

The hypothesis that TNFα can trigger pathological effects is supported by a number of recent findings. Besides TNFα being found in serum following injection of a lethal dose of LPS, infusion of TNFα into experimental animals produces effects similar to those manifested in Gram-negative sepsis. Furthermore, administration of a neutralizing monoclonal antibody against human TNFα to baboons, prior to a lethal dose of E.coli bacteria, has been found to prevent their deaths. In addition, the C3H HeJ strain of mice, which are genetically defective in TNFα production, are resistant to doses of LPS which are lethal in other strains. It is possible that prostaglandins and PAF are the direct mediators of cellular responses triggered by TNFα during endotoxaemia and shock, since inhibitors of the cyclooxgenase pathway, such as indomethacin or ibuprofen, prevent the injurious manifestations and potentially lethal outcome. IL-1, which has similar biological activities to TNFα, has also been shown to induce a shock-like state in rabbits. Combination of LPS and TNFα or IL-1 and TNFα produce more potent effects than any agent used alone. In fact, these cytokines or LPS may be used to induce cellular (delayed) hypersensitivity reactions in laboratory animals. For instance, if TNFα or IL-1 or LPS is injected intradermally and then the animals injected intravenously with LPS 18–24 hours later, they rapidly develop local and/or generalized haemorrhagic reactions. This is known as the Schwartzmann phenomenom or reaction. Interestingly, monoclonal antibodies to MuIFNγ have been shown to prevent an LPS-induced Schwartzmann reaction in mice, suggesting that IFNγ has an important role in this kind of delayed hypersensitivity response. Presumably, IFNγ activates macrophages to become more responsive to LPS in such situations, with resultant high levels of secretion of TNFα and subsequently of PAF, prostaglandins, and ROI.

It is probable, though frequently difficult to establish unequivocally, that TNFα is produced in response to Gram-positive bacteria and other microorganisms. Levels in blood are difficult to estimate generally, partly because of the very short half-life of TNFα and partly because of the presence of substances in serum and plasma that 'interfere' in the bio- and immunoassays used to detect TNF. Nor is it always clear how these other micro-organisms, which lack LPS, induce TNFα. Nevertheless, *Listeria monocytogenes*, a Gram-positive bacterium, induces serum levels of MuTNFα upon subcutaneous infection of mice. Neutralizing antibody against MuTNFα has been shown to convert an ongoing sublethal *Listeria* infection into a lethal one. This latter finding strongly suggests that TNFα normally has a protective function against infection with such bacteria. In contrast, *Listeria* injected intracerebrally into mice is associated with the production of very high levels of TNFα in CSF and the development of a fatal meningitis. (TNFα has also been detected in CSF of patients with pneumococcal or meningococcal meningitis, but not in any case of viral meningitis.) *Staphylococcus aureus*, another Gram-positive organism, which has been associated with 'toxic shock syndrome', a result of surgical wound infection or, infrequently, the use of a type of high-absorbency tampon during menstruation, also stimulates TNFα production. The exotoxin, toxic shock syndrome toxin 1 (TSST-1), produced by *S.aureus* is probably the inducer of TNFα in monocytes/macrophages. Toxic shock syndrome is characterized by high fever, hypotension, rashes, and other symptoms similar to those found for Gram-negative septicaemia, and it would appear possible that TNFα is a prime mediator of this condition. *S.aureus* and similar bacteria may also, through TNFα and IL-1 release and subsequent activation of cyclooxygenase pathways, be responsible for 'septic lung' and acute respiratory distress syndrome (ARDS).

Other infectious diseases where raised serum levels of TNFα have been reported include malarial and leishmanial parasitic infections. Malarial parasites may also induce TNFα production by macrophages *in vitro*. In a murine model, *Plasmodium berghei* induction of cerebral malaria, often a severe complication of human *Plasmodium falciparum* infection, was correlated with high circulating levels of TNFα. Polyclonal anti-TNFα antibodies were found to protect infected mice against development of cerebral malaria, thus implicating TNFα as playing an important role in the pathogenesis of this complication. Subsequently, it has been found that other anticytokine antibodies prevent cerebral malaria. For example, anti-IFNγ inhibited TNFα increase, as did a combination of anti-IL-3 and anti-GM-CSF; both treatments prevented cerebral malaria development. Such results suggest that IFNγ, which activates macrophages, and IL-3 and GM-CSF, which increase the production of monocytes/macrophages from haemopoietic precursors, are part of a cytokine cascade culminating in TNFα production involved in the pathogenesis of cerebral malaria.

In some infections, where raised serum levels of TNFα are not directly demonstrable, it may be possible to show that either components of the infectious agents stimulate TNFα production in PBMC or isolated macrophage cultures, or PBMC derived from infected individuals respond to LPS stimulation *in vitro* by increased TNFα production compared with those from healthy volunteers. For example, the purified lipoarabino-mannan, a major component of mycobacterial cell walls, has been shown to induce TNFα production by macrophages, comparable to that induced by LPS. Tuberculosis, caused by *Mycobacterium tuberculosis*, is often characterized by fever, weight loss, raised levels of acute-phase reactants, and necrotic lesions, and thus it is possible TNFα activity is involved since similar characteristics are manifested when TNFα is injected into laboratory animals. Again IFNγ may act as a proximal mediator for enhanced TNFα production by macrophages. In fulminant hepatic failure (FHF), which is caused by bacterial or fungal infections or possibly leakage of gut bacteria into the liver, patients' PBMC can be demonstrated to produce more TNFα and IL-1 following LPS-stimulation than control PBMC from healthy individuals, suggesting that TNFα and/or IL-1 might be involved in causing the massive liver necrosis and endotoxic shock-like symptoms of FHF. (FHF is a severe complication of prior chronic infections with hepatitis viruses, or paracetamol overdoses as in cases of attempted suicide.)

IL-6 is another cytokine produced by activated macrophages that might be expected to mediate inflammatory reactions, e.g. acute-phase protein release from the liver, and possibly therefore be involved in the pathogenesis of certain diseases. For instance, high levels of IL-6 have been found in the CSF of mice and patients with acute viral and bacterial meningitis, although whether these have a protective or pathophysiological role remains to be determined. Further, patients undergoing major bowel surgery may be shown to have raised serum IL-6 levels following their operation. This probably reflects release of bowel bacteria into the bloodstream which can then trigger IL-6 secretion, and presumably other cytokines, from circulating monocytes. Moreover, injection of LPS has been shown to elicit increased circulating IL-6 in healthy volunteers. Plasma IL-6 can synergize with TNFα and/or IL-1 in inducing the acute-phase reponse, and this may cause postoperative complications.

Cytokines in chronic illnesses

The borderline between acute and chronic illnesses is often blurred, and instances of acute phases or 'exacerbations' of chronic disease are numerous. For example, the complications associated with mycobacterial and parasitic diseases probably represent acute phases during disease progression. However, some illnesses do develop rather slowly and may be said to be chronic; examples are leprosy, multiple scelerosis, arthritis, and cancer. In some cases of chronic disease it is suspected that deficiencies in the cytokine network, particularly those activating the immune system, underlie the inability of the host to resolve the disease. In other cases, the chronic nature of a disease may be associated with long-term overproduction of certain cytokines and the resultant immunopathological effects. In all cases, there may be periods when the disease is inactive or latent, interspersed with periods of exacerbation and disease progression. Obviously, there are complex host mechanisms involved that both control the level of disease activity and potentially mediate pathology.

Despite the strong association of many cytokines with the cellular proliferative response, their 'true' roles in tumour progression and the pathological features of cancer remain difficult to ascertain. For the majority of cancers, no circulating levels of cytokines have been detected. This may not mean that they are entirely absent, however. The continuous low-level secretion of a particular cytokine may be insufficient to raise blood levels, and this probably is a reflection of the relatively short half-lives of cytokines (2–10 minutes) in the circulation. Nevertheless, there are a growing number of reports of cytokines being detected in cancer patients. One of the pathological signs of terminal cancer is weight loss or cachexia. TNFα, alternatively known as cachectin, has been shown to suppress lipid synthesis in fat cells and therefore has been suggested to cause weight loss. While injection of TNFα into experimental animals has been demonstrated to induce weight loss, this may be more a result of loss of appetite than a metabolic effect. However, strong suggestive evidence that TNFα does induce weight loss and progressive wasting has been obtained by constructing tumour cells with a inserted, constitutively expressed, TNFα gene and injecting these into nude mice. It was found that mice bearing tumours with the integrated TNFα gene developed progressive wasting and died more quickly than mice bearing tumours of the parental cell line without the TNFα gene. Nevertheless, that TNFα causes the 'cancer-associated cachexia' syndrome in some cancer patients remains controversial, and reports of circulating TNFα equally so. In all instances so far recorded, TNFα has been estimated in immunoassays only, and thus it is not clear whether this TNFα retains biological activity. The presence of immunoreactive TNFα, whether or not it is biologically active, may however suggest its continuous overproduction either by tumour-infiltrating macrophages and lymphocytes or by the tumour cells themselves in certain instances. The finding that PBMC from cancer patients with solid tumours release biologically active TNFα spontaneously (i.e. without addition of inducers) is supportive of this suggestion. Raised serum levels of immunoreactive TNFα have also been reported for some parasitic diseases, e.g. malaria, where there is also frequently an associated cachexia.

Reports of cytokines, other than TNFα, being present in raised amounts in the circulation of cancer patients are still relatively few. There is one report of IFNγ being found in the sera of patients with nasopharyngeal carcinoma, a cancer associated with Epstein–Barr virus, but there was no evidence for a pathogenic role of IFNγ in this disease. There are other unconfirmed reports of circulating IFNγ in haematological malignancies, and high production of IL-6 in bone marrow of multiple myeloma patients is also recorded. In contrast to this sparse literature, there are numerous reports on the presence and putative pathogenic roles of cytokines, particularly IFNs and TNFs, during auto-immune disease progression. Auto-immune diseases result usually from a breakdown in immunological tolerance to self-antigens and this can arise through either abnormal T_H-cell activity or lack of T-suppressor (T_S) cells, responsible for down-regulating immune responses. In the majority of auto-immune diseases the initial causative agent is unknown, although it is widely believed that viruses, bacteria, or mycoplasma, often infecting individuals years prior to the onset of disease, are responsible for lymphocyte sensitization to self-antigens. That certain auto-immune diseases, e.g. diabetes, may be induced by viruses, such as EMCV or Coxsackie virus B4, provides supportive evidence of the link between infection and initiation of auto-immune disease. Further, the involvement of IFNs in viral and microbial infections raises the possibility of associations between IFN activities and characteristics of auto-immune disease.

Systemic lupus erythematosus (SLE) is a complex autoimmune disease outwardly characterized by a bright red facial rash. SLE patients have circulating auto-antibodies to a number of self-proteins (e.g. IFNs) and nucleic acid (DNA), and characteristically there are kidney deposits of immune complexes as well as tubuloreticular or lupus inclusions in lymphocytes and certain other cell types. A further distinctive feature is the presence of a circulating acid-labile IFN, which antigenically appears to be of the IFNα type. This is unusual since most IFNα subtypes are described as being acid-stable, i.e. resistant to pH2 inactivation. The intrinsic acid-lability of IFNα in SLE has recently been disputed. The origin of 'acid-labile' IFNα in SLE is not known. Normally, IFNα production is suggestive of an ongoing viral infection, but so far no evidence of virus involvement has been obtained in SLE patients. The role of 'acid-labile' IFNα in SLE also remains uncertain. However, it is speculated that it could contribute to the pathogenesis of this auto-immune disease by

1   stimulating B-cell production of auto-antibodies,
2   increasing MHC expression and thus stimulating autoreactive T- and B-cells, and
3   interfering with immunological processes, e.g. disrupting T-cell functions.

Certain strains of inbred mice, e.g. New Zealand black (NZB), spontaneously develop an auto-immune disease which has several features, such as
auto-antibodies and glomerulonephritis, in common with those observed in
SLE. Although circulating levels of MuIFNα/β have not so far been detected,
injection of exogenous MuIFNα/β or MuIFNγ accelerates the onset of the
'SLE-like' disease in NZB mice. Moreover, treatment with neutralizing
anti-MuIFNγ antibodies has been found to retard disease progression and to
prolong survival. These findings suggest that IFNs have a pathogenic role in
auto-immune disease of NZB mice, possibly for the reasons speculated to
underlie the pathogenesis of SLE given above. The pathogenesis of lupus
nephritis in mice may also be correlated to the presence of other cytokines,
besides IFNs. For instance, increased TNFα and IL-1β gene expression has
been demonstrated in the kidneys of mice with lupus nephritis. In a rat
model, kidney glomerular injury caused by injections of antiglomerular
basement membrane (GBM) antibodies was found to be considerably increased by subsequent injection of low (sub-toxic) doses of TNFα, and
inhibited by neutralizing antibodies against TNFα. Therefore, TNFα is implicated as a mediator of glomerular damage, and may be envisaged to play a
similar pathogenic role in lupus nephritis in mice and SLE in humans. Again,
the induction of a cytokine cascade, as in experimental cerebral malaria,
involving T-lymphocyte IFNγ and macrophage TNFα may have relevance to
this class of autoimmune diseases.

   Insulin-dependent diabetes mellitus (IDDM) is a relatively common disease that appears to have a cell-mediated, auto-immune element. Following
onset, the pancreatic β-islet cells, which produce insulin, are destroyed with
the result that glucose uptake fails. It appears probable that both auto-
antibodies and CTL are involved in the lysis of β-cells. Raised levels of serum
IFNα have also been found in diabetics, especially soon after onset, and
immunoreactive IFNα has been demonstrated in immunohistochemically
stained sections of pancreatic tissue. The latter was closely correlated with
hyperexpression of MHC class I antigen expression in β-islet cells. The
presence of IFNα in the pancreas is suggestive of viral infection, but in most
cases the aetiology of IDDM is unknown. Nevertheless, it is clear that certain
viruses, e.g. mumps, rubella, Coxsackie B viruses, are capable of inducing
pancreatic disease and necrosis of endocrine cells, but not of β-cells, with
associated IFN production, and it is suspected that such viruses may provide
the initial trigger, possibly by viral protein mimicry of cell surface proteins,
for localized autoimmune responses. It is also known that β-cell MHC class II
antigen expression is increased following disease onset, and this is indicative
of T-cell recognition of β-cell surface molecules and secretion of IFNγ. The
latter may activate monocytes with ensuing synthesis of TNFα and IL-1β, and
it has been shown that IL-1β, but not IFNγ or TNFα, is cytotoxic to isolated
β-cells of rat or human origin. Thus, β-cells may be damaged by a combination of directly cytotoxic cytokines, autoreactive CTL, and cytokine-activated
ADCC by mononuclear phagocytes in the presence of auto-antibodies.

   Multiple sclerosis (MS) is another tissue-restricted, autoimmune disease of unknown aetiology, although again certain viruses, e.g. measles and retro-viruses, have been proposed as the initial causative agents. MS, which has a highly variable course, is a debilitating disease affecting limb movement and coordination that usually afflicts young adults, and is characterized by demyelination of white matter in the nervous system. This feature may be mimicked in Lewis rats by injecting myelin basic protein (MBP) in complete Freund's adjuvant, which induces a condition known as acute experimental auto-immune encephalomyelitis (EAE). The clinical symptoms of EAE, which include hind-limb paralysis, are manifested about 10–14 days following injection of MBP. The rats recover completely by day 18. It appears probable that IFNγ plays a pivotal role in the progression of EAE by inducing MHC class II antigen expression in rat astrocytes, thereby increasing presentation of tissue-specific antigens (e.g. MBP) to autoreactive T-lymphocytes. Recovery from EAE may result from inhibition of IFNγ production in 'effector' T-lymphocytes by suppressor T-cells with resultant down-regulation of MHC class II molecules and decreased self-antigen presentation. However, in MS there appears to be defective IFNγ synthesis in PBMC in response to mitogenic stimulation. Nevertheless, expression of MHC class I and class II antigens on astrocytes in brains from patients with MS has been observed and it has been suggested that the functionality of PBMC may be of little relevance to MS lesions which are primarily found in the brain. Indeed, there is a preliminary report of a perhaps more revelant imbalance of T_H subsets in the CSpF of MS patients such that IFNγ/IL-2 secreting T_{H1} subset is predominant, with the suggestion that IFNγ produced by these cells may enhance self-antigen presentation by astrocytes and Schwann cells. IFNγ has been shown to increase MHC class II antigen expression in astrocytes and Schwann cells *in vitro*, and its activity may be augmented when combined with TNFα. Furthermore, exacerbations of MS have been associated with IFNγ therapy in clinical trials. In contrast, intrathecal injection of IFNβ has led in some MS patients to a lessening of the frequency of exacerbations. How IFNβ acts in MS — whether by inducing immunosuppressive mechanisms, by antagonizing IFNγ induction of MHC class II, or by inhibiting latent virus reactivations — is quite unknown.

The biological activities of IL-1 and TNFα, including bone and cartilage resorption, induction of prostaglandins and collagenase from synoviocytes, and polymorphonuclear cell activation, appear to be directly relevant to the establishment of chronic inflammatory processes in arthritic diseases. Rheumatoid arthritis is a relatively common condition in older people, in which the synovial linings of joints between bones are chronically inflamed leading to tissue erosion and permanent damage. Such joints are often painfully swollen and the fluid they contain, the synovial fluid, is composed of a mixture of mucopolysaccharides and proteins. Leukocytes are also present and thus the synovial fluid has been examined for the presence of inflammatory mediators. IL-1 has been found in a high proportion of synovial fluids both from rheumatoid arthritis patients and from patients with other arthritic diseases. TNFα has also been found in synovial rheumatoid arthritis patients, but only in about 50 per cent of cases. In contrast, IFNα and IFNγ, which possibly could increase self-antigen expression through their effects on MHC antigen expression, appear to be present in very few synovial fluids. Despite the presence of IL-1 and TNFα in synovial fluids from rheumatoid arthritis patients, it has been very difficult to correlate disease progression and exacerbations with these cytokines. However, given the short half-lives of cytokines, sampling times may be criticial. In addition, the levels of inhibitors to IL-1 and TNF, which are also probably present in synovial fluids, may have a crucial bearing on the development of inflammation. A recent report suggests that serum levels of IL-1β correlate better with exacerbations than synovial fluid IL-1 levels.

Predisposition to many, if not all, auto-immune diseases is probably associated with the presence of certain 'susceptibility' genes. The identity of these latter is unknown, but may be reflected in the variable MHC gene locus of the human population. Certain diseases appear to be associated with particular HLA haplotypes, e.g. ankylosing spondylitis, a rheumatic disease, is associated with HLA-B27, an MHC class I antigen. There are also auto-immune disease associations with MHC class II molecules; for example, HLA-DR3 and HLA-DR4 have been linked to IDDM. In addition, the inclusion of TNFα and TNFβ genes within the MHC gene locus on chromosome 6 has suggested that their expression may be partly controlled by other genes within this complex. This may be important for the pathogenesis of some auto-immune diseases. In fact, such a connection has been made between TNFα production and lupus nephritis, an autoimmune disease that is strongly associated with MHC class II alleles in human and rodents, in an animal model system. Coeliac disease, a gluten inducible 'auto-immune' enteropathy in which there is flattening of the villi in the small bowel mucosa, also has a strong association with the HLA class II series of antigens, and there is preliminary evidence that TNFβ synthesis in the jejunum may contribute to the pathogenesis of the disease, e.g. in autodestruction of small bowel enterocytes leading to villous atrophy. (Gluten is known to be the important aetiological agent in coeliac disease since its exclusion from the diet leads to clinical remission and morphological improvement.)

There are a variety of other chronic inflammatory or auto-immune diseases in which cytokines have been implicated as playing pathogenic roles, and some examples are given in Table 8.2. In addition, the activity of the immune system and the biological activities of its mediators are involved in the rejection episodes following bone marrow, kidney, or heart allograft transplantation. Both TNFα and IFNγ, which may appear in detectable amounts in the circulation at certain stages following the transplantation operation, have been suggested to play pivotal roles in the rejection process. IL-6 has been found in the serum and urine of kidney transplant recipients. Moreover, elevated production of TNFα appears to be responsible for the skin and gut lesions of the acute phase of graft-versus-host disease (GVHD), a potentially lethal disease resulting from the introduction of allogeneic T-lymphocytes from a donor into an immunoincompetent host, as would occur for example

Table 8.2 Cytokines and disease associations

Disease	Cytokine	Putative pathogenic roles
Behçet's disease — eye lesions	Circulating acid labile IFNα/ IFNγ	Increased MHC class I/class II expression. Increased auto-antibody production
Graves' ophthalmopathy — immunological cytotoxicity against eye-muscle cells	IFNγ	Increased MHC class II expression. Increased ADCC killing of eye muscle cells
Sjögren's syndrome — chronic inflammatory disease of exocrine glands	Endogenous IFNα	Down-regulation of IFNα receptors in NK cells with resulting loss of NK cell activity
Kawasaki syndrome — panvasculitis with endothelial necrosis, plus prolonged fever, mucosal inflammation and rash	IFNγ, TNFα, IL-1	All induce target antigens in endothelial cells with resultant complement mediated lysis by circulating auto-antibodies
Aplastic anaemia — primary disorder of haemopoietic system	IFNγ, TNFα, (IFNα)	Inhibition of haemopoietic precursor proliferation
Pulmonary sarcoidosis — granulomatous inflammatory disease of lungs with cough, fever, and weight loss	TNFα	Increased IL-1 and inflammatory mediators by alveolar macrophages

in bone marrow allograft transplantation in an X-irradiated patient. In a mouse model of GVHD, anti-TNFα antibodies prevented the development of skin and gut lesions during the acute phase and markedly reduced overall mortality, strongly suggesting that TNFα is a pathogenic agent in GVHD.

Still other chronic diseases may be the result of primary immunodeficiencies, which can be inherited, congenital, or acquired. Affected individuals have disorders of humoral or cell-mediated immunity, and are markedly more susceptible to microbial infections than normals. Functional depression of T-lymphocytes is a common feature in several immunodeficiency diseases, e.g. ataxia-telangectasia and Wiskott–Aldrich syndrome, and it is clear that production of immunoregulatory cytokines such as IL-2 and IFNγ is severely affected, i.e. it is defective. On the other hand, IFNα production appears to be normal and in some cases raised levels have been found. However, the responses of certain leukocyte classes in immunodeficiency diseases may be defective, e.g. NK cells from severe combined immunodeficiency disease (SCID) patients have been shown to be unresponsive to IFNα, which usually activates the cytotoxic functions of NK cells. Such 'defectiveness' may arise through the lack of maturation factors, including cytokines, for leukocytes.

Much recent scientific and clinical attention has been focused on the epidemic of AIDS caused by infection with HIV. Many features of disease progression in AIDS are similar to those observed in primary immuno-deficiencies, e.g. disorders of humoral and cell-mediated immunity and defective T-cell functions. The latter correlates well with the progressive loss of the T_H lymphocyte subset, a well-characterized finding in AIDS patients. Several other immune defects, have also been reported in AIDS. They include: decreased NK cell activity, decreased cell-mediated cytotoxicity to certain virally infected cells, decreased B-cell proliferation to specific antigens but increased spontaneous B-cell proliferation and polyclonal increase in Ig, and decreased monocyte/macrophage functions. Impaired T-cell production of IFNγ, IL-2, other interleukins and CSFs probably in part accounts for these aberrant leukocyte functions. Production of other cytokines, e.g. IFNα from PBMC derived from AIDS patients in response to viral inducers *in vitro*, may also be markedly depressed. However, in otherwise symptomless HIV-infected individuals, the appearance of acid-labile IFNα in the circulation is prognostic of progression to ARC (AIDS-related complex) and to 'full-blown' AIDS. This acid-labile IFNα bears a striking resemblance to that found in SLE patients, and may have, as has been suggested for autoimmune diseases of the SLE-type, a pathogenic role. Further, it is widely believed that, while HIV-1 is directly cytopathic to T_H lymphocytes, the eventual depletion of the T_H subset has more to do with 'auto-immune' mechanisms. It has been proposed that HIV triggers a cell-mediated immunopathology involving either HIV-specific CTL or monocyte/neutrophil-mediated ADCC where HIV-infected T_H cells are specifically killed. Alternatively, HIV infection may generate auto-antibodies leading to the complement-mediated lysis of T_H cells. The presence of auto-antibodies may be relevant to the neurological complications, e.g. dementia, often accompanying other clinical symptoms of AIDS, such as opportunistic infections or Kaposi's sarcoma. In addition to the prognostic value of acid-labile IFNα for progression to AIDs, its presence in high levels in AIDS patients with Kaposi's sarcoma signified a poorer prognosis for progressive disease than if it were present in low levels. Symptoms such as fever, malaise, fatigue, and neutropenia commonly found in AIDS patients may be attributable to circulating high levels of acid-labile IFNα, as these are the same clinical features found following exogenous IFNα administration in cancer patients.

In summary, imbalances in the production and action of cytokines, particularly those affecting immunoregulation, resulting from the stimulation of autoreactive leukocytes or the depletion/absence of immunocompetent cells, can have profound influences on acute and chronic inflammation, may enhance autoimmune processes and ultimately may contribute to the pathogenesis of numerous diseases. Far from always having a protective or beneficial role, the presence of circulating or localized cytokines in high levels is often predictive of progressive disease in which they themselves may have a pathogenic role.

Further reading

Aderka, D., Fisher, S., Levo, Y., et al. (1985) Cachectin/tumour necrosis factor production by cancer patients. *The Lancet* **ii**, 1190.

Bachwich, P.R., Lynch, J.P., Larrick, J., et al. (1986) Tumour necrosis factor production by human sarcoid alveolar macrophages. *American Journal of Pathology* **125**, 421.

Balkwill, F., Osborne, R., Burke, F., et al. (1987) Evidence for tumour necrosis factor/cachectin production in cancer. *The Lancet* **ii**, 1229.

Barnes, D. and Sirbasku, D.A. (eds) (1987) *Peptide Growth Factors Parts I & II Methods in Enzymology* **146, 147**. Academic Press, San Diego.

Bate, C.A.W., Taverne, J., and Playfair, J.H.L. (1988) Malarial parasites induce TNF production by macrophages. *Immunology* **64**, 227.

Beck, J., Rondot, P., Catinot, L., et al. (1988) Increased production of interferon gamma and tumour necrosis factor precedes clinical manifestations in multiple sclerosis: do cytokines trigger off exacerbations? *Acta Neurologica Scandinavica* **78**, 318.

Bendtzen, K., Mandrup-Poulsen, T., Nerup, J., et al. (1986) Cytotoxicity of human pl7 interleukin-1 for pancreatic islets of Langerhans. *Science* **232**, 1545.

Bertani, T., Abbate, M., and Zoja, C. (1989) Tumour necrosis factor induces glomerular damage in the rabbit. *American Journal of Pathology* **134**, 419.

Billiau, A., Heremans, H., Vandekerchkhove, F., and Diller, C. (1987) Anti-interferon-gamma protects mice against the generalized Schwartzmann reaction. *European Journal of Immunology* **17**, 185.

Boswell, J.M., Yui, M.A., Burt, D.W., and Kelley, V.E. (1989) Increased tumour necrosis factor and IL-lbeta gene expression in the kidneys of mice with lupus nephritis. *Journal of Immunology* **141**, 3050.

Clemens, M.J., Morris, A.G., and Gearing, A.J.H. (eds) (1987) *Lymphokines and Interferons: A Practical Approach*. IRL Press, Oxford.

De Maeyer, E. and De Maeyer-Guignard, J. (1988) *Interferons and Other Regulatory Cytokines*. Wiley, New York. Chapter 16, p.380.

DiGiovine, F.S., Meager, A., Leung, H., and Duff, G.W. (1988) Immunoreactive tumour necrosis factor alpha and biological inhibitor(s) in synovial fluids from rheumatic patients. *International Journal of Immunopathology and Pharmacology* **1**, 17.

Di Sabato, G., Langone, J.J., and Van Vunakis, H. (eds) (1985) *Effectors and Mediators of Lymphoid Cell Functions. Methods in Enzymology* **116**, Academic Press, San Diego.

Eastgate, J.A., Symons, J.A., Wood, N.C., et al. (1988) Correlation of plasma interleukin-1 levels with disease activity in rheumatoid arthritis. *The Lancet* **ii**, 706.

Fast, D.J., Schlievert, P.M., and Nelson, R.D. (1988) Nonpurulent response to toxic shock syndrome toxin 1-producing *Staphylococcus aureus*: relationship to toxin-stimulated production of tumour necrosis factor. *Journal of Immunology* **140**, 949.

Fong, Y., Moldawer, L.L., Marano, M., et al. (1989) Endotoxemia elicits increased circulating IL-6 in man. *Journal of Immunology* **142**, 2321.

Foulis, A.K., Farquharson, M.A., and Meager, A. (1987) Immunoreactive alpha-interferon in insulin-secreting beta cells in type 1 diabetes mellitus. *The Lancet* **ii**, 1423.

Frei, K., Leist, T.P., Meager, A., *et al.* (1988) Production of B cell stimulatory factor-2 and interferon gamma in the central nervous system during viral meningitis and encephalitis. *Journal of Experimental Medicine* **168**, 449.

Gearing, A.J.H., and Hennessen, W. (eds.) *Cytokines: Laboratory and Clinical Evaluation* (1988) Developments in Biological Standardization **69** IABS Symposium, Karger, Basel.

Girardin, E., Grau, G.E., Dayer, J-M., *et al.* (1988) Tumour necrosis factor and interleukin-1 in the serum of children with severe infectious purpura. *New England Journal of Medicine* **319**, 397.

Grau, G.E., Fajardo, L.F., Piguet, P-F., *et al.* (1987) Tumour necrosis factor (cachectin) as an essential mediator in murine cerebral malaria. *Science* **237**, 1210.

Grau, G.E., Kindler, V., Piguet, P.-F., *et al.* (1988) Prevention of experimental cerebral malaria by anticytokine antibodies. *Journal of Experimental Medicine* **168**, 1499.

Havell, E.A. (1987) Production of tumour necrosis factor during murine listeriosis. *Journal of Immunology* **139**, 4225.

Hinterberger, W., Adolf, G., Aichinger, G., *et al.* (1988) Further evidence for lymphokine overproduction in severe aplastic anemia. *Blood* **72**, 266.

Hiromatsu, Y., Fukazawa, H., How, J., and Well, J.R. (1987) Antibody-dependent cell-mediated cytotoxicity against human eye muscle cells and orbital fibroblasts in Graves' ophthalmopathy — roles of class II MHC antigen expression and gamma-interferon action of effector and target cells. *Clinical and Experimental Immunology* **70**, 593.

Hopkins, S.J. and Meager, A. (1988) Cytokines in synovial fluid II. The presence of tumour necrosis factor and interferon. *Clinical and Experimental Immunology* **73**, 88.

Houssiau, F.A., Bukasa, K., Sindic, C.J.M., *et al.* (1988) Elevated levels of the 26K human hybridoma growth factor (interleukin 6) in cerebrospinal fluid of patients with acute infection of the central nervous system. *Clinical and Experimental Immunology* **71**, 320.

Jacob, C.O. and McDevitt, H.O. (1988) Tumour necrosis factor-alpha in murine autoimmune 'lupus' nephritis. *Nature* **331**, 356.

Jacob, C.O., Van der Meide, P.H., and McDevitt, H.O. (1987) *In vivo* treatment of (NZB × NZW) F_1 lupus-like nephritis with monoclonal antibody to gamma interferon. *Journal of Experimental Medicine* **166**, 798.

Jacobs, L., Salazar, A.M., Herdon, R., *et al.* (1987) Intrathecally administered natural human fibroblast interferon reduces exacerbations of multiple sclerosis: results of a multicenter, double-blinded study. *Archives of Neurology* **44**, 589.

Karzon, D.T. (1983) The immune basis for hypersensitivity to viral vaccines, in *Human Immunity to Viruses* (Ennis, F.A., ed.) Academic Press, New York, p.111.

Kingston, A.E., Bergsteinsdottir, K., Jessen, K.R., *et al.* (1989) Schwann cells co-cultured with stimulated T cells and antigen express major histocompatibility complex (MHC) class II determinants without interferon-gamma pretreatment: synergistic effects of interferon-gamma and tumour necrosis factor on MHC class II induction. *European Journal of Immunology* **19**, 177.

Klein, B., Zhang, X-G., Jourdan, M., *et al.* (1989) Paracrine rather than autocrine regulation of myeloma-cell growth and differentiation by interleukin-6. *Blood* **73**, 517.

Koshino, Y., Ryan, J., Cashman, S.J., *et al.* (1989) Direct evidence that tumour necrosis factor modulates antibody-mediated glomerular injury in rats. In preparation.

Kurane, I. and Ennis, F.A. (1988) Production of IFN alpha by Dengue virus-infected human monocytes. *Journal of General Virology* **69**, 445.

Kurane, I., Innis, B.L., Nisalak, A., *et al.* (1989) Human T cell responses to Dengue virus antigens: proliferative responses and IFN gamma production. *Journal of Clinical Investigation* **83**, 506.

Lakhdar, M., Oueslati, R., Ellouze, R., *et al.* (1989) High interferon titre and defective NK-cell activity in the circulation of nasopharyngeal carcinoma patients. *International Journal of Cancer* **43**, 543.

Leist, T.P., Frei, K., Kam-Hansen, S., *et al.* (1988) Tumour necrosis factor alpha in cerebrospinal fluid during bacterial, but not viral, meningitis. *Journal of Experimental Medicine* **167**, 1743.

Leung, D.Y.M., Geha, R.S., Newburger, J.W., *et al.* (1986) Two monokines, interleukin 1 and tumour necrosis factor, render cultured vascular endothelial cells susceptible to lysis by antibodies circulating during Kawasaki syndrome. *Journal of Experimental Medicine* **164**, 1958.

Levin, S. and Hahn, T. (1981) Evaluation of the human interferon system in viral disease. *Clinical and Experimental Immunology* **46**, 475.

McDonald, A.H. and Swanborg, R.H. (1988) Antigen-specific inhibition of immune interferon production by suppressor cells of autoimmune encephalomyelitis. *Journal of Immunology* **140**, 1132.

Malkovsky, M., Sondel, P.M., Strober, W., and Dalgleish, A.G. (1988) The interleukins in acquired disease. *Clinical and Experimental Immunology* **74**, 151.

Mathison, J.C., Wolfson, E., and Ulevitch, R.J. (1988) Participation of tumour necrosis factor in the mediation of gram negative bacterial lipopolysaccharide-induced injury in rabbits. *Journal of Clinical Investigation* **81**, 1925.

Meager, A., Leung, H., and Woolley, J. (1989) Assays for tumour necrosis factor and related cytokines. *Journal of Immunological Methods* **116**, 1.

Miyazu, M., Morishima, T., Hanada, N., *et al.* (1985) Types of interferons detected in cerebrospinal fluid from patients with viral infections of the central nervous systems. *Journal of Infectious Diseases* **152**, 1098.

Moreno, C., Taverne, J., Mehlert, A., *et al.* (1989) Lipoarabinomannan from *Mycobacterium tuberculosis* induces the proliferation of tumour necrosis factor from human and murine macrophages. *Clinical and Experimental Immunology* **76**, 240.

Movat, H.Z., Burrowes, C.E., Cybulsky, M.I., and Dinarello, C.A. (1987) Acute inflammation and Schwartzmann-like reaction induced by interleukin-1 and tumour necrosis factor. *American Journal of Pathology* **129**, 463.

Muto, Y., Nouri-Aria, K.T., Meager, A., *et al.* (1988) Enhanced tumour necrosis factor and interleukin-1 in fulminant hepatic failure. *The Lancet*, **ii**, 72.

Ohno, S., Kato, F., Matsuda, H., *et al.* (1982) Detection of gamma interferon in the sera of patients with Behçet's disease. *Infection and Immunity* **36**, 202.

Okusawa, S., Gelfand, J.A., Ikejima, T., *et al.* (1988) Interleukin 1 induces a shock like state in rabbits: synergism with tumour necrosis factor and the effect of cyclooxygenase inhibition. *Journal of Clinical Investigation* **81**, 1162.

Oliff, A., Defeo-Jones, D., Boyer, M., *et al.* (1987) Tumours secreting human TNF/cachectin induce cachexia in mice. *Cell* **50**, 555.

Paganelli, R., Capobianchi, M.R., Ensoli, B., *et al.* (1988) Evidence that defective gamma interferon production in patients with primary immunodeficiencies is due to intrinsic incompetence of lymphocytes. *Clinical and Experimental Immunology* **72**, 124.

Panitsch, H.S., Hirsh, R.L., Haley, A.S., and Johnson, K.P. (1987) Exacerbations of multiple scelerosis in patients with gamma interferon. *The Lancet* **i**, 893.

Pestka, S. (ed.) (1981), (1986) *Interferons*, Parts A, B, and C. *Methods in Enzymology* **78, 79, 119** Academic Press, San Diego.

Piguet, P.F., Grau, G.E., Allet, B., and Vassalli, P. (1987) Tumour necrosis factor/ cachectin is an effector of skin and gut lesions of the acute phase of graft-vs-host disease. *Journal of Experimental Medicine* **166**, 1280.

Pomerantz, R.J. and Hirsch, M.S. (1987) Interferon and human immunodeficiency virus infection, in *Interferon 9* (Gresser, I. ed.) Academic Press, New York, p.113.

Richie, H.R., Manogue, K.R., Spriggs, D.R., et al. (1988) Detection of circulating tumour necrosis factor after endotoxin administration. *New England Journal of Medicine* **318**, 1481.

Rook, G.A.W., Taverne, J., Leveton, C., and Steele, J. (1987) The role of gamma-interferon, vitamin D_3 metabolites and tumour necrosis factor in the pathogenesis of tuberculosis. *Immunology* **62**, 229.

Rothstein, J.L. and Schreiber, H. (1988) Synergy between tumour necrosis factor and bacterial products causes hemorrhagic necrosis and lethal shock in normal mice. *Proceedings of the National Academy of Sciences USA* **85**, 607.

Scuderi, P., Sterling, K.E., Lam, K.S., et al. (1986) Raised serum levels of tumour necrosis factor in parasitic infections. *The Lancet*, **ii**, 1364.

Seeger, W. and Lasch, H.G. (1987) Septic lung. *Reviews of Infectious Diseases* **9**, *Supplement* 5, S270.

Shiozawa, S., Yoshikawa, N., Iijima, K., and Negishi, K. (1988) A sensitive radio-immunoassay for circulating alpha-interferon in the plasma of healthy children and patients with measles virus infection. *Clinical and Experimental Immunology* **73**, 366.

Shoenfeld, Y. and Isenberg, D.A. (1989) The mosaic of autoimmunity. *Immunology Today* **10**, 123.

Socher, S.H., Martinez, D, Craig, J.B., et al. (1988) Tumour necrosis factor not detectable in patients with clinical cancer cachexia. *Journal of the National Cancer Institute* **80**, 595.

Spruance, S.L., Green, J.A., Chiu, G., et al. (1982) Pathogenesis of herpes simplex labialis: correlation of vesicle fluid interferon with lesion age and virus titer. *Infection and Immunity* **36**, 907.

Takeda, A., Minato, N., and Kano, S. (1987) Selective impairment of alpha-IFN-mediated natural killer augmentation in Sjögren's syndrome: differential effects of alpha-interferon, gamma interferon, and interleukin 2 on cytolytic activity. *Clinical and Experimental Immunology* **70**, 354.

Taylor, P., Meager, A., and Askonas, B.A. (1989) Influenza virus-specific T cells lead to early interferon gamma in lungs of infected hosts: development of a sensitive radioimmunoassay. *Journal of General Virology* **70**, 975.

Teppo, A.M. and Maury, C.P.J. (1987) Radioimmunoassay of tumour necrosis factor in serum. *Clinical Chemistry* **33**, 2024.

Torseth, J.W. and Merigan, T.C. (1986) Significance of local gamma interferon in recurrent herpes simplex infection. *Journal of Infectious Diseases* **153**, 979.

Tracey, K.J., Beutler, B., Lowry, S.F., et al. (1986) Shock and tissue injury induced by recombinant human cachectin. *Science* **234**, 470.

Tracey, K.J., Lowry, S.F., and Cerami, A. (1988) Cachectin: a hormone that triggers acute shock and chronic cachexia. *Journal of Infectious Diseases* **157**, 413.

Van Oers, M.H.J., Van Der Heyden, A.A.P.A.M., and Aarden, L.A. (1988) Interleukin 6 (IL-6) in serum and urine of renal transplant recipients. *Clinical and Experimental Immunology* **71**, 314.

Waage, A., Espevik, T., and Lamvik, J. (1986) Detection of tumour necrosis factor-like cytotoxicity in serum from patients with septicaemia but not from untreated cancer patients. *Scandinavian Journal of Immunology* **24**, 739.

Waage, A., Halstensen, A., and Espevik, T. (1987) Association between tumour necrosis factor in serum and fatal outcome in patients with meningococcal disease. *The Lancet*, **i**, 355.

Williams, B.R.G., Read, S.E. and Gelfand, E.W. (1984) *In vitro* hyporeactivity to alpha-IFN in children with severe combined immunodeficiency disease. *Clinical and Experimental Immunology* **56**, 34.

Yee, A.M.F., Buyon, J.P., and Yip, Y.K. (1989) Interferon-alpha associated with systemic lupus erythematosus is not intrinsically acid labile. *Journal of Experimental Medicine* **169**, 987.

Zinkernagel, R.M. (1988) Virus-triggered AIDS: a T-cell-mediated immunopathology. *Immunology Today* **9**, 370.

9

Clinical applications of cytokines

9.1   Introduction

The potent biological activities of cytokines, particularly those that mediate cytotoxicity and microbicidal effects, have strongly suggested that cytokines will be useful therapeutic or prophylactic agents for a wide spectrum of diseases. Cytokines are multi-activity mediators, and therefore have complex biological actions within the host. This means that it is usually difficult to predict what effect(s) individual cytokines will elicit when administered alone in high doses to patients with particular diseases. In the case of hormone treatment, often the injection of exogenous hormone simply replaces the lack of circulating levels of that hormone, e.g. insulin in IDDM, human growth hormone in dwarfism, etc. Such 'replacement therapies' have on the whole been very successful. It is clear also that hrEPO, which regulates erythrocyte production, may replace the deficit of natural EPO in severely anaemic patients, for example those with kidney disease. However, in most cases of proposed cytokine treatment it is not known whether there are endogenous deficits of particular cytokines in the body and thus such therapy does not apparently generally constitute a replacement therapy.

In medicine, cytokines are often classified with a broader group of biologically active substances, loosely referred to as 'biologicals'. Many of the latter have come to be known as 'biological response modifiers' (BRMs). Thus, treatment with BRMs has been called 'biotherapy', and where a BRM specifically affects the immune system, as 'immunotherapy'. It is probably true that cytokines can behave as BRMs, but it is not obvious that this capacity is always what achieves the beneficial therapeutic effect. In some cases, cytokines are used in very large amounts and may act in a manner similar to chemical drugs. For instance, the anticancer activity of high-dose IFNα may have more to do with its direct cytotoxic action on tumour cells than with modifying biological responses, e.g. augmentation of NK cell activity or enhancement of MHC protein expression. The information available in the literature suggests that it is also true to say that cytokines are adminstered mostly in high-dosage formulations, often close to the maximum tolerated dose (MTD), and thus such treatment is frequently associated with toxicity. In fact, toxic side-effects may be so severe that patients are unable to continue such cytokine treatment for long. It may be fairer then to view cytokine treatment as a novel kind of therapy which may incorporate features of both chemotherapy and biotherapy.

Cytokine therapy was developed in the 1980s, although it had its origins in the availability of leukocyte IFN from large-scale human PBMC and lymphoblastoid cell systems and the subsequent molecular cloning of HuIFNα subtypes in around 1978. Since then, a growing number of cytokines have been isolated, characterized, molecularly cloned, and expressed in high yield in genetically engineered organisms, thus becoming available as rDNA products for clinical evaluation. Virtually every novel cytokine that has been discovered in the 1980s has been thought to be of potential clinical importance, and this has led to a 'rash' of new recombinant cytokines being developed as experimental medicinal products. By far the majority of recombinant cytokines are produced by *E.coli* into which a human cytokine cDNA coding sequence has been inserted and in which the cytokine is expressible in high yield. Cytokine proteins from this source may differ structurally from those produced by human cells in that, while they have the correct amino acid sequence, they lack specific post-translational modifications, e.g. glycosylation, normally carried out in mammalian cells. Lack of these structural modifications may have little or no apparent effect on the biological activity of certain cytokines *in vitro*, as has been mentioned in passing in previous chapters, but could affect their biology, distribution, stability, and immunogenicity *in vivo*. Even when cytokines are produced from mammalian or other eukaryotic cells, e.g. yeast or insect cells, they in most cases will still be non-identical to natural human cytokines because of the variability of post-translational modification processes. Furthermore, site-specific mutagenesis or chemical synthesis of the genetic material coding for cytokines raises the possibility for deliberate structural modification. All sorts of modifications from single amino acid substitutions to consensus sequence and hybrid cytokines, e.g. the N-terminal half of one cytokine joined to the C-terminal half of another, are now possible. Obviously, there are many molecular variations which will be of relevance to biological activity, pharmacological activity, efficacy, and safety issues. In addition, methods of production and purification may affect the quality and safety of the end product. For example, mammalian cells used for production may contain adventitious micro-organisms, endogenous viruses, and potentially oncogenic DNA. Purification procedures may introduce undesirable chemicals. Clearance of unwanted contaminants such as DNA, viruses, and chemicals is necessary, together with evidence of product consistency, before recombinant cytokines may be used in patients. Similar criteria now apply to cytokines produced in large-scale human cell cultures.

9.2 The clinical potential of cytokines

Interferons

The potent antiviral and antiproliferative activities of IFNs *in vitro* have suggested their potential prophylactic and therapeutic use in a number of virally mediated and malignant diseases. In addition, host defence mechanisms including NK-cell cytotoxicity and ADCC, macrophage activation, and expression of histocompatibility antigens, are increased by IFNs. This suggests that IFNs could have therapeutic value for the treatment of disease. In fact, in the 1970s rather too high hopes were raised that IFN would be a panacea for all ills. Now in the light of hundreds, possibly more than a thousand, clinical trials in which IFN has been pitted against a diversity of human diseases, it is apparent the early optimism has all but vanished. There is only a disappointingly meagre tally of diseases in which IFN can truly be said to provide a durable beneficial effect. Complete responses with IFN are rare, and it is probably unwise to say that it is curative. Nevertheless, there has been significant progress and even breakthroughs in the treatment of a handful of diseases with IFN, and it cannot be written off yet. Furthermore, much has been learnt about the scheduling, dosage, and route of administration of IFN in relation to particular patient groups, disease stages, and toxic side-effects. Such information has not only significantly aided the development of more efficacious therapeutic regimes with IFN, but will probably also aid clinicians in their handling and use of other cytokine products.

The types of HuIFNs available for clinical evaluation have been fairly restricted. Human leukocyte IFN, produced from virally induced PBMC, was available in relatively small amounts at approximately 1 per cent purity from the early 1970s. Human lymphoblastoid IFN from the B-cell line Namalwa was introduced in the late 1970s. Both leukocyte and lymphoblastoid IFNs contain mixtures of HuIFNα subtypes, but differ significantly from one another in the proportions of subtypes. Early phase I clinical trials, in which leukocyte and lymphoblastoid IFNs were administered to terminally ill cancer patients to study their pharmacological activity quickly established that high doses (3–10 million units) were reasonably well tolerated, although there were a number of unexpected, reversible side-effects associated with parenteral treatment. The main noticeable side-effect is a 'febrile reaction complex' including fever, headache, malaise, etc., but there are also suppressive effects on bone marrow, liver, and kidney functions (Table 9.1). At extremely high repeated doses (30 million units) effects on the CNS leading to the patient becoming disorientated, confused, and comatose, have been observed (Table 9.1). Originally, it was thought that such toxicity was due to impurities contained in IFN preparations, but when highly purified (>95 per

Table 9.1   Side-effects of IFNα therapy

Observed clinical responses
Fever
Chills
Malaise
Myalgia
Headache
Fatigue
Anorexia/weight loss

Pharmacological toxicity
Liver toxicity
Kidney toxicity, e.g. proteinuria and glomerulonephritis (rare)
Inhibition of haemopoiesis, e.g. thrombocytopenia and granulocytopenia
CNS toxicity, e.g. EEG changes, confusion, altered mental states
Heart disturbances, e.g. arrhythmia, ischaemia

Immunological responses
Depressed NK cell activity and ADCC on prolonged therapy
Induction of autoantibodies

cent) preparations of recombinant HuIFNα2 became available in the early 1980s it became clear that the 'flu-like' febrile reaction and the other side-effects were due to the actions of the IFN protein itself.

Besides leukocyte IFN, relatively large quantities of highly purified lymphoblastoid (Namalwa) IFN and recombinant HuIFNα2 have been available throughout the 1980s. HuIFNα1 (also designated αD) was also available for a short time, but none of the other dozen or more α subtypes have been developed for clinical studies. In addition, various natural and recombinant HuIFNβ and HuIFNγ preparations have been produced. Recombinant IFNβ and IFNγ derived from *E.coli* are non-glycosylated, although these can also be prepared as glycoproteins from mammalian cells, e.g. Chinese hamster ovary cell lines. In one variety of non-glycosylated HuIFNβ the cysteine residue at position 17 has been replaced by a serine, and this apparently gives a more stable product from *E.coli*. The majority of clinical trials to date have been carried out with preparations containing HuIFNα since they are more readily produced than either HuIFNβ or HuIFNγ, particularly as the natural products, e.g. from Namalwa lymphoblastoid cells.

In one of the early clinical trials of IFN in 1973, the 'world's entire supply' of leukocyte IFN at that time was tested against rhinovirus (common cold) and influenza virus infections in volunteers at the Common Cold Research Unit, Salisbury, UK. In this trial, leukocyte IFN was applied intranasally in drops before and after infection, but clinical improvement, though statistically significant, was marginal. Since those early days, IFNs have been tested over and over again in many clinical trials to assess whether they can prevent or cure virus infections. It is now clear that IFNα formulations administered in the form of an intranasal spray can prevent, but not cure, rhinovirus infections. Such prophylactic application is, however, less effective against influenza virus infections. Also, repeated daily spraying eventually produces stuffiness and nasal erosions making the treatment unattractive for mass usage. Other topical local applications of IFNα in the form of creams or ointments to genital herpes virus lesions and warts (*Condylomata acuminata*) have also been used with limited beneficial effect.

Most clinical investigations with IFNs have used the parenteral, intra-muscular, or intravenous, route of administration, even when in the case of certain viral infections the lesions are exteriorized. For example, herpes zoster infection, which is often a complication in immunosuppressed patients, may be treated with daily intramuscular injections of IFNα or IFNβ. Some improvement in lesion healing time and resolution of the infection has been recorded for many such patients. Similar beneficial effects have been found in herpes labialis infections and *Condylomata acuminata*, genital warts associated with papillomaviruses, following parenteral administration of IFNα. Perhaps, the most potentially important application of IFNα in virally mediated disease is in the control of hepatitis B virus (HBV) infections. The latter are endemic in many countries, and affect hundreds of millions of people worldwide. Chronic active hepatitis B has been shown to respond to INFα treatment by the disappearance of viral infectivity markers, e.g. clearance of viral DNA, and the possibility of seroconversion in many patients, although when treatment is terminated the hepatitis infection frequently recurs. It is of interest to note in HBV infections that endogenous IFNα production may be suppressed by viral activity, and thus the administration of exogenous IFNα may in this case constitute a replacement therapy. Unlike herpes virus infections where there are as good or better alternative therapeutic drugs, e.g. acyclovir, HBV infections respond to little else other than IFNα, and so it may eventually be used as the preferred treatment, at least in the West, to control HBV disease. An interesting use of IFNα in the therapy of a virally caused disease has been in the treatment of the very rare juvenile laryngeal papilloma where benign laryngeal warty outgrowths associated with papillomaviruses obstruct the airways and can be life-threatening. This condition was, before IFN became available, treatable only by surgical removal of the warts. This had to be repeated every time the warts re-grew until puberty, when the warts tended to regress spontaneously. IFNα treatment has been found to induce regression of such warts, and their growth may be controlled if IFN is given over several months. When IFN is stopped, however, the warts begin to grow again. Nevertheless, suitable maintenance therapy using low-dose IFNα formulations may prevail against wart growth until such time as they no longer pose a problem. Rather disappointingly, recent results from a multicentre randomized clinical trial indicate that leukocyte IFN is neither curative nor of substantial value as an adjunctive agent in the long-term management of this disease. Both IFNα and IFNβ inhibit HIV-1 replication *in vitro*, but it is not yet clear whether they have any lasting antiviral effects *in vivo*. IFNα has been shown to induce regression of Kaposi's sarcoma in a proportion of AIDS patients with this complication, but that may be more to do with its antitumour than its antiviral activity. There are also preliminary reports that IFNα may act as an 'immune booster' in AIDS patients to prevent the occurrence of opportunistic infections.

Where IFNβ has been used in the treatment of virally mediated disease, its effects have been shown to be similar to those of IFNα, and it is not clear whether it has any particular advantage over the latter. When injected intramuscularly, IFNβ tends to remain localized whereas IFNα readily enters the circulation. The lower 'bioavailability' of IFNβ may therefore mean that it is less efficacious than IFNα generally. However, IFNβ treatment may be of clinical use in auto-immune diseases such as MS, where intrathecal injections of purified natural IFNβ have already been shown to reduce the frequency of exacerbations in some patients (see p. 254). Other auto-immune diseases, e.g. rheumatoid arthritis, may, paradoxically, respond positively to IFNγ treatment. In several auto-immune diseases IFNγ is suspected of having a pathogenic role because of its capacity to induce MHC class II proteins and thus enhance 'self-antigen' presentation (see Chapter 8). Thus, the observation that IFNγ induces remissions in rheumatoid arthritis is quite surprising. Needless to say, the mechanism underlying the beneficial effect of IFNγ is unknown, but may be associated with cortisol release (see p. 238). Other conditions such as asthma and chronic granulomatous disease (CGD) may also be treatable with IFNγ. In asthma, the allergic-type reaction may be reduced by the action of IFNγ on Ig isotype synthesis and secretion by plasma cells; IFNγ inhibits IgE production and stimulates IgG 2a (see p. 152). In certain types of CGD, IFNγ probably acts by stimulating and thus correcting respiratory burst activity of macrophages and neutrophils to increase killing of bacteria.

The use of IFN as a potential anticancer agent has probably excited most interest from clinicians in the past decade. However, despite the intense interest shown by the media, there was never any particular reason to believe that IFN was going to be more effective than other conventional forms of cancer treatment, e.g. chemotherapy and radiotherapy. By and large the results of numerous clinical trials have borne out the belief of many scientists and clinicians that IFN would be of rather limited usefulness in cancer therapy. Perhaps predictably, IFNs have been found to be of some use in the treatment of haematological malignancies, where tumour cells are more accessible than in carcinomas (solid tumours).

Early phase I clinical trials showed that even with terminally ill cancer patients, objective responses regarding tumour burden could be demonstrated in approximately 10 per cent of patients. Clinicians measure the effect of IFN, or other potential antitumour agents, by assessing the size of the tumour(s) or the number of tumour cells present following treatment. If there is 100 per cent resolution of all measurable disease, this is termed a complete response (CR), and if there is greater than 50 per cent decrease in all measurable disease, a partial response (PR). There can also be minor responses (MR) amounting to less than 50 per cent decrease in all measurable disease, and stable disease (SD) where the tumour burden remains more or less consistent for a prolonged period. In most cancers, the course and outcome of the disease is highly variable and 'spontaneous remissions' are sometimes observed. Therefore, clinical trials should be set up as randomized, 'blinded' trials with two groups of patients, only one of which receives IFN. In practice, this clinical trial procedure has not always been adhered to. This has given rise to unsatisfactory, and in some cases anecdotal, results from uncontrolled trials leading to false optimism. Nevertheless, a number of properly conducted phase II clinical trials, in which IFNs are targeted against particular types of cancer, have revealed the extent to which different IFNs are effective against particular malignancies.

IFNα has been most successful in the treatment of a very rare B-cell malignancy known as hairy-cell leukaemia (HCL) with CR plus PR amounting to around 80 per cent of patients treated. In the majority of HCL patients the 'hairy cells' invade the spleen and bone marrow. IFNα treatment, if continued for several months, leads to greatly decreased numbers of hairy cells and improvement in normal cell counts. In the case of CR, the bone marrow is cleared of hairy cells. Although the treatment of HCL patients with IFNα has only been going for five years or so, it is certain that this form of therapy is at least as effective and durable as chemotherapy using for example the drug pentostatin (2-deoxycoformycin), an inhibitor of purine metabolism. A problem that has been encountered, particularly with high-dose recombinant IFNα2, is the induction of anti-IFNα2 antibodies. The neutralizing activity of these may negate the beneficial effects of IFNα2 therapy in HCL. However, treatment with IFN may be 'salvaged' by switching to lymphoblastoid or leukocyte IFN, which contain mixtures of IFNα subtypes and thus are not so readily neutralizable by endogenous anti-IFNα2. It should be pointed out that this problem is not peculiar to IFNα2 treatment of HCL, and anti-IFNα2 antibodies have been induced in patients with other types of cancer, e.g. renal cell carcinoma, following high-dose therapy regimes. Probably lymphoblastoid and leukocyte IFNs are less immunogenic than either of the two varieties of recombinant HuIFNα2 currently used. It is also interesting to note that development of auto-antibodies, e.g. antinuclear and antithyroid antibodies, has been reported in patients with carcinoid tumours receiving IFNα2, suggesting the latter can cause auto-immune disease (see p. 252).

IFNα treatment of chronic myelogenous leukaemia (CML) has also been extremely successful. In CML there is an initial chronic phase in which the leukaemic cells grow slowly and persist for two to four years, followed by a dramatic blast crisis where the myeloid leukaemia cells proliferate rapidly leading to a fatal outcome. Treatment of CML in the chronic phase with IFNα by daily intramuscular injection of 3–9 million units has achieved up to 80 per cent haematological responses, with about 70 per cent of patients having a complete haematological remission. Patients with a complete remission have a greater projected three-year survival rate than those who do not. These results strongly suggest that IFNα can be used for effective control of CML in a high percentage of patients, and may improve their long-term survival. In low-grade, indolent, or non-aggressive, lymphomas there have been a reasonable number of good responses using IFNα therapy. This has been particularly so in the rare T-cell lymphoma, mycosis fungoides. However, the higher-grade, aggressive lymphomas respond much more poorly.

There are a number of solid tumours for which treatment with IFN has induced some PRs, but with very few CRs. These include renal cell carcinoma, multiple myeloma, malignant melanoma, and AIDS-related Kaposi's sarcoma. Response rates up to 40 per cent have been achieved in clinical trials, but overall the response rate is below 20 per cent. In renal cell carcinoma better responses have been reported if IFNα treatment is given following surgical removal of 'bulky' disease, but further evidence of efficacy is required to substantiate these observations. Early results from a multiple myeloma trial in 1980 using leukocyte IFN suggesting a high incidence of responses have not been substantiated in later clinical studies of this disease. IFNα therapy of multiple myeloma appears to be inferior to chemotherapy with melphalan-prednisone. Metastatic malignant melanoma is an extremely difficult cancer to treat by any means, and the overall response rate with recombinant IFNα2 of around 18 per cent compares favourably with chemotherapy and encourages further investigation. IFNα has also shown activity against AIDS-related Kaposi's sarcoma, but response rates have been found to be better in AIDS patients who were free of prior opportunistic infections and had a good lymphocyte count. It is speculated that the anti-angiogenic activity of IFNα may contribute to remission of this angiogenic tumour.

IFNα therapy has had little activity against the common cancers, such as those of the lung, breast, and colorectal tissues, which are the major killers. A few patients with these cancers have had responses following IFNα treatment, but by and large it does not seem that IFNα as a single agent will have a major impact in therapy of these solid tumours. The results of clinical trials using IFNα against a range of cancers is summarized in Table 9.2. It is thought likely that in future clinical trials IFNα will be combined with other forms of cancer treatment in the hope that such 'combination therapy' will prove more effective. IFNβ has given similar results in clinical trials to those obtained with IFNα in certain types of cancer. For instance, the Ser[17] form of IFNβ, which has been the most used 'variety', has limited activity in renal cell carcinoma. However, [Ser[17]] IFNβ has invariably been found to be immunogenic, inducing anti-IFNβ antibodies, and this may restrict its usefulness. In contrast to IFNα and IFNβ, IFNγ appears to have extremely limited antitumour activity, despite its enhancing effects on immune functions. Nevertheless, while IFNγ as a single agent is demonstrably ineffective against a range of cancers, it may still, in combination with other cytokines such as TNFα, or cytotoxic drugs, emerge as a useful BRM in this area by inducing synergistic activities.

Table 9.2 Clinical trials with IFNα against malignant diseases (adapted from Foon, 1989)

Tumour	No. of evaluable patients	Responses			CR + PR responses (%)
		CR	PR	MR	
Haematological malignancies					
Hairy cell leukaemia	158	22	86	44	68
Non-Hodgkin's lymphoma (low grade)	107	12	37	6	46
Intermediate and high-grade lymphoma	61	1	8	2	15
Hodgkin's disease	21	0	4	2	19
Cutaneous T-cell lymphoma	42	8	14	3	52
Chronic lymphocytic leukaemia	73	0	12	—	16
Multiple myeloma	224	3	41	—	20
Chronic myelogenous leukaemia (pre-blast crisis)	68	8	46	7	79
Solid malignancies					
Osteogenic sarcoma	15	0	1	—	7
Malignant melanoma	185	7	14	2	11
Breast carcinoma	187	0	14	10	7
Renal cell carcinoma	252	6	37	28	17
Kaposi's sarcoma (AIDS related)	120	14	22	—	30
Colorectal carcinoma	65	0	2	—	3
Carcinoid tumour	29	0	16		55
Lung — small cell	10	0	0		0
— non-small cell	70	0	1	1	1
Ovarian cancer	42	5	3	—	19
Bladder cancer	55	20	16	—	65
Head and neck (squamous)	11	4	6	—	91
Nasopharyngeal	13	0	2	2	15
Cervical cancer	14	3	3	—	43

CR, complete response (absence of disease); PR, partial response (>50 per cent decrease in disease); MR, minor response (<50 per cent decrease in disease)

As a tailpiece to the therapeutic uses of IFNs, it appropriate to point out the common finding of thrombocytopenia, a marked decrease in platelet counts, as an 'unwanted' side-effect of IFN therapy. This IFN-induced side-effect has now been put to positive use in the treatment of thrombocytosis (markedly elevated platelet numbers) associated with various myeloproliferative diseases. IFNα therapy may thus continue to find new diseases to control in the future, and the extent of its usefulness may never be fully known.

Interleukin-2

The stimulating activity of IL-2 on the cytotoxic function of NK cells, and more importantly of LAK cells against tumour cells *in vitro*, suggested that IL-2 had potential as an anticancer agent. Rather little was known about the activities of IL-2 *in vivo* before the advent of recombinant IL-2 in the early 1980s. Nor was it known whether there would be toxic side-effects associated with administration of IL-2. Human IL-2, like most HuIFNs, is fairly species specific and therefore very high doses of HuIL-2 or IL-2s of other species, e.g. mouse, were required to test the effects of IL-2 in laboratory animals. Early phase I clinical trials predominantly employed intravenous bolus administration of recombinant HuIL-2 (rHuIL-2) in high dose, and this quickly established that IL-2 would induce severe toxic side-effects. The latter include hypotension, oliguria, fluid retention, progressive dyspnoea (difficulty in breathing), atrial arrhythmias, and thrombocytopenia. The most serious and dose-limiting side-effect is an increase in vascular permeability ('vascular leak syndrome') which leads to fluid extravasation and subsequent oedema (swelling), ascites, pulmonary oedema, and pleural effusions. It is probably caused by IL-2-activated lymphocytes adhering to vascular endothelial sites. Similar toxicity has been demonstrated in rodents, including mice and rats. Patients receiving rHuIL-2 not unexpectedly feel rather unwell and suffer fever, nausea or vomiting, and alterations in mental status. Despite the seriousness of these side-effects, as expected IL-2 induces lymphoid hyperplasia, e.g. increases in mature T-cells, neutrophilia, and eosinophilia which could contribute to antitumour mechanisms. Infusion of rHuIL-2 by intravenous bolus has thus been shown to be active against a limited number of cancer types, including renal cell carcinoma, melanoma, and non-Hodgkin's lymphoma. However, overall response rates with rHuIL-2 as a single agent are disappointingly low. Therefore, new strategies are being employed in an attempt to improve IL-2 activity, e.g. by combining it with other cytokines (IFNs, TNF), monoclonal antibodies, or cytotoxic drugs. A response rate of approximately 30 per cent has been reported for the combination of IL-2 and IFNβ in renal cell carcinoma, for example. Although such combinations may lead to some improvements in the treatment of certain cancers, by far the greatest advance has been in the use of IL-2 to stimulate leukopherized LAK cells of cancer patients *in vitro*. After several days in the presence of IL-2 these activated leukocytes are infused back into the patients. This is known as 'adoptive cellular therapy'. In most cases, activated LAK cells are combined with high doses of IL-2, and it has been demonstrated that such therapy can induce tumour regression in cancers, e.g. colorectal cancer, that respond poorly to other forms of treatment. This form of aggressive antitumour therapy is again complicated by the seriousness of toxic side-effects, which are similar to those observed with IL-2 alone. It is apparent that IL-2 stimulates LAK cells to produce a range of other cytokines including TNFs and these may be responsible for many of the side-effects, e.g. increased vascular permeability. Renal cell carcinoma is probably the most responsive to this type of adoptive cellular therapy, but an overall response rate of 22 per cent has been recorded for the 'difficult to treat' malignant melanoma. Complete responses (CRs) are rare, however, and, despite initial tumour regressions, in many cases remission is not durable.

Tumour infiltrating lymphocytes (TIL) have been shown to be 50 to 100 times more cytotoxic to autologous tumour cells *in vitro* than LAK cells. This has suggested a modified approach in which TIL, rather than LAK, are harvested from solid tumours, e.g. melanoma, renal, or head and neck tumours, expanded and activated *in vitro* in the presence of IL-2 and then infused back into the cancer patient. Preliminary clinical trials using TIL are underway and the results so far are promising. A combination therapy involving TIL, IL-2, and cyclophosphamide has recently been reported to induce responses in 60 per cent of 15 malignant melanoma patients. It is clear that this kind of therapeutic approach deserves further exploration.

IL-2 has also been used in AIDS patients, where it was hoped that it would restore T_H-lymphocyte numbers. However, it was quickly ascertained that IL-2 provided no beneficial effect in AIDS, and on the contrary may have made matters worse by stimulating HIV replication in activated T_H-lymphocytes.

Tumour necrosis factors

Observations that TNFs can induce haemorrhagic necrosis of certain transplantable tumours in mice, together with their proven direct cytotoxicity to a range of tumour cells *in vitro*, have strongly suggested that they could be used therapeutically in cancer patients. Clinical trials to investigate the activity of TNFs against different cancers did not however take place until hrTNFα became available in the mid-1980s. To date some dozen or more such clinical trials involving over 300 cancer patients have been carried out, but the number of responses reported has been disappointingly small. Toxicity again has been found to be a serious and difficult obstacle, since this often approaches the level found in endotoxaemia and endotoxic shock following high-dose TNFα administration. Short infusions of hrTNFα are associated with a variety of undesirable side-effects including fever, headaches, general malaise, lethargy, rigors, etc., with hypotension being the dose-limiting effect. 'Vascular leak syndrome', a feature of IL-2 infusion, and subsequent oedema is also found in patients treated with hrTNFα. Prolonged infusions lead to marked myelosuppression, with a progressive decrease in circulating leukocytes and platelets, and to liver toxicity.

The toxicity of TNFα is well described, but the central question is whether this cytokine has antitumour efficacy. This has been difficult to demonstrate and may reflect the inability to produce a systemic level of TNFα high enough to be efficacious, owing to dose-limiting toxicity. Nevertheless, results from phase I clinical trials indicated a poor response rate, although patients entered into such trials have probably had 'heavy' prior therapy and are therefore unlikely to give good responses. Phase II trials are now getting under way, but it is too soon to predict their outcome. Anti-inflammatory drugs such as indomethacin are being used to control toxic side-effects, but it is not clear whether these will also negate putative antitumour activities. Combination approaches, e.g. TNFα plus IFNγ, are also being explored. The development of TNFβ as an anticancer agent has lagged far behind that of TNFα, but it is possible that TNFβ may unexpectedly be the more efficacious of these two related cytokines and this remains to be tested.

Haemopoietic growth factors

It is unlikely that CSFs such as GM-CSF and G-CSF will have any direct therapeutic actions against solid tumours, but they will probably be useful in cancer treatment for the reason that they increase circulating numbers of leukocytes (Table 9.3). Thus, in patients with malignant melanoma or breast cancer receiving high-dose, myelotoxic, chemotherapy, an accelerated granulocyte recovery has been demonstrated if they are given infusions of recombinant human GM-CSF following autologous bone-marrow transplantation. Toxicity of rGM-CSF appears to be much more limited than that of either IL-2 or TNFα and in most cases is restricted to slight fever, headaches, phlebitis, and flushing. There are however some indications that monocyte/macrophage-mediated toxicity may be problematical in patients receiving GM-CSF. For this reason, more interest recently has centred on hrG-CSF which appears to be completely without toxic side-effects. For instance, hrG-CSF increased neutrophil counts to three times higher than controls without toxicity in a group of patients with sarcoma of the bladder once they had completed a combination chemotherapy course. It has also been shown to reduce neutropenia in patients receiving chemotherapy. This has suggested a further potential role for hrG-CSF. For example, it might be used prior to chemotherapy or radiotherapy to boost granulocyte counts and thus permit higher than 'normal' doses of chemotoxic drugs or radiation to be given, with the expectation that such increased doses will be more efficacious and lead to more durable responses (Table 9.3).

M-CSF, which is not very effective in stimulating human monocyte progenitor proliferation *in vitro*, has been more difficult to assess in terms of its clinical potential. It is a strong inducer of monocyte toxicity, which may point to adverse effects *in vivo*. However, increased monocyte functions such as ADCC could be important in the lysis of tumour cells and thus a combination of M-CSF and antitumour-specific antigen moab might provide an efficacious therapy for certain tumours.

Generally speaking, haemopoietic growth factors have both growth-promoting and differentiating roles in leukaemic cells. Possibly, their dif-

Table 9.3   Potential clinical uses of haemopoietic growth factors (adapted from Devereux and Linch, 1989)

To boost haemopoietic processes:

Following chemo/radiotherapy

Before chemo/radiotherapy to permit high-dose treatment

Following bone marrow transplantation

In aplastic anaemia and other cytopenias

In anaemia of chronic renal failure and other anaemias of diseased states (EPO only)

As an adjunct to autologous blood transfusion (EPO only)

To stimulate leukaemia cells:

To induce terminal differentiation of leukaemic cells in myelodysplasia

To stimulate leukaemic cells into growth cycle before chemotherapy

To stimulate mature phagocytic cell function:

In microbial infections

In malignancies

---

ferentiating effects could be used to 'differentiate out' leukaemic cells so that they lose their proliferative capacity. Alternatively, growth factor stimulation of leukaemic cells into a replicative phase, e.g. S-phase of the cell cycle when DNA synthesis occurs, may sensitize them to the actions of chemical drugs (Table 9.3).

Haemopoietic growth factors may also find therapeutic uses in various myeloproliferative disorders. For example, patients with aplastic anaemia may benefit from GM- or G-CSF therapy. Such treatment would not only restore leukocyte counts but also reduce the risk of microbial infections (Table 9.3).

It is clear that the haemopoietic growth factors, especially GM- and G-CSF and including EPO, have great potential for the therapy of many diseases. Future clinical trials should provide interesting and important data over the next few years.

Other cytokines

It is difficult to say yet whether the 'clinical promise' of cytokines other than those already discussed will be fulfilled. While data from *in vitro* experiments and animal model systems support the belief that many cytokines have potential therapeutic or prophylactic roles in disease, the often unpredicted activities and toxicity of cytokines *in vivo*, as already encountered with IFNs, TNF, and IL-2, makes it hard to speculate on whether they will turn out to be clinically useful. IL-1, for example, has been shown to enhance cellular proliferative and immune responses, but like TNFα, with which it shares many biological activities, it may be too profoundly toxic for use as an anticancer agent. IL-4 also can act as a stimulator of leukocyte proliferation and function, but its augmentation of IgE secretion and thus potential for inducing allergic responses may preclude much clinical use. Nevertheless, there is a growing list of cytokines that remain to be clinically evaluated. Some, like TGFβ and PDGF, could be useful in wound healing. Others, e.g. TGFα or FGF, acting as angiogenic factors, might find roles in re-vascularization of damaged tissues and organs. Further, TGFβ, which antagonizes the actions of TNFα, might be employed in disease situations where the induction of TNFα is likely to cause problems, as in allograft rejection. Novel cytokines such as oncostatin M and AR with antitumour cell activity *in vitro* also await clinical assessments. Obviously there remains much to be done in order to learn whether or not such cytokines are of lasting clinical value.

Further reading

Anderson, T.D. and Hayes, T.J. (1989) Toxicity of human recombinant interleukin-2 in rats. *Laboratory Investigation* **60**, 331.

Bartsch, H.H., Pfizenmaier, K., Rausching, W., and Nagal, G.A. (1988) Tumour necrosis factor alpha administered IM or intratumoral in patients with advanced cancer. *Journal of Cancer Research and Clinical Oncology* **114**, 44.

Billiau, A. (1985) The interferon system as a basis for antiviral therapy or prophylaxis. *Antiviral Research Supplement* **1**, 131.

Bissett, J., Eisenberg, M., Gregory, P., *et al.* (1988) Recombinant fibroblast interferon and immune interferon for treating chronic hepatitis B virus infection: patients' tolerance and the effect on viral markers. *Journal of Infectious Diseases* **157**, 1076.

Blick, M., Sherwin, S.A., Rosenblum, M., and Gutterman, J. (1987) Phase I study of recombinant human tumour necrosis factor in cancer patients. *Cancer Research* **47**, 2986.

Bloom, M. (1987) Cancer M.D.'s clash over interleukin therapy. *Science* **235**, 154.

Browning, J. (1987) Interferons and rheumatoid arthritis: insight into interferon biology. *Immunology Today* **8**, 372.

Creagen, E.T., Kovach, J.S., Moertel, C.G., *et al.* (1988) A phase I clinical trial of recombinant human tumour necrosis factor. *Cancer* **62**, 2467.

Devereux, D. and Linch, D.C. (1989) Clinical significance of the haemopoietic growth factors. *British Journal of Cancer* **59**, 2.

Douglas, R.M., Moore, B.W., Miles, H.B., *et al.* (1986) Prophylactic efficacy of intranasal alpha-2 interferon against rhinovirus infections in the family setting. *New England Journal of Medicine* **314**, 66.

Feinberg, B., Kurzrockm, R., Talpaz, M., *et al.* (1988) A phase I trial of intravenously administered recombinant tumour necrosis factor alpha in cancer patients. *Journal of Clinical Oncology* **6**, 1328.

Ferro, T.J., Johnson, A., Everitt, J., and Malik, A.B. (1989) IL-2 induces pulmonary edema and vasoconstriction independent of circulating lymphocytes. *Journal of Immunology* **142**, 1916.

Figlin, R.A., Dekernion, J.B., Mukamel, E., *et al.* (1988) Recombinant interferon alpha-2a in metastatic renal cell carcinoma: assessment of antitumour activity and anti-interferon antibody formation. *Journal of Clinical Oncology*, **6**, 1604.

Foon, K.A. (1989) Biological response modifiers: the new immunotherapy. *Cancer Research* **49**, 1621.

Gisslinger, H., Ludwig, H., Linkesch, W., *et al.* (1989) Long term interferon therapy for thrombocytosis in myeloproliferative diseases. *The Lancet* **i**, 634.

Goldstein, D. and Laszlo, J. (1986) Interferon therapy in cancer: from imaginon to interferon. *Cancer Research* **46**, 4315.

Golomb, H.M. (1987) The treatment of hairy cell leukaemia. *Blood* **69**, 979.

Guidelines on the production and quality control of cytokine products derived by modern biotechnological processes (1988) *Trends in Biotechnology* **6**, G9–G12.

Guidelines on the preclinical biological safety testing of medicinal products derived from biotechnology (1989) *Trends in Biotechnology* **7**, G13–G16.

Hawkins, M.J., Borden, E.C., Merritt, J.A., *et al.* (1984) Comparison of the biologic effects of two recombinant human interferons alpha (rA and rD) in humans. *Journal of Clinical Oncology* **2**, 221.

Healy, G.B., Gelber, R.D., Trowbridge, A.L., *et al.* (1988) Treatment of recurrent respiratory papillomatosis with human leukocyte interferon. *New England Journal of Medicine* **319**, 401.

Jacobs, S.K., Wilson, D.J., Kornblith, P.L., and Grimm, E.A. (1986) Interleukin-2 or autologous lymphokine-activated killer cell treatment of malignant glioma: phase I trial. *Cancer Research* **46**, 2101.

Kradin, R.L., Kurnick, J.T., Lazarus, D.S., *et al.* (1989) Tumour-infiltrating lymphocytes and interleukin-2 in treatment of advanced cancer. *The Lancet* **i**, 577.

Krown, S.E. (1988) Interferons in malignancy: biological products or biological response modifiers. *Journal of the National Cancer Institute* **80**, 306.

Kuhls, T.L., Sacher, J., Pineda, E., *et al.* (1986) Suppression of recurrent genital herpes simplex virus infection with recombinant alpha2 interferon. *Journal of Infectious Diseases* **154**, 437.

Lane, C.H., Kovacs, J.A., Feinberg, J., *et al.* (1988) Antiretroviral effects of interferon-alpha in AIDS-associated Kaposi's sarcoma. *The Lancet* **ii**, 8622.

Lotze, M.T. and Rosenberg, S.A. (1988) Interleukin 2 as a pharmacologic reagent, in *Interleukin 2* (Smith, K.A., ed.) Academic Press, San Diego, p. 237.

Mihich, E. (1985) Biological response modifiers: their potential and limitations in cancer therapeutics. *Cancer Investigation* **3**, 71.

Morstyn, G. and Burgess, A.W. (1988) Hemopoietic growth factors: a review. *Cancer Research* **48**, 5624.

Oberg, K., Alm, G., Magnusson, A., *et al.* (1989) Treatment of malignant carcinoid tumours with recombinant interferon alpha-2b: development of neutralizing interferon antibodies and possible loss of antitumour activity. *Journal of the National Cancer Institute* **81**, 531.

Oldham, R.K. (1985) Biologicals and biological response modifiers: new approaches to cancer treatment. *Cancer Investigation* **3**, 53.

Oldham, R.K. (1985) Interferon: a model for future biologicals, in *Interferon 6* (Gresser, I., ed.) Academic Press, New York, p. 127.

Oldham, R.K. (1986) Biotherapy: the fourth modality of cancer treatment. *Journal of Cellular Physiology Supplement* **4**, 91.

Orkin, H. (1989) Molecular genetics of chronic granulomatous disease. *Annual Review of Immunology* **7**, 277.

Ozer, H., Golomb, H.M., Zimmerman, H., and Spiegal, R.J. (1989) Cost-benefit analysis of interferon alpha-2b in treatment of hairy cell leukaemia. *Journal of the National Cancer Institute* **81**, 595.

Platzer, E. (1989) Human haemopoietic growth factors. *European Journal of Haematology* **42**, 1.

Remick, D.G. and Kunkel, S.L. (1989) Toxic effects of cytokines *in vivo*. *Laboratory Investigation* **60**, 317.

Rinehart, J.J., Young, D., Lafarge, J., *et al.* (1987) Phase I/II trial of interferon-beta-serine in patients with renal cell carcinoma: immunological and biological effects.

Cancer Research **47**, 2481.

Schneider, A., Papendick, U., Gissmann, L., and De Villiers, E.M. (1987) Interferon treatment of human genital papilloma virus infection: importance of viral type. *International Journal of Cancer* **40**, 610.

Scott, G.M., Philpotts, R.J., Wallace, J., *et al.* (1982) Prevention of rhinovirus colds by human interferon alpha-2 from *E.coli. The Lancet* **i**, 186.

Selby, P., Hobbs, S., Viner, C., *et al.* (1987) Tumour necrosis factor in man; clinical and biological observations. *British Journal of Cancer* **56**, 803.

Sieff, C.A. (1988) Haemopoietic growth factors: *in vitro* and *in vivo* studies, in *Recent Advances in Haematology* **5** (Hoffbrand, A.V., ed.) Churchill Livingstone, Edinburgh, p. 1.

Silberstein, D.S., Schoof, D.D., Rodrick, M.L., *et al.* (1989) Activation of eosinophils in cancer patients treated with IL-2 and IL-2-generated lymphokine-activated killer cells. *Journal of Immunology* **142**, 2162.

Smalley, R.V. and Borden, E.C. (1986) Interferons: current status and future directions of this prototypic biological. *Springer Seminars in Immunopathology* **9**, 73.

Smedley, E., Katrak, M., Sikora, K., and Wheeler, T. (1983) Neurological effects of recombinant human interferon. *British Medical Journal* **286**, 262.

Smith, C.I., Weissberg, J., Bernhardt, L., *et al.* (1983) Acute Dane particle suppression with recombinant leukocytes A interferon in chronic hepatitis B virus infection. *Journal of Infectious Diseases* **148**, 907.

Spriggs, D.R., Sherman, M.L., Frei, E. III, and Kufe, D.W. (1987) Clinical studies with tumour necrosis factor, in *Tumour Necrosis Factor and Related Cytotoxins*, (Brock, G. and March, J. eds) CIBA Foundation Symposium **131**. Wiley, Chichester, p. 206.

Strander, H. (1984) The interferon system in antitumour therapy — some personal views, in *The Biology of the Interferon System 1984* (Kirchner, H. and Schellekens, H., eds) Elsevier, Amsterdam, p. 489.

Talpaz, M., Kantarijian, H.M., McCredie, K.B., *et al.* (1987) Clinical investigation of human alpha interferon in chronic myelogenous leukaemia. *Blood* **69**, 1280.

Treanor, J.J., Betts, R.F., Erb, S.M., *et al.* (1987) Intranasally administered interferon as prophylaxis against experimentally induced influenza A virus infection in humans. *Journal of Infectious Diseases* **156**, 379.

Turner, R.B., Felton, A., Kosak, K., *et al.* (1986) Prevention of experimental coronavirus colds with intranasal alpha-2b interferon. *Journal of Infectious Diseases* **154**, 443.

Tyrrell, D.A.J. (1976) *Interferon and its Clinical Potential.* Heinemann, London.

Urba, W.J., Clark, J.W., Steins, R.G., *et al.* (1989) Intraperitoneal lymphokine-activated killer cell/interleukin-2 therapy in patients with intra-abdominal cancer: immunologic considerations. *Journal of the National Cancer Institute* **81**, 603.

Yamazaki, S. (1984) Further studies on clinical trials of interferon in Japan. *Japanese Journal of Medical Science and Biology* **37**, 209.

Appendix

A.1 Glossary

Allerge normally harmless substance to which certain individuals are sensitized leading to inflammatory and anaphylactic reactions on exposure.

Angiogenesis the process of blood vessel growth.

Antibody complex protein (immunoglobulin) released by plasma cells which is capable of binding to a particular antigen.

Antigen substance which produces an immunological response leading to antibody production and cell-mediated immunity.

Autoantibody antibody binding to self-antigens, to which the host is normally tolerant.

Autocrine manner of stimulation by a cellular factor acting on the cells producing it.

Autoimmune disease wide spectrum of diseases caused by dysregulation of the immune system.

B-lymphocyte (B-cell) a type of white blood cell capable of being activated to proliferate and differentiate into an antibody-producing plasma cell.

Biological responses modifier (BRM) substance inducing specific biological effects *in vivo*.

Cachexia weight loss and severe tissue wasting associated with chronic invasive diseases.

CD-antigens a nomenclature system relating to cellular differentiation antigens, principally of leukocytes.

Colony stimulating factor one of a group of cytokines capable of stimulating the proliferation and differentiation of certain haemopoietic cell lineages.

Complementary DNA (cDNA) DNA formed by reverse transcription of messenger (m)RNA.

Complementary DNA library set of cDNAs from a particular cell type.

Cytokine one of a class of inducible, water-soluble, heterogeneous proteinaceous mediators of animal origin with molecular weight greater than 5000 that exercise specific, receptor-mediated effects in target cells and/or in the mediator-producing cells themselves.

Cytotoxin a cell-derived substance capable of inducing cell death in target cells.

Domain part of a protein, referring in particular to a receptor.

Endothelial cell polygonal cell found lining the inner surfaces of blood vessels and other tissues.

Endotoxin the lipopolysaccharide (LPS) component of Gram-negative bacterial cell walls which can activate macrophages.

Erythrocyte red blood cell.

Erythroblast an erythrocyte stimulated into DNA synthesis.

Exon gene segment encoding a polypeptide

Fibroblast a 'spindle'-shaped cell found in various tissues, which can be cultured *in vitro*.

G-protein one of a heterogeneous class of intracellular signal transducing proteins.

Genome the complete set of genes of an organism.

Glycosylation a process of adding carbohydrate groups onto a protein immediately after synthesis in eukaryotic cells.

Granulocyte phagocytic polymorphonuclear leukocyte with large numbers of granules. Includes neutrophils, eosinophils, and basophils.

Growth factor one of several different cytokines capable of inducing mitogenesis.

Haemopoiesis the process of populating and replacing circulating erythrocytes and leukocytes from stem cells contained within the fetal liver and bone marrow.

Haemopoietic growth factor one of several different cytokines including colony stimulating factors which regulate the proliferation and differentiation of haemopoietic cell lineages.

Homology degree of structure similarity.

Interferon one of a group of cytokines with antiviral activity.

Interleukin one of several different cytokines acting between leukocytes and other cell types, which has a variety of stimulatory activities.

Intron gene segment which interrupts a protein coding sequence.

Kilodalton (kDa) a molecular weight of 1000.

Kinase enzyme capable of phosphorylation of particular substrates.

Leukocyte generic name for white blood cells.

Lymphoblastoid cell transformed lymphocyte capable of infinite growth capacity.

Lymphokine one of a subset of cytokines produced by lymphocytes and lymphoblastoid cells.

Macrophage phagocytic leukocyte found in various tissues which is important in non-specific cellular immunity and antigen presentation.

Major histocompatibility complex (MHC) variable complex cell-surface glycoproteins which distinguish self from non-self and which are involved in antigen presentation.

Mitogen substance inducing mitosis and cell division.

Monocyte macrophage precursor found in the circulation.

Monokine one of a subset of cytokines produced by monocytes or macrophages.

Nuclear transcription factor protein capable of binding to the regulatory elements of genes to induce transcription.

Oncogene dysregulated or mutated proto-oncogene producing protein products, oncoproteins, mediating loss of cellular growth control and oncogenesis.

Oncogenesis the process of neoplastic cellular transformation leading to the development of tumorigenic (tumour) cells.

Paracrine manner of stimulation by a cellular factor acting on cells close to the cells producing it.

Plasma cell antibody-producing cell of the B-cell lineage.

Phospholipase A enzyme of the cyclooxygenase pathway involved in the formation of arachidonic acid metabolites, e.g. prostaglandins.

Phospholipase C several isoenzymes catalysing the breakdown of phosphatidyl inositol to produce secondary messengers within the cytoplasm.

Pleiotropic acting on many different cell types.

Pleiotypic having many different activities.

Pluripotential (multipotential) inherent characteristic of stem cells whereby through differentiation many different cell types may be produced.

Protein kinase C phosphorylating enzyme associated with the inner surface of the plasma membrane which is involved in signal transmission from receptors and cellular activation processes.

Reverse transcriptase enzyme catalysing reverse transcription.

Reverse transcription the synthesis of complementary DNA (cDNA) from mRNA.

Signal sequence short N-terminal hydrophobic amino acid sequence present in the precursors of secreted proteins which is cleaved off prior to exit from the cell.

Synergy combined activities of cytokines which are greater than the sum of their individual activities.

T-lymphocyte (T-cell) a type of white blood cell capable of responding to foreign antigens and thus of mediating cellular immunity.

Thymocyte precursor of T-lymphocyte undergoing development in the thymus.

Transgenic an animal that has been implanted with genes from some other species.

Transformed cell cell which has undergone immortalization and phenotypic changes *in vitro* and which may or may not be tumorigenic.

Tumour cell cell capable of producing a tumour which is unresponsive to mediators of normal cell growth control.

Virion a complete virus particle.

A.2   Abbreviations

aa	amino acid
ACTH	adrenocorticotrophic hormone
ADCC	antibody-mediated cellular cytotoxicity
ADP	adenosine diphosphate
aFGF	acidic FGF
Ag	antigen
AGE	advanced glycosylation end-product
AIDS	acquired immunodeficiency syndrome
ALL	acute lymphocytic leukaemia
AML	acute myeloid leukaemia
AMP	adenosine monophosphate
ANLL	acute non-lymphocytic leukaemia
AP	acute phase
AR	amphiregulin
ARC	AIDS-related complex
ARDS	acute respiratory distress syndrome
ATL	adult T-cell leukaemia
ATP	adenosine triphosphate
BCDF	B-cell differentiation factor
BCG	bacille Calmette-Guérin
BCGF	B-cell growth factor
BCL	B-cell leukaemia
bFGF	basic FGF
BFU-E	erythroid burst forming units
BMP	bone morphogenetic protein

Bo	(prefix) bovine
BPA	burst-promoting activity
BRM	biological response modifier
BSF	B-cell stimulating factor
c-FMS	M-CSF-R
cAMP	cyclic AMP
CD	cellular differentiation antigen
cDNA	complementary DNA
CFU	colony forming unit
CFU-E	CFU-erythroid
CGD	chronic granulatomous disease
CIF	cartilage-inducing factor
CML	chronic myeloid leukaemia
CNS	central nervous system
ConA	concanavalin A
CR	complete response
CSF	colony stimulating factor
CSpF	cerebrospinal fluid
CTL	cytotoxic T-lymphocyte
CTX	cytotoxin
DH	delayed hypersensitivity
DIA	differentiation inhibitory activity
DNA	deoxyribonucleic acid
DPP-C	decapentaplegic gene complex
DTH	delayed type hypersensitivity
E-CSF	eosinophilic CSF
EAE	experimental autoimmune encephalomyelitis
EBV	Epstein-Barr virus
EDF	eosinophil differentiating factor
EEF	exoerythrocytic form
EGF	epidermal growth factor
EGF-R	EGF receptor
ELAM-1	endothelial leukocyte adhesion molecule-1
EMCV	encephalomyocarditis virus
EP	endogenous pyrogen
EPO	erythropoietin
ES	embryonic stem (cells)
FcR	cell-surface receptor for the Fc fragment of immunoglobulin
FGF	fibroblast growth factor
FHF	fulminant hepatic failure
FITC-A	fluorescein-conjugated avidin
FSH	follicle stimulating hormone
G-CSF	granulocyte-colony stimulating factor
GBM	glomerular basement membrane
GDP	guanosine diphosphate
GEMM-CFU	granulocyte-erythroid-macrophage-megakaryocyte-CFU
GH	growth hormone
GM-CSF	granulocyte-macrophage-colony stimulating factor
GP	granulocyte pyrogen
GTP	guanosine triphosphate
GVHD	graft-versus-host disease
H-1	haematopoietin-1

HBV	hepatitis B virus
HCGF	haemopoietic cell growth factor
HCL	hairy-cell leukaemia
HILDA	human interleukin for DA cells
HIV	human immunodeficiency virus
HLA	human cell surface antigen of the major histocompatibility complex
hr	(prefix) human recombinant
hrEPO	human recombinant EPO
hrIFN	human recombinant IFN
HSF	hepatocyte-stimulating factor
Hu	(prefix) human
ICAM-1	intercellular adhesion molecule-1
IDDM	insulin-dependent diabetes mellitus
IDO	indoleamine 2,3-dioxygenase
IF	initiation factor
IFN	interferon
IFNa/b-R	IFNα/β receptor
IFNg-R	IFN gamma receptor
Ig	immunoglobulin
IGF	insulin-like growth factor
IGF-IR	IGF-I receptor
IGF-IIR	IGF-II receptor
IL	interleukin
IRE	IFN gene regulatory elements
IRP	international reference preparation
IS	international standard
ISRE	IFN-stimulated regulatory element
K_d	dissociation constant
LAF	lymphocyte activating factor
LAK	lymphokine activated killer (cells)
LCMV	lymphocytic choriomeningitis virus
LEM	leukocyte endogenous mediator
LGL	large granular lymphocytes
LIF	leukaemia inhibitory factor
LPS	lipopolysaccharide
LR	leukoregulin
LT	lymphotoxin
M-CSF	macrophage-colony stimulating factor
M-CSF-R	M-CSF receptor
MAb	monoclonal antibodies
MAF	macrophage activating factor
MBP	myelin basic protein
MCAF	monocyte chemotactic and activating factor
MCGF	mast cell growth factor
MCP	monocyte chemoattractant protein
MDNCF	macrophage-derived neutrophil chemotactic factor
MEL	murine erythroleukaemia
MHC	major histocompatibility complex
MIF	macrophage migration inhibition factor
MIP	macrophage inflammatory protein
MIS	Müllerian inhibitory substance
MM	multiple myeloma

MMTV	mouse mammary tumour virus
moab	monoclonal antibody
MR	minor response
mRNA	messenger RNA
MS	multiple sclerosis
MSH	melanocyte-stimulating hormone
MTD	maximum tolerated dose
Mu	(prefix) murine
MW	molecular weight
Mx	Murine protein induced by IFNα
NC	natural cytotoxic (cells)
NGF	nerve growth factor
NK	natural killer (cells)
NKCF	natural killer cytotoxic factor
NRK	normal rat kidney (cells)
NRL	neuroleukin
NZB	New Zealand Black (strain of mouse)
OAF	osteoclast-activating factor
OKM1	monocyte/macrophage marker
oTP-1	ovine trophoblastic antiluteolytic protein
PAF	platelet activation factor
PBMC	peripheral blood mononuclear cells
PDGF	platelet-derived growth factor
PDGF-R	PDGF receptor
PGE_2	prostaglandin
PGI_2	prostacyclin
PHA	phytohaemagglutinin (plant lectin)
PHI	phosphohexose isomerase
pI	isoelectric point
PIK	phosphoinositide kinase
PKA	protein kinase A
PKC	protein kinase C
PLC	phospholipase C
PMA	phorbol myristate acetate
PR	partial response
PSF	persisting cell-stimulating factor
rDNA	recombinant DNA
rIL	recombinant IL
RESV	respiratory syncytial virus
RNA	ribonucleic acid
ROI	reactive oxygen intermediates
RSV	Rous sarcoma virus
RTK	receptor tyrosine kinase
SCID	severe combined immunodeficiency disease
SCLC	small cell lung cancer
SD	stable disease
SLE	systemic lupus erythematosus
SM-FeSV	Susan McDonough strain of feline sarcoma virus
SSV	simian sarcoma virus
T_H	T-helper cell
tANLL	therapy-induced ANLL
TCGF	T-cell growth factor (interleukin-2)

TGF	transforming growth factor
TIL	tumour-infiltrating lymphocytes
TNF	tumour necrosis factor
TNF-R	TNF receptor
TRF	T-cell replacing factor
TSH	thyrotropin
Vg	vegetalizing protein
VGF	vaccinia growth factor
VSV	vesicular stomatitis virus

A.3   Single-letter code for amino acids

A	alanine
C	cysteine
D	aspartic acid
E	glutamic acid
F	phenylalanine
G	glycine
H	histidine
I	isoleucine
K	lysine
L	leucine
M	methionine
N	asparagine
P	proline
Q	glutamine
R	arginine
S	serine
T	threonine
V	valine
W	tryptophan
Y	tyrosine

Index